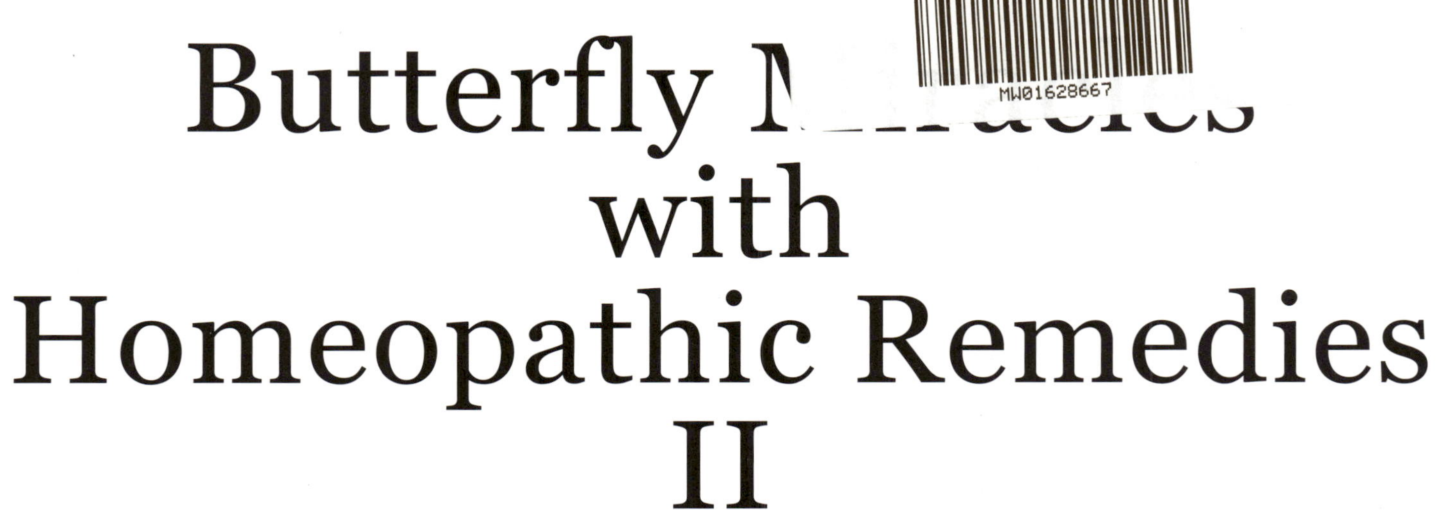

Butterfly Miracles with Homeopathic Remedies II

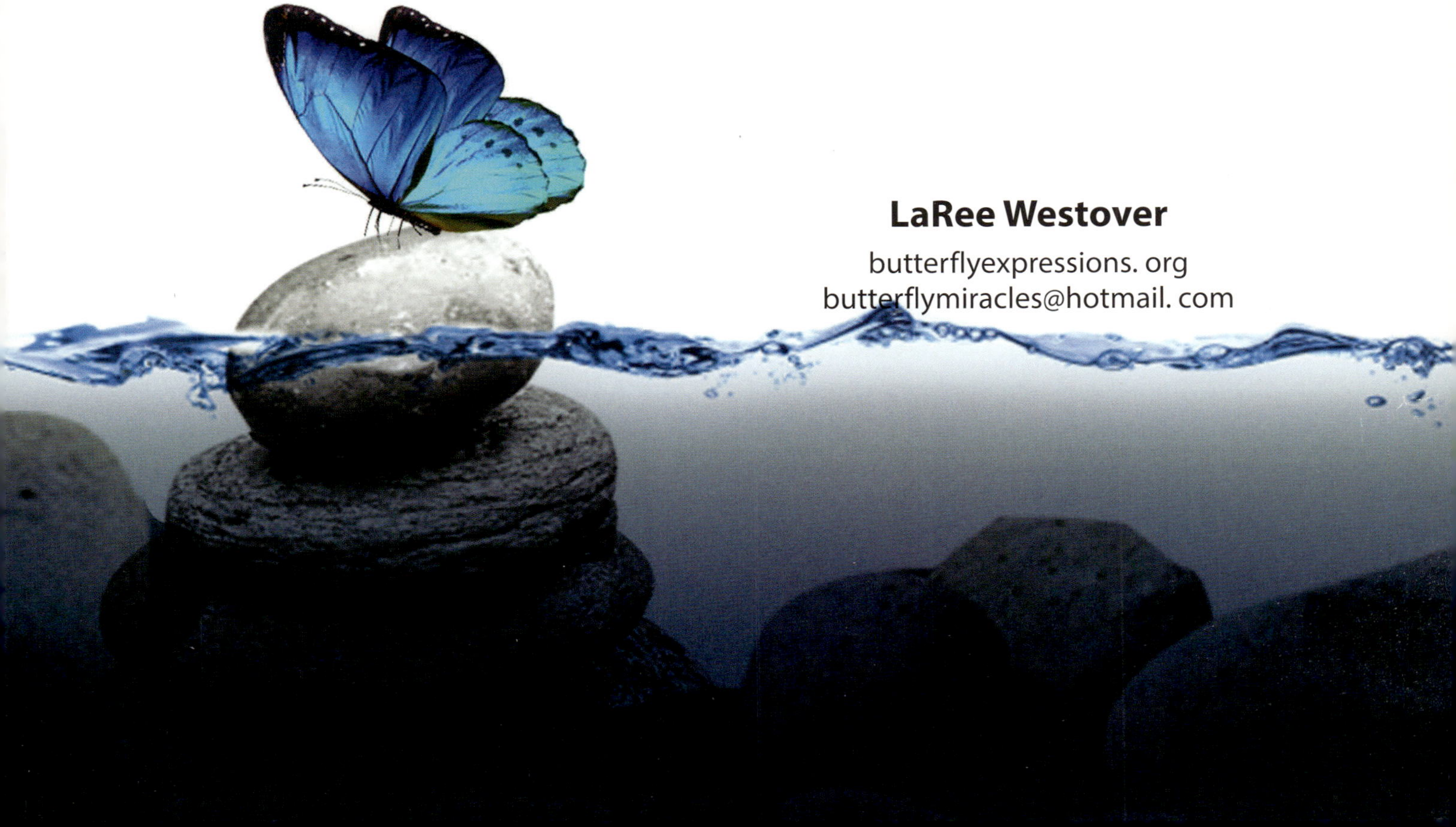

LaRee Westover
butterflyexpressions. org
butterflymiracles@hotmail. com

Hope Renewed

Homeopathic theory and practice differ greatly from any other healing modality, past or present, in several very basic ways.

First: Since the beginning of time, mankind has attempted to find methods to restore good health and proper functioning of the body following accidents or illnesses. Healing without causing harm has always been the goal of good men in medicine. Homeopathy can be, for everyone who is willing to make an effort, the answer to that quest.

When Samuel Hahnemann (considered the father of homeopathic theory) created his first remedy according to homeopathic protocols, he showed us a way to heal without side effects. He, and others like him, illuminated the path to the utilization of the many diverse substances found on this earth, even very toxic ones, to bring about positive changes in health without the destruction of delicate tissues or negative effects on the mind or emotions.

Second: Followers of homeopathic theory believe that every ailment of the physical body had its beginning in the vital energy of the body. Homeopathic theory also teaches that because the systems of the body are so interconnected by the vital energy, ailments cannot confine themselves to only one area of the body at a time. It is impossible to have just a pain in the head (or just a break in a bone) without having symptoms which range over many, if not all, of the systems of the body and into the emotions and mental processes. A corollary of this understanding is that all substances utilized for healing purposes (or for any other purpose) also affect a variety of body systems and go into the energy itself to reestablish (or disrupt) health.

Homeopathic remedies are studied and their effects recorded in this manner. When a remedy is given, symptoms throughout the whole body and mind are observed and the remedy is chosen to care for and restore balance to all of these areas.

Last and very important: In homeopathy, its history as well as its present-day usage, we have a graphic illustration of the goodness of God in inspiring and providing for His children. From the variety of substances whose healing properties have been discovered and utilized in homeopathy, a person can see that every creation of God found on this earth must be of benefit for the use of man. We can see that God has provided methods by which healing can be accomplished without destructive side-effects.

What more could a loving Father have done for His children? Every time I reach for a homeopathic remedy—whether it is plant, animal, mineral, or noxious substance based—I feel touched by Heaven's concern and caring for me. As the remedy brings health to my physical body or perspective to my mind or emotions, I feel the additional healing benefits of gratitude and reverence.

It takes some study and effort to become proficient in the use of homeopathic remedies. It is well worth whatever effort required! In addition, the accepting of responsibility for our own and our family's health, coupled with gratitude to the Creator, blesses and strengthens us in a myriad of ways.

May you find as much joy and success with homeopathic remedies as I, and many others, have done!

The "Butterfly Miracles" Bookshelf

ESSENTIAL OILS
History of Essential Oils
Schools of Thought
Tests and Standards
Shelf Life
Safety Guidelines
Women and Children
Methods of Use
Plant Families
Meridians and Chakras
Single Oils
Blended Oils

HERBAL REMEDIES
Nutrition and Your Body
Vitamin Absorption
Food and Nutrients
Vitamin Bandits
Drugs and Nutrition
Sub-clinical Malnutrition
Herbs as Nutrition
Doing a Cleanse Right
Use of Herbal Remedies
Basic Herbal Knowledge
Recipes: Tinctures, Teas, Salves

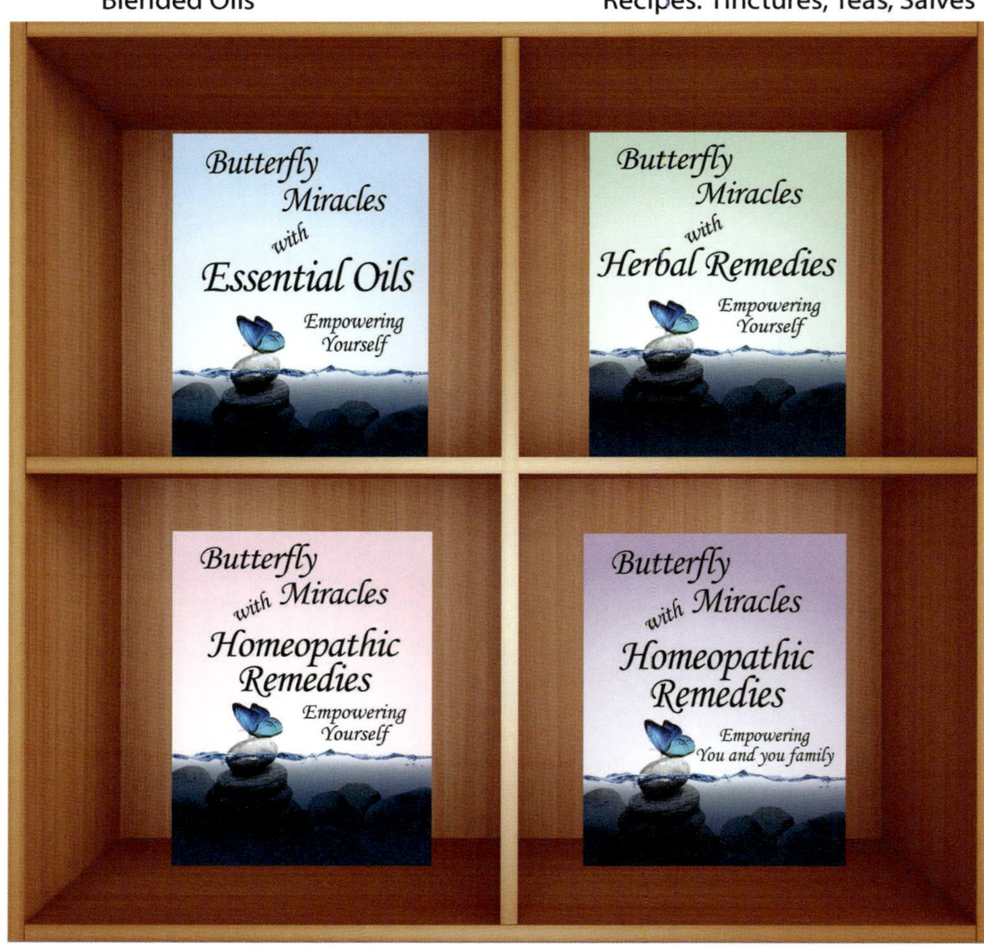

HOMEOPATHIC I
Principles of Homeopathy
Types of Remedies
Dilution and Potency
Taking Homeopathic Remedies
The Symptom Picture
Taking a Case History
Biochemic or Cell Salts
Flower Essence Remedies
Energetic Remedies
Remedies by Classification

HOMEOPATHIC II
Families - Children
Pregnancy
Labor and Delivery
Postpartum
Women's Health
Infant Care
Chronic Fatigue
Glandular Support
Headaches
Weakness

Legalese

There is absolutely no substitute for caution and common sense!

This book is written for general information and education only. It is not my intent to diagnose or prescribe for any ailment whatsoever. Your use of the information contained in this book is entirely at your own discretion and is, also, entirely your own responsibility. My goal is, simply, to bring to your attention things that, when I became aware of them, seemed to make significant changes in the quality of my life. It is not meant to be training in psychology, psychotherapy or medicine of any kind. You are advised to apply the techniques and information along with the assistance of competent professionals.

You have managed this far in your life without that homeopathic remedy you are considering and you can manage another day or two while you start slowly to determine the correct remedy, potency, and dosages for your own needs. It is my recommendation that you start slowly, with a remedy or two, determining what is best for your own needs.

There are details concerning the safe use of homeopathic remedies that cannot be contained in any book. Before using a homeopathic remedy the reader is advised to seek the assistance of a competent professional.

The statements and products mentioned in this book have not been evaluated by the FDA. They reflect traditional and anecdotal usage and data from recent scientific studies.

I hope you come to enjoy and love homeopathic remedies as much as I do

ISBN-10

0-9971993-3-8

ISBN-13

978-0-9971993-3-8

May 2016 Printing

Printed in the United States of America

Table of Contents

SECTION ONE: Homeopathic Formulas (Low Potency Combinations)

Introduction: Some Homeopathic Philosophizing .... p 1

CHAPTER 1 LOW POTENCY COMBINATION REMEDIES .... p 3

Abscess .... p 3
***ACNE* .... *p* 3**
Acne .... p 3
***ADDICTIONS* .... *p* 4**
Addictions #1 .... p 4
Addictions #2 .... p 5
Addictions #3 .... p 5
***ADRENAL GLANDS* .... *p* 6**
Adrenal Support .... p 6
Allergies #1 .... p 6
Allergies #2 .... p 6
Allergies #3 .... p 7
Allergies #4 .... p 7
Allergies #5 .... p 7
Allergies #6 .... p 8
Allergies #7 .... p 9
Allergies #8 .... p 9
Anger .... p 9
Anxiety #1 .... p 10
Anxiety #2 .... p 10
***ARTIFICIAL SWEETENERS* .... *p* 11**
Artificial Sweeteners .... p 12
Backache #1 .... p 13
Backache #2) .... p 13
Backache #3 .... p 13
Bacteria .... p 14
Bed-wetting .... p 14
Bioplasma .... p 15
***CANDIDA* .... *p* 15**
Candida #1 .... p 15
Candida #2 .... p 16
Candida #3 .... p 16
Cardio Arythmia #1 .... p 16
Cardio Arythmia #2 .... p 17
Chronic Fatigue Syndrome Information .... p 17
CFS #1 .... p 20
CFS #2 .... p 20
CFS #3) .... p 21
CFS #4 .... p 21
CFS #5 .... p 22
***A FINAL WARNING* .... *p* 22**

Colds #1 . . . . p 23
Colds #2 . . . . p 23
Congestion #1 . . . . p 24
Congestion #2 . . . . p 24
Coxsakie Information. . . . . p 25
Coxsakie . . . . p 25
Decongestion . . . . p 26
Detox #1 . . . . p 26
Detox #2 . . . . p 27
Detox #3 . . . . p 27
Detox #4 . . . . p 27
Detox #5 . . . . p 28
ALDICARB and the FDA and EPA. . . . . p 29
Detox #6 . . . . p 29
Detox #7 . . . . p 30
Detox #8 . . . . p 31
Detox #9 . . . . p 32
Detox #10 . . . . p 32
Detox #11 . . . . p 33
Detox #12 . . . . p 33
Detox #13 . . . . p 33
Diarrhea #1 . . . . p 34
Diarrhea #2 . . . . p 34
Digestive #1 . . . . p 35
Digestive #2 . . . . p 35
Digestive #3 . . . . p 36
Digestive #4 . . . . p 36
Dioxins . . . . p 37
Energy Alignment. . . . . p 37
ER 911. . . . . p 38
Essiac. . . . . p 39
Exhaustion #1 . . . . p 40
Exhaustion #2 . . . . p 40
Exhaustion #3 . . . . p 40
Eye Irritation #1. . . . . p 41
Eye Irritation #2. . . . . p 41
Fatigue #1 . . . . p 41
Fatigue #2 . . . . p 42
Fatigue #3 . . . . p 43
Fatigue #4 . . . . p 43
Fatigue #5 . . . . p 44
Fever . . . . p 44
Five Flower Formula. . . . . p 44
Flu Symptoms #1. . . . . p 44
Flu Symptoms #2. . . . . p 44
Fungus #1 . . . . p 45
Fungus #2 . . . . p 46

Gallbladder Distress ....p 46
Glandular/Lymph #1 ....p 46
Glandular/Lymph #2..................................p 47
Glandular Support #1 ....p 48
Glandular Support #2 ....p 48
Glandular Support #3 ....p 49
Glandular Support #4 ....p 50
Hair/Nails..................................p 51
Headache #1..................................p 51
Headache #2..................................p 52
Hormone Balancer ....p 52
Incontinence ....p 53
Indigestion #1 ....p 53
Indigestion #2 ....p 54
Infection Fighters #1..................................p 54
Infection Fighters #2..................................p 55
Infection Fighters #3..................................p 55
Infection Fighters #4..................................p 56
Infection Fighters #5..................................p 56
Injuries ....p 57
Insomnia #1 ....p 58
Insomnia #2 ....p 58
Intestinal Cleanse ....p 59
Intestinal/Stomach Distress #1 ....p 60
Intestinal/Stomach Distress #2 ....p 61
Intestinal/Stomach Distress #3 ....p 61
Intestinal/Stomach Distress #4 ....p 62
Intestinal/Stomach Distress #5 ....p 62
Intestinal/Stomach Distress #6 ....p 62
Kidney #1 ....p 63
Kidney #2 ....p 63
Kidney #3 ....p 63
Kidney #4 ....p 64
Kidney #5 ....p 64
Kidney #6 ....p 65
MERIDIAN BALANCING COMBINATION ....p 65
Governing Vessel..................................p 66
Central Vessel ....p 67
Gallbladder..................................p 69
Liver ....p 70
Kidney..................................p 71
Urinary Bladder..................................p 72
Large Intestine..................................p 73
Lung ....p 74
Stomach ....p 75
Spleen ....p 76

Triple Warmer....p 77
Pericardium....p 78
Small Intestine....p 80
Heart....p 81
Miasms....p 82
Migraine #1....p 83
Migraine #2....p 84
Muscle Aches and Pains #1....p 85
Muscle Aches and Pains #2....p 85
Muscle Weakness....p 86
Nerve #1....p 86
Nerve #2....p 87
Nerve #3....p 87
Neuralgia....p 88
Pain Remedy #1....p 88
Pain Remedy #2....p 89
Pancreatic Distress....p 89
PARASITES....p 89
Parasites #1....p 90
Parasites #2....p 90
Parasites #3....p 91
Pregnancy....p 91
Rescue Remedy....p 92
Respiratory Distress #1....p 92
Respiratory Distress #2....p 93
Respiratory Distress #3....p 93
Respiratory Distress #4....p 93
Respiratory Distress #5....p 94
Scars/Adhesions....p 94
Sinus....p 95
Skin Eruptions....p 95
Sleep....p 95
Teething....p 96
Tension #1....p 96
Tension #2....p 97
Traumatic Experiences....p 97
Vaginitis....p 98
Venous Congestion....p 98
Warts....p 99
Weakness #1....p 99
Weakness #2....p 100
Weakness #3....p 101
Weakness #4....p 102
Weakness #5....p 102
Yeast....p 103

SECTION TWO Remedies for Pregnancy, Childbirth, and Infant Care

CHAPTER TWO MATERIA MEDICA .... p 107
(FOR PREGNANCY CHILDBIRTH, AND INFANT CARE)

CHAPTER THREE PRENATAL PROBLEMS.. p 127
(PREGNANCY, CHILDBIRTH, WOMEN'S HEALTH, INFAN)

CHAPTER FOUR MISCARRIAGES .... p 137

CHAPTER FIVE PREPARATION FOR LABOR AND DELIVERY .... p 139

CHAPTER SIX LABOR—ONSET THROUGH SECOND STAGE .... p 141

CHAPTER SEVEN LATE LABOR, DELIVERY, AND POST-PARTUM .... p 149

CHAPTER EIGHT POST CESAREAN DELIVERY .... p 157

CHAPTER NINE INFANT CARE.. p 159

CHAPTER TEN BREAST FEEDING .... p 169

CHAPTER ELEVEN BASIC DOSAGE GUIDELINES .... p 173

Section One

Homeopathic Formulas (Low Potency Combinations)

Some Homeopathic Philosophizing

In the fifth century B. C. , Hippocrates, the "Father of Medicine," wrote that there were two methods of healing: by contraries or by similars. There are still, today, only 2 basic methods of healing: by contraries and by similars, with sub-sets of nutrition, prevention and the surgical removal of the offending part.

An example of healing by contraries, or antidotes as they are known in today's terminology, is the giving of a laxative to correct constipation. The underlying problem with this form of healing is three-fold. First, most of the substances prescribed are toxic and must be given in unhealthy doses in order to bring about a result. The result achieved is too often a palliation of symptoms, rather than a cure. Second is the problem of stopping the action of the "cure"—alleviating the constipation without creating diarrhea, for example. The third problem is the development of dependency on the drug for the body to accomplish a normal function.

The "law of similars" on which homeopathy is based states that when an imbalanced state (given a "dis-ease" name in today's parlance) exists, we seek a remedy that would create the same symptoms of distress in a healthy body. Put very simply, the remedy brings that particular symptom pattern to the attention of the energy system, or immune function, which then focuses on the imbalance and handles it in the most efficient manner possible. The result is often the putting of the system to rights, instead of just masking the symptom without any re-balancing or correcting of the underlying problem.

Samuel Hahnemann, considered the originator of this school of thought and the modality of homeopathy, began his search for a way to administer medicines safely, effectively, and without side-effects in 1810. He developed a method of dilution and succussion to produce varying levels of potency while creating remedies that were safe. This method is still used today in the production of homeopathic remedies. The paradox of homeopathy is that the more diluted a solution is the more potent and deep-acting it becomes.

Hahnemann used, in the early days of his work, only low-potency remedies one at a time—no combining of remedies as is often done today. Work with the higher potencies was still in early stages of development even at the time of his death. Among homeopathic physicians today, there is a split between those who use only low potency remedies given in quick succession and those who use the higher potencies given less frequently. The low potency group is again divided between those who use a single remedy at a time and those who combine several remedies in a "shotgun" approach.

Lower potency remedies are believed to be especially effective with children and with people who have particularly strong constitutions and whose innate self-healing capacities are still at high levels. However, they are often used on the elderly and the infirm because they are unable to sustain the "nudge" given the immune system by the higher potencies.

The premise of higher potency prescribing is to stimulate the body's healing mechanism to eradicate the problem entirely and permanently. All homeopathic remedies work on the emotional and psychological underpinnings of a malady, but the higher potencies reach a deeper level and have a greater likelihood of bringing about permanent changes.

There seems to be a time and a place for both methods, but I am often astonished at the healing capacities of the higher potency remedies. People whose constitutions are weaker, or who have suffered long with a chronic condition, often seem to need a "slow start" with the lower potencies, however. At low potency a slow process of overall strengthening and alleviating of symptoms is begun. Real improvement, and the complete re-balancing of both the physical and mental spheres, occurs when the higher potencies can finally be utilized.

Every homeopathic remedy has a "picture" of the symptoms it would produce in a well person. In order to be effective, this "symptom picture" must match the person's symptoms very closely. Time and care should be taken to understand the nature of the malady as well as the nature of the person—what are their likes and dislikes, what makes things better or worse for them, etc.

The drawback of homeopathic remedies is that if the wrong remedy is given—the symptom pictures do not match closely enough—those symptoms not already found in the person can be created energetically. In those areas of health where the symptoms do not match, the person is "well" and the remedy eventually produces the matching symptoms in those "well" aspects. The severity of the energetic symptoms and the rapidity with which they develop is in direct proportion to the potency of the remedies given.

Combination remedies are always low potency because there will be aspects of the various symptom pictures of the remedies (since they are often quite opposite to each other—dry cough as opposed to wet cough, dull headache on left side or piercing pain on the right, etc.) which would be produced very quickly at higher potency. Low potency combination remedies should be taken for only a few days at a time. These interruptions keep symptom pictures (or provings, as they are known) from developing.

The beauty of low-potency combination remedies (remedies containing several single remedies that apply to some aspect of a problem in some way) is that some measure of relief—often quite a lot—can be attained without the in-depth study of the person and the problem that would be required for higher potency usage. Nor do you need encyclopedic knowledge about the symptom picture of hundreds of remedies so that you can find just the right one. The small list of single remedies contained in the combination that brought some relief could then be studied individually, their symptom pictures matched to the remaining (or returning) symptoms, and a single remedy chosen for use at a higher potency. The result should be a deeper level of re-balancing, both emotionally and physically.

With this program of using a low potency combination followed by use of a higher potency single in mind, this book of information about some common (and a few rather unusual) combination remedies has been created. Information as to what particular symptoms each single remedy in the combination has been placed there to address is given in some detail. We hope you will find this information useful in planning your homeopathic strategies and in learning about the remedies.

Remember, all remedies in liquid form contain some alcohol—at Butterfly Express, LLC, this amount is less than 10%. Remedies also contain distilled water or reverse osmosis water.

Chapter One

LOW POTENCY COMBINATION REMEDIES

ABSCESS

Abscesses are accumulations of pus in tissues, organs, or any confined space in the body. Abscesses may be located externally or internally and may be the result of injury, lowered resistance to infection, or sluggishness of the lymphatic system. The infected part, whether internal or external, becomes swollen, inflamed, and tender. The sufferer may also experience fatigue, loss of appetite, weight loss along with alternating sensations of fever and chills.

Infections are a common human disease and can be produced by bacteria, viruses, fungi, and parasites. An abscess can form in the brain, lungs, teeth, gums, abdominal wall, gastrointestinal tract, ears, tonsils, sinuses, breasts, kidneys, prostate gland and along any muscle or in any tissue anywhere in the body.

ABSCESS (6X)

PINUS SYLVESTRIS (Scotch pine) Pinus has in its symptom picture pain, swelling, inflammation, and mucus in any location throughout the body. The action of Pinus has a heavy emphasis on glandular distress and the inguinal (groin) area.

CADMIUM OXIDATUM (cadmium oxidate) Cadmium is indicated for dull achiness all over, chills, and fever with great sweat. The pain and pressure being experienced because of the inflammation is greatly relieved when the eruption finally begins to form.

ACNE

The exact cause of acne varies from individual to individual, but contributing factors include heredity, oily skin, androgens (male hormones), allergies, stress, the use of certain drugs, and overconsumption of junk foods including saturated and hydrogenated fats. Nutritional deficiencies, exposure to industrial pollutants, and the overuse of cosmetics and skin care products often play a role in outbreaks. The pores of the skin need to be kept clean, allowing the skin to breathe. Exercise, which results in cleansing of the pores by sweat, and exposure of the skin to the bacteriostatic action of sunlight can be very helpful.

The skin is the largest eliminative organ of the body. When the colon and kidneys are not functioning optimally, the skin is often used to eliminate accumulated poisons. Acne is always a signal that work on the eliminative organs and the liver needs to be done immediately.

ACNE (9X)

KALI MURIATICUM (potassium chloride) This cell salt enhances the integrity of the cells in the epidermis. The symptom picture includes eruptions containing thick, white or cream-colored pus on forehead, face, lips and chin. This type of acne often indicates improper digestion of rich or fatty foods and sluggish action of the liver. Restless, anxious sleep, discontent, irritability and anger are some of the emotional symptoms. (Sounds like a teenager or a person suffering from hormonal imbalances to me!)

SILICA TERRA (pure flint) This is the #1 remedy for expelling foreign objects and infections from the body. The remedy picture includes unhealthy skin and constant suppuration. The mental/emotion symptoms include loss of self-confidence, performance anxiety, and complaints brought on by anticipation of failure. The person is usually prone to procrastinate.

ADDICTIONS

One definition of addiction could be becoming so accustomed to a substance that the body no longer functions properly if that substance is withdrawn. An addicted person experiences intense desires and cravings as the body sends out messages attempting to fill its "needs." Withdrawal symptoms include headache, insomnia, sensitivity to light and noise, diarrhea, hot and cold flashes, sweating, deep depression, irritability, irrational thinking, and disorientation.

Drug use and substance abuse of any kind depletes the body of nutrients! The body links toxic chemical substances to nutrients in an attempt to pass them through the system with as little damage to organs and tissues as possible. Attempts to detox the body must be accompanied with nutritional support and support to the eliminative organs and systems.

ADDICTIONS #1 (6X)

This compound is comprised of Scutellaria laterifolia and 7 flower essence remedies. Each of these may be helpful in overcoming addictive cravings, especially the ones that are accompanied by mood swings and erratic physical responses.

AGRIMONY (flower essence) Agrimony personalities exhibit outward confidence and good cheer, but this is only a mask covering deep anguish of the soul. There is often a strong attraction to drugs or other addictive substances as a means of keeping the mask in place and the pain at a distance. This remedy is meant to aid in finding true inner peace by transforming pain into growth and coming to an understanding of one's own feelings.

CALIFORNIA POPPY (flower essence) The pattern of imbalance for this remedy includes searching outside of oneself for false forms of enlightenment and peace, often through addictive substances. This remedy can aid a person in the development of a solid spiritual life and great inner strength.

MORNING GLORY (flower essence) This remedy is important for overcoming addictive habits and coping with the "hung over" feelings that substance abuse creates. This remedy is especially helpful in overcoming erratic sleeping and eating habits and in strengthening the nerves and the immune response.

RED POPPY (flower essence) Red Poppy is for the development and strengthening of inner spiritual guidance and good sense.

SELF-HEAL *(flower essence)* Self-heal brings a sense of responsibility for one's own healing and a lessening of the need for external people and things to find happiness and fulfillment. This remedy can help a person achieve faith in the possibility, even probability, of complete wellness and wholeness.

WALNUT (flower essence) Brings the courage to follow one's own path, utilizing the best aspects and lessons of family/community values and past experiences. This remedy is important for times of transition such as leaving behind addictive behaviors.

MOUNTAIN IRIS (flower essence) The focus of this remedy is to find balance and harmony in the midst of the struggles and battles of our daily lives.

SCUTELLARIA LATERIFOLIA (skullcap) Skullcap, in any form, is always a nervine. In this homeopathic blend, it is meant to help quiet the mind when it is full of nervous fear or restlessness. This remedy is excellent for promoting sleep and helping focus the mind on the task at hand.

ADDICTIONS #2 (7X)

GENTIANA AMARELLA (gentian) For those who—for the moment, at least—lack inner stamina, willpower, and faith. Lack of physical stamina may also be present. This gentle combination is meant to accelerate healing in persons who are full of doubts and discouragement about the process of cure or their ability to ever completely heal and move on. Gentian is especially useful for those who magnify setbacks into a profound sense of discouragement that causes them to give up.

GUACO MIKANIA (climbing hemp weed) Guaco has an affinity for the nervous system, particularly the spine and lower limbs, although it has been used historically for mental incapacities and circulation problems to the head, especially in heavy drinkers.

KALI HYPOPHOSPHORICUM (hypophosphate of potassium) Great fatigue and debility with atrophy of muscular tissues. Used historically for the effects of excessive tea drinking. May prove useful for the effects of overuse of other alkaloids and for toxic chemical poisonings.

CROCUS SATIVUS (saffron) Picture includes rapid changing of mental conditions—anger and violence followed by sorrow and repentance, laughter quickly followed by tears and despondency, etc. This remedy is helpful with fainting spells and the after-effects of surgery and surgical anesthesia.

ADDICTIONS #3 (7X)

Helps with emotionally driven eating and food cravings. (This remedy, new for us, excites me!)

IODUM PURUM (Iodine) Provings for Iodum indicate appetite disorders that bring about malnutrition, emaciation, and physical debility. The flip side of these behaviors is ravenous hunger with great thirst. Naturally, with Iodum, there are thyroid disorders including goiter. Emotional symptoms include impulsive behavior, physical ill effects of nervous shock, anxiety when quiet or things are quiet around them, and general depression. There is often great restlessness. Pancreatic disease is also listed.

LYCOPODIUM CLAVATUM (club moss) Lycopodium is a great polycrest with a large list of symptoms available for study. The symptoms most likely to apply to addictions are probably emotional ones such as dyslexia, loss of self-confidence, fear of public speaking, melancholy, and panic attacks. Other symptoms include acidity, colitis, allergies, gallstones, indigestion, malnutrition due to weakness of digestion. The person usually has many food allergies, reacts poorly to sugar (sweets of any kind, really) and bread. A Lycopodium personality will have had colic as a baby and be prone to hypoglycemia as an adult.

PHOSPHORUS (the element) With Phosphorus, there is always great sensitivity to the struggles of other people. The Phosphorus personality is excitable, impressionable, prone to great anxiety and constant fear that something is about to go wrong. There may an oppressive feeling in the chest, as if there were a great weight laid on it. A particular keynote is a craving for ice cold drinks. The joints suddenly give way and gastritis with heartburn is a common symptom.

SEROTONIN (a brain neurotransmitter) Insufficient amounts of serotonin create a massive list of problems. Among them are compulsive disorders, bulimia, insomnia, restlessness, learning disorders, anxiety, and other mood disorders, nervous tension, twitching, heart palpitations, and water retention. Excess serotonin creates a form of depression that has been linked, quite thoroughly, to irritable bowel syndrome and several diseases that doctors have previously considered to be psychosomatic in origin.

BACOPA MONNIERI (water hyssop) Symptoms include being better able to handle difficult mental tasks and is useful for memory disorders and stress related anxiety. Bacopa has many symptoms related to the digestive tract including diarrhea, irritable bowel syndrome, gastric ulcers, and anemia.

ADRENAL GLANDS

The adrenal cortex helps maintain salt and water balance in the body. It is also involved in the metabolism of carbohydrates, the regulation of blood sugar, and the balance of hormones throughout the body. In addition, the adrenal glands supply us with adrenaline when we feel the need to either "fight" or "flee."

ADRENAL SUPPORT (6X)

SEPIA SUCCUS (cuttlefish ink) Sepia has been placed in this remedy because of its action on hormones. It is a common (polycrest) remedy for women. In fact, Sepia is the #3 polycrest remedy for women (and is among the top 10 remedies for men). The most important keynotes of Sepia are laxness of tissues, prolapse of organs, feeling as if everything is falling out the bottom, and being overwhelmed by the responsibilities of family.

IGNATIA AMARA (St. Ignatius bean) Ignatia is a hormone balancing remedy, known for its specific action against mood swings, PMS, and ailments brought on by grief. Grief and loss are always a part of this remedy and are the trigger for a great many of the physical ailments being displayed by the person.

CALCAREA CARBONICA (calcium carbonate) Overworked and exhausted are the most obvious symptoms here. There will be hormonal and menstrual problems, as well as kidney/bladder irritations

GUNPOWDER (black gunpowder) This remedy is specific to glandular system disorders and compromised immune systems with constant infections, septicemia, and hormonal imbalances.

EUPHORBIA PILULIFERA (pill-bearing spurge) Euphorbia has a dramatic action on the heart and is indicated for "pale, delicate and sensitive women" (Murphy).

ALLERGIC REACTIONS

An allergy is an inappropriate response by the body to any substance that is not harmful to most people. The immune system, which is supposed to protect us from toxins and pathogens, wrongly identifies a substance as harmful to us and goes into action. The response can be anywhere from mildly annoying to symptoms severe enough to create anaphylactic shock. These types of allergies grow worse with each reaction; they are NOT something that a person typically grows out of.

ALLERGY RELIEF #1 (7X)

GRINDELIA ROBUSTA (rosin-wood) The symptoms here are a full range of allergic responses such as lung disorders, respiratory distress, asthma, rashes, and itching eyes.

URTICA URENS (stinging nettle) This polycrest remedy has a wide range of severe allergic reactions in its symptom picture and is especially suited for use with bee stings and for the *ill effects of eating shellfish*. Unusual and noteworthy symptoms include chronic gout, joint pain, hives, itchy blisters on fingers and hands, and burning pain in the throat.

HYDROPHYLLUM VIRGINICUM (Virginia waterleaf) Hydrophyllum's range of action includes symptoms relating to the eyes. Among them will be swollen eyelids, eye inflammation, itching, and sensitivity to light.

ALLERGIES #2 (6X)

GUACO (climbing hempweed) Guaco grows in tropical areas and has a local reputation for relief from the bites of scorpions and snakes. This remedy acts predominantly on the nervous system. Outstanding symptoms are pain along the spine and constriction and feeling of paralysis in the throat.

CADMIUM METALLICUM (cadmium metal) Cadmium markedly affects the eyes with light sensitivity, burning, and inflammation ocurring. There may be extreme neuralgic headaches, difficult respiration with coughs that are mucus filled—sometimes blood-streaked—with bronchial and pulmonary distress. Chronic dermatitis is often seen.

EUPHORBIUM OFFICINARUM (gum euphorbium) The symptom picture includes hay fever, headache, inflammation of the eyelids with itching, constant dry cough with a hollow sound, dryness of the mouth with a white-coated tongue, and ringing in the ears—especially when sneezing and at night.

ALLERGIES #3 (9X)

APIS MELLIFICA (honey bee) Allergy symptoms of Apis include burning, itching and inflammation of serous membranes, excessive swelling with edema, kidney distress, and heart troubles. Apis can be useful for both mild situations and serious allergic shock reactions.

ALLIUM CEPA (red onion) Allium covers more symptoms of common colds and hay fever than any other remedy. The eyes feel as though you are cutting up raw onions at the moment. There will be increased secretions from mucus membranes, hacking cough, dripping nose, sneezing, fever with thirst, hoarseness, and a sensation of a lump in the throat.

ALLERGIES #4 (6X)

Specifically for allergies to animal hair but often useful for other allergies when the symptom picture fits the allergies the person is experiencing.

GRINDELIA ROBUSTA (rosin-wood) The symptoms here are a full range of allergic responses such as lung disorders, respiratory distress, asthma, rashes, and itching eyes.

PINUS SYLVESTRIS (Scotch pine) The picture of Pinus is predominantly lung symptoms similar to what is experienced with bronchitis. A lot of mucus but the accompanying cough is short and dry. There are feelings of tightness in the chest with impaired ability to breathe.

VERATRUM ALBUM (white hellebore) Veratrum symptoms always include profound prostration, and near total collapse with extreme coldness and weakness. There may be spasmodic contractions of the muscles of the chest. With veratrum type symptoms everything comes on suddenly.

GELSEMIUM SEMPERVIRENS (yellow jasmine) The most notable symptom of Gelsemium is burning in the larynx and chest when coughing. There will be extreme itching of the skin but there may or may not be any eruptions. The person will be trembling with weak, aching muscles as the reaction progresses.

PSORINUM (scabies nosode) Psorinum is specific for allergies and hay fever which are a family inheritance related to the Psora miasm. Offensive, foul-smelling discharges of all sorts. Hot sensation in chest with a great deal of pain. The keynote Psora pattern of remedies working well for a time but then failing to produce effective results with the need to find another remedy and then another in order to keep healing progressing will be present.

ALLERGIES #5 (8X)

Particularly for reactions to mold, yeast, or dust.

SILICA TERRA (pure flint) Bruised pain in chest when coughing or breathing deeply. Itchy eruptions, mostly on the chest area and chronic skin rashes appearing at any time. Asthma-like symptoms as a result of allergies, usually worse in the early fall. Violent cough, especially when lying down. Chronic catarrh and coryza in the nose and sinuses.

PHOSPHORUS (the element) Phosphorus ailments can be insidious—gradually increasing in their effect on the entire system. The allergic reactions of Phosphorus consist of irritation, inflammation, and degeneration of the mucus membranes. There may be a feeling of a great weight on the chest, with difficulty breathing and feelings of heat throughout the body. There is frequent itching and burning of the eyes with sensitivity to wind.

HISTAMINUM MURIATICUM (histamine) Allergic reactions with asthma-like symptoms, including bronchial and respiratory irritation keynote Histaminum. There will be dryness of the mucus membranes of the nose and throat. Other symptoms include edema, hives, itching, and redness of the eyelids.

RANUNCULUS SCELERATUS (marsh buttercup) Look for the characteristic mapped or peeled looking tongue with rawness and burning that extends into the throat. The person will be experiencing fluent coryza with much sneezing.

This formula also contains remedies made from a variety of molds, yeasts, and dusts not identified specifically by the manufacturer.

ALLERGIES #6 (6X)

This remedy was formulated for use when there has been an allergic reaction to chemical inhalants/ inhalers. It is also useful for related allergy symptoms brought on by the liver toxicity created by the use of these chemicals regularly.

EUPHRASIA OFFICINALIS (eyebright) Euphrasia is specific for allergic reactions with a pronounced action on the eyes. Symptoms include eye irritation with discharge and copious watering, glandular swellings, and very offensive sweat as the body attempts to detoxify from the inhaled poisons.

WYETHIA HELENOIDES (poison weed) With Wyethia, there are reactions which target the throat but have a history of dropping quickly into the chest. There is swelling of the glands in the right side of the neck with a characteristic itching of the upper palate.

NAPTHALINUM (tar camphor) Napthalinum is said to reduce the suffering from the inflamed, bloodshot eyes of the hay fever season. Other symptoms include attacks of sneezing, skin rashes, eczema and psoriasis.

HISTAMINUM MURIATICUM (histamine) Symptoms of Histaminum include allergic reactions with asthma-like symptoms including bronchial irritation and dryness of the mucus membranes of nose and throat. Other symptoms include edema, hives, itching, and redness of the eyelids.

NATRUM MURIATICUM (sodium chloride) Natrum displays the usual symptoms of hay fever and allergies with the additional discomfort of blinding headaches, fluttering and palpitations of the heart with constriction of the chest and high blood pressure.

TABACUM NICOTIANA (tobacco) This remedy is for the more serious, advancing toward anaphylactic shock, symptoms of severe allergic reactions. There will be high tension of the coronary arteries with intermittent pulse. As the reaction worsens, the person will experience icy coldness with sweat, fainting and nausea. Complete prostration of the entire muscular system and severe mental confusion is a possibility if things are allowed to get worse without intervention.

ARSENICUM ALBUM Arsenicum is the first remedy to reach for in any acute ailment whether it is a cold, hay fever, influenza or food poisoning. Shortness of breath is a keynote symptom with extreme restlessness, or anxiety and restlessness, presenting alternately.

ALLERGIES #7 (6X)

Predominantly for tree pollen allergies.

CARDUUS MARIANUS (St. Mary's thistle) The major focus of this remedy is for liver dysfunction which, of course, often plays a role in allergic reactions. Other keynote symptoms are pressure in eyelids and eyeballs, pressing pain in the throat on speaking or swallowing. Swallowing is usually very painful with a painful burning sensation.

EQUISETUM HYEMALE (horsetail) Horsetail, herbally, is a remedy for kidney issues and the same is true for the homeopathic form of this wonderful herb. When the kidneys are eliminating properly and maintaining proper water levels in the body, allergic reactions are less likely and less severe if they do occur. Sharp pain in the outer angle of the eye—more often in the right one. There may also be a sharp sticking pain in the throat.

IRIS VERSICOLOR (blue flag) Symptoms include burning of the mouth, tongue and throat, redness and inflammation of the eyelids with burning in the inner canthuses, and vision disturbances with headache.

RANUNCULUS SCELERATUS (marsh buttercup) The focus of Ranunculus for allergies is pain in chest/lung area that is worse for deep breathing and a raw and burning tongue with pain in the throat.

ZINCUM PHOSPHORICUM (zinc phosphide) With Zincum allergies there will be foggy vision. Zincum is also a tonic for the kidneys and useful for lung issues and asthma-type symptoms.

ALLERGIES #8 (6X)

EUPHRASIA OFFICINALIS (eyebright) Allergic reactions with a specific action on the eyes are typical. There will be eye irritation with discharge and copious watering. There may also be glandular swellings and very offensive sweat as the body attempts to detoxify from the poisons that have been inhaled.

PSEUDO-NARCISSUS (daffodil) The Pseudo-narcissus picture includes allergy symptoms such as watery eyes, frontal headache, increased pulse, increased flow of saliva, severe coryza of the nose and the opposite symptoms of dryness in the throat rather than an increased flow of saliva.

RANUNCULUS SCELERATUS (marsh buttercup) A keynote of Ranunculus sceleratus is the severe burning and scraping sensations in the throat. There may be fluent coryza with attacks of sneezing accompanied by headaches in which the head feels as if it were too large.

SULPHURICUM ACIDUM (Sulphuric acid) Various types of coryza from the nose with a copious flow that is thin, watery discharge that is a bit lemony is a major symptom here. Alternatively, as so often happens in the symptom pictures of homeopathic remedies, the symptoms may present the opposite pattern of dryness in the nose with loss of the senses of smell and taste. The symptoms that respond to Sulphuric acidum often include itching all over with boils or abscesses on the skin.

ANGER (3X)

GENTIAN AMARELLA (gentian) Emotionally Gentian personalities, in an out of balance state, tend to exaggerate the small setbacks and tiny "molehills" in life and relationships into major events and calamities. Viewing life in this way sets them up for doubts and discouragement, angry outbursts, and often prevents them from enjoying their lives and their relationships.

ALPINE LILY (flower essence) For balancing the interaction between Yin (feminine/passive) and Yang (male/aggressive) energies. This interplay is basic to our mental and physical health and governs our personality style.

STICKY MONKEYFLOWER *(flower essence)* In today's society violence, anger, and manipulation are often portrayed as positive attributes (or at least acceptable, maybe he will change behavior), especially in relationships between men and women. This essence addresses these inappropriate emotions and behaviors, helping us feel and express deep feelings of love and togetherness. Promotes genuine love and compassion, particularly in the expression of sexuality.

LARKSPUR (flower essence) In this personality is seen the polar opposites of leadership characterized by joyful service with contagious enthusiasm and leadership that is distorted by burdensome dutifulness with self-centeredness and self-aggrandizement.

LARCH (flower essence) Larch is particularly healing to the throat (communication and creativity) chakra and can help us communicate our needs effectively, appropriately, and with confidence. Larch is suited for those whose poor self-esteem causeS them to appear hostile or judgemental in their relationships with others. Larch can alleviate expectations of failure and fear of trying or even beginning to try.

ANXIETY #1 (9X)

This remedy is specific for panic attacks, anxiety from injury, or fear of upcoming events.

PIPER METHYSTICUM (kava-kava) This remedy is used as a stimulant by the natives in Polynesia before undertaking important business or religious ceremonies because it excites the mind and sharpens the faculties making them capable of more intense mental labor without fatigue. Symptoms include mental tension, constrictive feelings of the chest and stomach, heavy sensation behind upper part of the sternum, insomnia, neuralgias, and nerve pains after dental work. Symptoms are worse when reading or thinking but better from movement and open air.

HYPERICUM PERFORATUM ***(St. John's Wort)*** St. John's Wort has been used for many, many years in the treatment of a wide range of nervous disorders. These disorders include, among others, general depression and depression following wounds and injury to nerve rich areas of the body such as fingers, toes, the spine, and the coccyx. Hypericum is indicated whenever there is excessive pain or acute sensitive to pain and is especially useful when there are shooting pains from the injured part. From the descriptions, I would suggest this for learning disabilities that include omitting letters, mistakes in speaking, using words out of order or incorrectly and for the anxiety that such problems create. A great remedy for those who suffer from Seasonal Affective Disorders.

ACONITUM NAPELLUS (monkshood) Aconite is a polycrest remedy for accidents or illnesses that were sudden enough or severe enough to induce fear, shock, or great anxiety. The anxiety and fear is often accompanied by a fear of death or fear of the future. There will likely be tingling, with coldness and numbness all over the body. This is an excellent remedy for nightmares, phobias, insomnia with thrashing about, despair from pain, and panic attacks The symptoms are usually worse at night.

ANXIETY #2 8X

SECALE CORNUTUM Secale is a remedy for restlessness, anxiety, extreme debility and prostration, stinging neuralgic pains which burn like fire, numbness, and twitching and spasms of muscles. Contraction and then dilation of blood vessels with palpitations and erratic pulse may develop making the person feel sad, suspicious and afraid. Symptoms are worse from heat but better for cold applications or open air.

TUBERCULINUM BOVINUM is the nosode of the Tuberculosis miasm. Keynotes are deep feelings of being unfulfilled, with a desire to travel or take a new job. There will be a sensation of suffocation and depression with malicious behavior. Physical symptoms include heaviness and pressure over the heart with palpitations on taking a deep breath. Things get worse in a small room and in the evening.

ARTIFICIAL SWEETENERS

ASPARTAME

Robin Murphy, ND, a renowned homeopath, discusses aspartame in his Materia Medica and says that:

> Aspartame is an artificial sweetener and *neurotoxin.* It chemically breaks down into very toxic by-products, including formaldehyde, formic acid, and methanol.* The homeopathic indications are based on aspartame's many toxic side effects. There is certainly enough experience with the side-effects of this substance to form a clear picture of its effects on the human body!

*Methanol is another name for wood alcohol and is known to be poisonous even when consumed in relatively modest amounts. Disorders caused by toxic levels of methanol include blindness, brain swelling, and inflammation of the pancreas and inflammation of the heart muscle.

The FDA in 2007 published a Board of Inquiry Report revoking the petition for approval of aspartame. This report listed 92 nasty symptoms of ingesting aspartame which were used as the basis of an attempt to have the manufacturer, Searle, indicted for fraud. Result? Donald Rumsfeld, CEO of Searle, *somehow* not only avoided prosecution but got this deadly poison approved to market for human consumption!

Symptoms for the homeopathic version of Aspartame taken from the FDA's list of nasty symptoms (Remember, there were 92 symptoms—I won't try to list them all here) include headache, dizziness, problems with balance, mood swings, vision disturbance, seizures (including Grand Mal and Petit Mal) and convulsions, memory loss, fatigue, weakness, neurological disorders, changes in heart rate and other cardiovascular disturbances, numbness, difficulty breathing, difficulty swallowing, speech impairment, muscle tremors, wheezing, constipation, unsteady gait, coughing blood, glucose disorders, hallucinations, shortness of breath on exertion, ***death***, and ***developmental retardation in children.***

The list has, of course, been withdrawn. (Reference, Dr. Betty Martini, Founder of Mission Possible World Health International and the Aspartame Toxicity Center.) There is a short, but very educational, film entitled "Sweet Misery: A Poisoned World" that I believe you will find interesting. Aspartame is a hidden ingredient in many pharmaceutical drugs. I credit aspartame with the heart problems which have plagued my life for many years

SACCHARIN

Quoting Robin Murphy, ND on saccharin:

> This substance is a derivative of benzoic acid, and is made synthetically from coal-tar. Saccharin is not recommended for children with "sulfa drug" allergies, and has been linked to short-term problems with infant muscle tone, "lazy" eye, irritability, and insomnia. Saccharin has been implicated in the development of photosensitive skin eruptions in humans, and as a hypoglycemic agent in animals. Increased incidences of bladder cancer and tumors have been found in toxicity studies.

Saccharin, like aspartame, remains on the market today and is not always listed on labels. If it is on labels it may be a slightly altered version and be listed under another brand name altogether.

The basis for the proposed ban of saccharin in the past was a study that documented an increase in cancer in rats being fed saccharin. The "Delaney clause" of the Food Additive Amendments to the Federal Food, Drug, and Cosmetic Act states that no substance can be deemed unsafe if it causes cancer only in animals, but sometimes animal studies are all that we have to go on. When studies were conducted on humans they did not have, in my opinion, sufficient length to adequately allow time for much of anything, certainly not cancer, to show up.

In suspending the proposed saccharin ban, Congress ordered that products containing the popular sweetener must carry a warning about its potential to cause cancer. The FDA formally lifted its proposal to ban the sweetener in 1991 based on new studies, and the requirement for a label warning was eliminated by the Saccharin Notice Repeal Act in 1996. I can find no good science for the refusal of congress to ban, or at least label, this stuff but I do wonder if the "paper or money trail" of this legislation might make interesting reading!

HOMEOPATHY AND ARTIFICIAL SWEETENERS

Detoxifying the body from these alarming substances (and avoiding them as much as possible in the future) seems like a good idea when you consider the great amount of evidence that exists as to their potential for great harm to the body and mind. This remedy may be a good first step in such a program.

Homeopathic theory includes the doctrine that "a homeopathic version of the substance that produces certain symptoms in a well person will stimulate the body to "throw off" those same symptoms when a person is ill. " This is called the " law of similars." Taking aspartame or saccharin in homeopathic form does not exactly follow this protocol. This protocol would be more of an "exact working against an exact poison" protocol rather than the use of a "similar." In homeopathic parlance, this is referred to as the "prescribing of a nosode". A nosode MUST be given INTERCURRENTLY with another remedy. Recent thought is that flower essences are wonderful intercurrent remedies and I would certainly support the kidneys as the body cleanses itself from these toxic substances.

It is a good idea, after completing a regimen of a nosode and intercurrent remedies, to pay close attention to the remaining symptoms and follow up with a remedy or remedies that match those symptoms. For more information on working with nosodes, please see Butterfly Miracles with Homeopathic Remedies, Book One, which is a more comprehensive work on homeopathic thought and treatment.

ARTIFICIAL SWEETENERS REMEDY (9X)

ASPARTYL-PHENYLALANINE ISODE (aspartame) The following is a partial list of the possible side-effects of aspartame—in addition to the FDA's list of problems on the previous page. According to homeopathic principles, side-effects becomes the things for which a remedy might be useful whether or not the problem was caused by aspartame. Epilepsy, seizures and convulsions, auto-immune diseases, increased susceptibility to infections, allergic reactions, lupus, hypertension, major blood sugar issues, vision disturbances, weariness, mental confusion with headache, poor concentration, poor memory, anxiety attacks, depression, ***marked personality changes***, rapid heart beat, palpitations, numbness and tingling of limbs, asthmatic reactions, chronic cough, constipation and/or diarrhea, vertigo.

Makes me wonder how many of the things we call "disease" in this day and age are related to this one chemical and how many other "diseases" are the results of other chemicals that have become part of our lives every day.

SACHARINUM ISODE (sacharin) There are very few provings of this remedy and none that I could find contained much depth. This short list includes, short-term problems with infant muscle tone, lazy eye, irritability, insomnia, the development of photosensitive skin eruptions, breathing difficulties, diarrhea and hypoglycemia (in animal studies), An increased incidence of bladder cancer and tumors were also found in toxicity studies.

Site after site on the web will tell you that saccharin is perfectly safe. All I can tell you, for sure, is that it is NOT safe for me! The negative impact (literally) on my heart and nervous system has always been almost instantaneous!

Remedies A-C

BACKACHE #1 (6X)

TUBERCULINUM BOVINUM (tuberculosis nosode) The symptom picture includes backache which includes tension in the nape of the neck and down the spine. There is a feeling of chilliness between the shoulders or up the back. The pain in the back may be accompanied by heart palpitations. Keynote mental symptoms are dissatisfied and restless with a desire to travel, move about or change jobs.

PSORINUM (scabies nosode) Severe backache with difficulty in straightening the back is a common symptom of this remedy, as is painful stiffness of neck with swelling of glands at nape. The backache is often accompanied by weakness and debility and has malnutrition or improper eating habits at the core of the cause. The pain of this remedy is made worse by walking or standing and there will be a marked despair of ever recovering from this pain.

LYCOPODIUM CLAVATUM (club moss) Back and bone pain which has an underlying causation in malnutrition from improper eating habits or ***weakness of the digestive system***. The pain is best described as throbbing and pulsating and may involve the neck as well as the back. There is a keynote symptom of headache that is worse if the person is not eating regularly.

BACKACHE #2 (6X)

PHOSPHORUS (the element) The phosphorus picture includes a variety of back and sacral pain with none of them listed as keynotes of the remedy. Keynotes of Phosphorus are often mental and must be present for this remedy to be effective. These symptoms include sensitivities to lights, odors, noise, and the pain and suffering of others. The symptoms may be brought on by any type of bad news, by horror stories, thunderstorms, the dark, and just about everything else—a remedy for very sensitive people.

CIMICIFUGA RACEMOSA (black cohosh) This is a polycrest remedy for women in labor, back pain during labor in childbirth, especially if the pain is in the sacral region, moving through the hips and down the thighs, and is accompanied by nausea and vomiting.

SEPIA SUCCUS (cuttlefish ink) This is predominantly a women's remedy. A keynote is lack of muscle tone. The lack of muscle tone in the abdominal area causes a backache in the lumbar (small of the back) region. This can be really nasty during labor. The back pains will be sudden and feel as if the back is being struck by a hammer with the pain made worse by stooping or kneeling. After the initial few attacks, the pain settles in to a dull throbbing and feeling of weakness in the lumbar area.

CALCAREA FLUORATA (calcium fluoride) The backache of Calcarea florata is a chronic back pain, usually from a strain or other injury. The backache gets worse initially with any movement, but improves with continued gentle motion and simple exercises.

BACKACHE #3 (6X)

HYPERICUM PERFORATUM (St. John's Wort) Hypericum is for damage and injury to nerves. The pain, no matter where in the body it is located, is usually a shooting nerve pain coming in spasms. This remedy is particularly useful for tailbone (coccyx) injuries.

UVA URSI (bearberry) Uva ursi is for backache due to bladder or kidney disorders. The backache will be better for lying on the back because this position relieves the pressure on the bladder. There may be shooting pain from hip to hip and the backache may be accompanied by headache.

ZIZIA AUREA (meadow parsnip) There is lower back pain with dragging sensation in both hips. There is a tired feeling in legs after slightest exertion. The pain is made worse from movement and the back is sensitive to touch.

BACTERIA (9X)

GUACO (climbing hempweed) The diarrhea of Guaco is extreme with aching in sacrum and loins and pain and rumbling in the bowels. In the provings, rice-water stools occurred along with difficult swallowing. There will be pain along the spine and pain in the hip joints, ankle joints, and the soles of the feet. The legs will feel very heavy. Symptoms will be worse from bending, from motion, and at night.

PULSATILLA NUTTALIANA (American pulsatilla) Symptoms of Pulsatilla include a dark stool that is covered with mucus. There is constipation with sudden attacks of diarrhea. The tongue is coated white, and covered with a tough slime. The center of the tongue has a yellowish cast becoming unusually red and dry after eating. There is a feeling of weight and pressure in the stomach after eating. Faintness and aching pain in chest are also common symptoms. Sleep is restless with frontal headache.

EUPHORBIA IPECACUANHAE (Ipecacuan spurge or American ipecac) This remedy is said to be a more active emetic than Ipecacuanha. Symptoms include long-continued vomiting with a sense of heat, vertigo, blurry vision, fatigue, and prostration.

VERVAIN (flower essence) Bach listed this remedy in the category of "Over Care for Other's Welfare". Other mental and emotional characteristics might include enthusiasm over fixed ideas with somewhat offensive zeal in trying to persuade others to your point of view. The result is escalating tension in relationships and within oneself. The excessive drive leads to a gradual depletion of reserve energy. This is a remedy for those prone to manic states followed by depressive ones. I am not completely sure why this remedy would be included in a bacteria fighting remedy except that this emotional pattern might lead on to increased susceptibility to infections.

PYROGENIUM (rotten meat pus) Pyrogenium symptoms include high fevers with sore limbs. The fever produces great sweat but sweating does not cause a drop in temperature. There is diarrhea with fever and excruciating, throbbing headache, heart palpitation, and horribly offensive discharges.

BED-WETTING (9X)

Bed-wetting can occur in any age group and have a number of varying causes. This combination seems to be targeting physical bladder irritation with an underlying emphasis on nervousness and fearfulness.

EUPHRASIA OFFICINALIS (eyebright) Euphrasia is a wonderful remedy for the kidneys and the bladder. There will be nocturnal bladder irritability with dribbling urine.

KALI SULPHURICUM (Potassium sulphate) Inflammation of the basin-shaped area of the kidney. There is high oxalate (oxalic acid) count in the urine. High oxalate count is implicated in the formation of kidney stones and is found in people suffering from chronic candida infections. Studies have also shown that children with autism have particularly high levels of oxalates in their urine. A connection has been drawn between a lack of lactobaccilus in the intestine and high oxalates. It is believed that vitamin C, if not absorbed properly, converts to oxalic acid. (Choose vitamin C supplements with care—ascorbate, not ascorbic acid.) Be careful with hybrid citrus fruits. There will be a strong craving for sweets.

RED CHESTNUT (flower essence) This remedy is in the group "For Those who Have Fear" and is specific for physical nervousness with tightening of muscles in the stomach and abdominal regions.

VIOLA ODORATA (sweet-scented violet) Viola odorata is of particular benefit to bed-wetting in nervous children. The urine will be milky with a strong smell. This remedy is also indicated for the removal of parasites. That is a very helpful thing since parasites are involved in bed-wetting more often that one would think.

BIOPLASMA (4X)

A combination of all 12 of the Schuessler biochemic tissue salts

CALCAREA FLUORATA (calcium fluoride)
CALCAREA SULPHURICA (calcium sulphate)
KALI MURIATICUM (potassium chloride)
KALI SULPHURICUM (potassium sulphate)
NATRUM MURIATICUM (sodium chloride)
NATRUM SULPHURICUM (sodium sulphate)
CALCAREA PHOSPHORICA (calcium phosphate)
FERRUM PHOSPHORICUM (phosphate of iron)
KALI PHOSPHORICUM (potassium phosphate)
MAGNESIA PHOSPHORICA (Magnesium phosphate)
NATRUM PHOSPHORICUM (sodium phosphate)
SILICA TERRA (pure flint)

Information about Schuessler's biochemic tissue salts is available on the web and in many books and booklets with excellent descriptions of each one.

In 1858, the now famous idea was postulated that the body is merely a collection of cells, and that medical treatment should be directed towards the individual cell. Dr. Schuessler recognized that certain "cell salts" were of paramount importance to the over-all health of individual cells. His work led to the making of these 12 homeopathic, or biochemic, remedies. The study of them is both fascinating and informative!

I can find no indication in the literature that Dr. Schuessler ever combined all 12 of his remedies into one combination remedy, nor do I know who first tried this or marketed it, or who first gave this remedy to me. I only know that over the years I have used this combination for many things with great success and it is now for sale on any site that sells tissue salt remedies.

Of particular note is Bioplasma's ability to coagulate the blood in a serious, deep cut where bleeding is profuse. Bioplasma is nearly miraculous in its ability to stop a hemorrhage in women.

Bioplasma is useful in stimulating the body to uptake and utilize the trace minerals that are so necessary to optimal health of muscle, nerve, organ, and tissue cells. Bioplasma also has a stabilizing influence on nerves and nerve tissue and promotes healing in any type of wound or injury.

CANDIDA

Candida albicans is a naturally occurring yeast-like fungus that lives in various mucus membranes of the body and in the intestinal tract. Under certain conditions natural balance is upset and the candida multiply and travel through the bloodstream to many parts of the body. Because it is found, when it shouldn't be, in many parts of the body, this remedy is characterized by many symptoms. Nevertheless, the root cause of all of the symptoms is the out-of-balance state in the intestinal mucosa.

CANDIDA #1 (6X)

Candida #1 targets many symptoms and can prove helpful in reestablishing healthy intestinal function. It is not a substitute for proper diet, exercise, or proper use (or elimination altogether) of antibiotics.

FERRUM METALLICUM (iron metal) There is a sensation that the bowels have been bruised with cramp-like pain in the region of the spleen and chronic catarrh of the bladder. There will be a great desire for sweets,but sweets are the worst possible food for an overgrowth of candida.

NATRUM ARSENICUM (sodium arsenate) The keynote symptom is abdominal pain with a feeling of shifting through the bowels. The discomfort and stomach pain is made better by the passage of gas.

ZINCUM PHOSPHORICUM (zinc phosphide) Some alternative medical personnel believe that candida overgrowth is made possible, in part, by a lack of the trace mineral, zinc. Symptoms include abdominal pain, backache, constipation and diarrhea by turns, with mental depression and fatigue.

CANDIDA #2 (6X)

The focus is on abdominal and digestive issues where candida begins and, sometimes, remains.

CHIONANTHUS VIRGINICA (fringe tree) Physical symptoms include liver congestion or obstruction, menstrual or liver-based headaches (frontal headache), enlarged spleen, paroxysms of abdominal pain, loss of appetite, nausea, alternating constipation and diarrhea, listlessness and apathy. The person is nervous and restless but wants to be left alone. They may find relief from lying on the abdomen.

ALUMINUM PHOSPHORICA (aluminum phosphate) Diarrhea and/or constipation. Many foods sound good to the person but aggravate symptoms all over the body. Mental prostration with confusion of the mind and apathy is listed. Phosphorica always indicates extreme weariness and fatigue.

CANDIDA #3 (6X)

This remedy focuses mainly on thrush symptoms in the mouth and throat.

CANDIDA ALBICANS NOSODE (thrush fungus) This is the nosode of the thrush fungus so it displays all of the various candida symptoms. Used with other remedies, as in this combination, should aid in reestablishing a proper balance of candida bacteria throughout the body.

NATRUM MURIATICUM (sodium chloride) Symptoms appropriate to this remedy include increased salivation with thrush ulcers in the mouth and burning when food touches the mouth or throat.

RANUNCULUS SCELERATUS (marsh buttercup) Rawness with burning pain in the mouth and a mapped-looking tongue.

CARDIO ARRYTHMIA #1 (9X)

EPHEDRA VULGARIS (ma huang) This remedy is for damage done by diet pills containing a laboratory-reduced (drug) form of ma huang. Symptoms include extreme apathy and fatigue, violent headache, nausea, and general weakness. The heartbeat will be strong but there will be weakness of the pulse. Respiration will be accelerated, with retention of urine. There will be heaviness in all of the limbs in the evening and numbness of entire left arm (causing some concern) and a great longing for sleep.

IPECACUANHA (ipecac root) Dryness of mouth and great thirst are indications as is chest pain with shortness of breath The pulse is accelerated but weak. One side of the face is hot, the other side is cold. There will likely be migraine or headache of gastric origin with persistent nausea and vomiting.

MANCINELLA VENENATA (manganeel apple) Pressure and needle-like pains in the chest, heart related, with palpitations in the evening are part of the Mancinella picture. Violent coughing from exertion is seen. The person may be forgetful with suddenly vanishing thoughts. There is painful stiffness of lower back and neck when walking. Everything is worse from cold, damp, and from cold drinks.

NATRUM SULPHURICUM (sodium sulphate) The chest feels empty and all gone or there is pressure on the chest as if a heavy load is lying there with stitches in the left side of the chest. The eyes are very sensitive to light and there are violent pains at the nape of the neck and at the base of the brain.

THUJA OCCIDENTALIS (arborvitae) This is a full scale heart remedy. There are anxious palpitations on waking in the morning with cramp in the heart with violent pulsations in evening. The pulse will be full and accelerated in the evening, slow and weak in the mornings with persistent swelling of veins. There is always an intense desire for dark chocolate and salt (Oh, those wonderful new bars that they make!) This is the leading remedy, in former generations, for adverse reaction to vaccinations and is still a polycrest for these types of reactions.

CARDIO ARRYTHMIA #2 (9X)

CRATAEGUS OXYACANTHA (hawthorn berries) Another great heart remedy. Symptoms include anxiety with palpitations, cardiac insufficiency with the heart muscle seeming flabby and worn out, aortic congestion, weakness, and valvular incompetence. This remedy can sustain the heart during infectious disease and aid in recovery from heart attacks because it increases heart strength. This is a very useful remedy for congestive heart failure and enlarged heart. This type of impending heart failure is recognized by symptoms arising from the slightest exertion. There is usually, but not always, high blood pressure.

CAPSICUM ANNUUM (cayenne pepper) Symptoms of this remedy include a sensation of constriction in the chest with difficult breathing and sluggish circulation. The poor circulation creates extreme sensitivity to cold and damp along with capricious and changeable moods. The face may be red but will feel cold. The muscles will ache and, perhaps, jerk at times. Muscle pain will be felt in various places such as the legs, arms, shoulders, or back and be extremely painful and violent. There will be a burning sensation as though the muscle has been terribly overworked.

CHRONIC FATIGUE SYNDROME (CFS)—A CONDENSED OVERVIEW

Chronic fatigue syndrome is a condition that has become so widespread in the United States as to qualify as a rising epidemic. The cause, or causes, of chronic fatigue syndrome are not well understood. It is sometimes referred to as chronic Epstein-Barr syndrome because of the high incidence of the presence of Epstein-Barr virus in people who suffer from this syndrome. However, just as many people test positive for this virus without exhibiting the symptoms of the syndrome. This has led some experts to conclude that the condition may be triggered by any viral attack that the body did not handle well, not just by the Epstein-Barr virus.

Another claimed, or suspected, cause is chemical poisoning from one source or another, including dental fillings and prescription drug use. Yet other experts suspect an unidentified immune system dysfunction, or a defect in the mechanisms that regulate blood sugar or that blood pressure issues may be the culprit. Other proposed causes include anemia, diabetes, hypoglycemia, hypothyroidism, a Candida albicans overgrowth, food or chemical allergies, or intestinal parasites.

In other words, the cause is unknown and the symptoms vary widely from person to person. Actually, that is the definition of a "syndrome" as compared to a disease—having no idea what is causing it.

Symptoms and Determining if This Could Be What's Wrong with You

Chronic fatigue syndrome does not manifest the same way in any two people. It is more a matter of having an array of many of the typical symptoms. It is helpful in obtaining a diagnosis (if you want one) if the Epstein-Barr virus is found to be present. A family history of mononucleosis or hepatitis is an indicator of exposure.

A family history of other infectious diseases, multiple allergies, asthma, and certain cancers may indicate an underlying immunological problem and a predisposition to this condition. Recurring sore throats and/or swollen glands, frequent colds or other infections, and various hormonal imbalances are also considered pre-indicators.

Dietary habits are extremely important, as is the need to eliminate the ingestion of chemical poisons such as alcohol, tobacco, carbonated beverages, and recreational drugs. "Current medications, or medications taken in the past, may also be significant. For example, prolonged and multiple antibiotic use, steroids, birth control pills, chemotherapy (just about any drug, really) can have a suppressive effect on the immune system." (Jesse Stoff, MD, Chronic Fatigue Syndrome, The Hidden Epidemic).

The list of symptoms includes abdominal bloating, migratory aching muscles and joints with increasing stiffness and loss of motion, marked irritability or personality changes, anxiety, depression, difficulty concentrating, significant loss of stamina an hour or so after meals, cravings for sugar or caffeine, sudden episodes of dizziness, rapid onset of fatigue at odd times, intermittent fever of no apparent cause, headaches, digestive and/or intestinal problems, mood swings, muscle spasms, recurrent upper respiratory infections, sensitivity to light and temperature, food and environmental sensitivities, sleep disturbances, temporary memory loss, and—finally—extreme and often disabling fatigue.

Chronic Fatigue Syndrome (CFS) affects the entire person (every organ and system is a potential target for trouble) and the entire person must be considered in looking for symptoms and finding a treatment modality that will be effective. It is not the presence of any one symptom that indicates CFS. It is the presence of a constellation of symptoms including any combination of the above list.

An unusual phenomenon: From time to time, in the midst of the disabling fatigue, a CFS sufferer will hit upon an idea (they were often very creative and dynamic people before the overwhelming fatigue of CFS) and suddenly the energy just flows for a time—until the project is completed, *or nearly so*. This is remarked on time and time again in the literature and is not really understood. I can only tell you that it is not that the person is lazy the rest of the time, and it is not necessarily an indication that they are suddenly getting better.

The best description of CFS I have ever found is in the chapter entitled Footprints: The Diagnostic Dilemma in the book Chronic Fatigue Syndrome, The Hidden Epidemic, by Jesse A. Stoff, MD, and Charles R. Pellegrino, Ph. D. This book is a wealth of excellent information and it is written in a very readable and entertaining style. The information in this book was the basis for the creation of the first four of the following CFS homeopathic remedies listed in this book.

Homeopathy and the Treatment of CFS

Treating homeopathically is treatment following "the law of similars." The specific name of the disease (or syndrome) is not relevant. What matters is that your symptom picture and the symptom pictures of the remedies you intend to use match each other!! A struggling adrenal cortex always manifests in certain ways, as does a clogged liver or colon. Disease names are only a "left-brained," categorical way of describing symptoms. Disease names are pretty much ignored by competent homeopathic prescribers if they wish to be effective at solving the "case."

Symptoms are what matters!! And symptom-picture methodology is where homeopathic remedies shine!!

Stress and CFS

A quote from Science News, September 12, 1987, and re-quoted in Chronic Fatigue Syndrome, The Hidden Epidemic by Stoff and Peligrino:

> *Tending to a relative with Alzheimer's disease is not just psychologically stressful over the long run, say researchers at Ohio State University College of Medicine in Columbus, it can undermine the caregiver's immune responses. . . Subjects caring for an Alzheimer victim reported more distress and poorer mental health than individuals with no such responsibilities. Caregivers also had indications of poor immune function: lower percentages of T-lymphocytes and helper T-lymphocytes than controls, as well as a lower ratio of antibody-stimulating cells to anti-body-supressing cells.* ***In addition, there was evidence of poorer immune system control of the latent Epstein-Barr virus among caregivers.***

The following is a quote from Norman Cousins in Anatomy of an Illness, and requoted in Chronic Fatigue Syndrome, The Hidden Epidemic by Stoff and Pelegrino:

> *Adrenal exhaustion could be caused by emotional tension, such as frustration or suppressed rage . . . the negative effects of the negative emotions on body chemistry. The inevitable question arose in my mind: what about the positive emotions? If negative emotions produce negative chemical changes in the body, wouldn't the positive emotions produce positive chemical changes? Is it possible that love, hope, faith, laughter, confidence, and the will to live have therapeutic value? Do chemical changes occur only on the downside?*

Stress, and its relationship to physical and mental health, is an elusive subject to study or to treat. It is not so much a matter of what stresses are in our lives, but it matters very much how we handle the stresses under which we live. Our responses to stress should be very carefully considered—and chosen.

There are 4 main ways of responding to the daily stresses of living and to the major disasters of our lives:

1. We ***surrender*** to the flow of circumstances in our lives fatalistically, as though we have no control and, therefore, no say in the direction our lives take. This makes us either victims or martyrs and is one of the most destructive things that we can do to ourselves.

2. We ***ignore*** the struggles of life as we pass through them, pretending that all is well and there is nothing to be concerned about or dealt with. This inevitably leads to an accident or an illness as our body tries to make us consciously aware of our own needs.

3. We attempt to ***resist***, which often wastes energy, adds fuel to the destructive processes of stress, and usually gets us nowhere very fast.

4. We ***learn*** from our circumstances and use them as stepping stones and catalysts for our growth and for the achievement of our goals. Needless to say, this last one—learning from the experiences of our lives—is the only appropriate response to stress if we wish to be well and happy.

In order to discover a possible psychological underpinning for any chronic illness, there are several difficult questions that need to be asked—and thought about deeply. Some examples are:

1. Am I using my illness to get the care and/or the attention that I felt I deserved or needed and wasn't getting?
2. Do I enjoy not having to deal with people and situations that I dislike or find overwhelming?
3. Am I using my illness to avoid the possibility of failure, or even the possibility of success, with the attendant stresses of either situation?
4. Do I feel sorry for myself and see myself as either a victim or a martyr?

Nutrition, Supplements, Herbs and CFS

This can be summed up very simply. You need all of the nutrition that you can get to put your entire system—every organ and cell— back on track, and you cannot afford to take very many of the things that rob your body of nutrients—junk food, drugs and medications, to name just a few.

Do your homework on what is available to supply the nutrients you need and what you can do to maximize your body's absorption of these nutrients. Bear in mind that overloading on supplements that you are not absorbing creates its own kind of stress in the body, and can quickly become a major contributor in the escalation of the problem rather than being part of finding a solution.

THE CHRONIC FATIGUE SYNDROME REMEDIES

Consider the use of Glandular Support #3 and Detox #1 along with the following remedies as the symptoms indicate the need for them.

CFS #1 (12X)

ECHINACEA ANGUSTIFOLIA/PURPUREA (purple coneflower) Echinacea stimulates the immune response and is a tonic for the blood. The symptom picture includes many of the physical and mental symptoms of CFS and has strong indications for the support of liver function. Great fatigue and prostration are keynotes of both the remedy and chronic fatigue syndrome, making a good match.

Echinacea should be considered to be taken as an *herbal* supplement, also, as it is known to be a protection against bacterial and viral infections and to eliminate chemical toxins.

ARGENTUM NITRICUM (silver nitrate) The physical description of this remedy includes colic with much gas and distension of the abdomen, great lassitude, and weariness. Emotional patterns include many fears, a list of phobias, a lot of anxiety—especially about personal performance, with a great fear of failure (or success) and a fear that something bad is about to happen. The person is usually impulsive—always wants to do things in a hurry. An especially strong and important keynote is an almost overwhelming craving for sweets.

FERRUM PHOSPHORICUM (iron phosphate) The combination of the two great polycrests, Ferrum and Phosphoricum, creates an outstanding remedy for extreme debility, exhaustion and anemia. This remedy is said to increase hemoglobin levels in the blood by instructing various organs and systems as to their tasks in this regard. This remedy is indicated for the first stage of all inflammatory disorders.

Ferrum phos is an outstanding example of synergy, the combining of remedies so that the sum is greater than the total of the parts, in the best healing sense. In this case, the Argentum nitricum and the Ferrum phosphoricum greatly enhance the immune strengthening properties of the Echinacea. This remedy helps in the regenerative process in the individual cells of organs, tissues, and nerves.

CFS #2 (6X)

APIS MELLIFICA (honey bee) Based on anecdotal evidence, a few doctors have used the sting of the honey bee in the treatment of nerve and immune system disorders such as multiple sclerosis. Chronic fatigue certainly qualifies as a nerve and immune system disorder! This is interesting in light of the symptom picture of this remedy. It matches the symptoms of MS very closely.

Apis has an unusually slow action and must not be discontinued too soon. The increased flow of urine produced by this remedy indicates that it is having a favorable effect and is detoxifying the body as intended. A keynote is hot, stinging, burning sensations, the location of which may be anywhere in the body. Other keynotes are extreme tenderness in the abdominal region, nervousness, and great restlessness.

BELLADONNA (deadly nightshade) Belladonna acts on the brain, nerve centers, glandular and lymphatic systems. The symptoms are notable because of their sudden onset. Abdominal symptoms include extreme sensitivity to touch, with tenderness and swelling. There is also several kinds of insomnia and other sleep disorders.

Together these two remedies make an awesome combination for use with nerve disorders, abdominal distress, and insomnia. I have found them very effective.

The use of ***HYPERICUM PERFORATUM (St. John's Wort)*** with CFS remedy #2—even added to the combination—should be considered, if the symptom pictures match. Hypericum is listed for nervous depression following injury or chronic illness, as well as for a host of other mental and physical symptoms that describe the chronic fatigue sufferer.

CFS #3 (6X)

This remedy targets the liver, pancreas, adrenal cortex, and digestive function.

HEPAR SULPHURIS CALCAREUM (Calcium sulphide) Mental symptoms include oversensitiveness to impressions, people, and places with extreme irritability, impulsiveness, and sometime a ferocious temper. Sadness and depression to the point of a desire for death are not uncommon symptoms. There is a definitive action on the liver, the lymphatic, and the glandular systems.

MERCURIUS SOLUBILIS (mercury vivus) People needing this remedy are often described as human thermometers. That's mercury!—up and down and constantly changing, especially in moods and energy levels. There will be dejection and discouragement. Mercurius also has an action on the lymphatic system and increases glandular activity. Both of these functions are sorely needed when coping with CFS. Physically and mentally, the symptom picture includes many of the symptoms of CFS and fatigue in general. Other physical symptoms include tinnitus, pancreas dysfunction, and liver enlargement.

SPONGIA TOSTA (roasted sponge) This remedy is specific to the adrenal glands and acts as a stimulant to the liver. Physical symptoms include severe exhaustion and a feeling of heaviness after exertion. Watching them walk up a short incline is enough to make the observer tired! Their clothes feel uncomfortable and whenever possible, they will undo their pants, loosen their tie and unbutton their shirt a bit. Stiffness in the muscles and severe constipation are absolutes. There will be fear of the future.

TARAXACUM OFFICINALE (dandelion) Deficiency of liver and bladder with liver clogging and the attendant front headache are part of this picture. Gastric distress with feelings of bubbles bursting in the abdomen. There will be impatience, irritability, and much grumbling going on under the breath.

This remedy seems to stimulate the anabolic metabolism of the liver. Doing so supports the immune system, takes stress off the pancreas and adrenal glands, and improves digestive function. The abdominal pains and bloating noted by CFS sufferers often subside with the use of this remedy.

CFS #4 (6X)

With this compound you should notice, over several weeks, a lessening of both fatigue and irritability and a clearing of the dark circles under the eyes.

SEPIA SUCCUS (cuttlefish ink) Sepia symptoms include a sluggish liver with the sensation of something twisting in the stomach and intestines. The person will be mentally and physically worn out, irritable, overwhelmed, and averse to the company of those they love—family for whom they feel responsibility.

IGNATIA AMARA (St. Ignatius bean) Ignatia is always about the physical effects of grief and worry. Some physical symptoms seen in CFS include spasms and cramps in the back and other muscles, sciatic pain in back and hips, joints feeling as if they have been dislocated, much flatulence, and insomnia due to the mind focusing on griefs, disappointments, or worries.

CALCAREA CARBONICA (calcium carbonate) Extreme fatigue due to mental or physical overwork. The person is constantly worrying about all their responsibilities and duties. They have nightmares and poor sleep patterns with frequent sourness and nausea in the stomach.

CFS #5 (6X)

CALCAREA MURIATICA (calcium chloride) The symptoms of Calcarea muriatica include anxiety with weakness and trembling and is also indicated for the relief of glandular swelling and gastric pain.

KALI PHOSPHORICUM (potassium phosphate) Symptoms include fatigue, insomnia, nervous prostration, increased sensitivity to all impressions, and weakened state from mental or physical stresses.

RESERPINUM (alkaloid of Rauwolfia serpentina) Reserpinum symptoms include the slowing down of mind and body, lassitude and aversion to work in the evening, nervous depression, alarming fatigue symptoms in normally hyperactive and aggressive persons, spasmodic attacks of pain in the colon, constipation followed by diarrhea, the need for sleep or period of rest after meals, and gastric and duodenal ulcers.

ZINCUM MURIATICUM (zinc chloride) Zincum and Muriaticum together indicate great fatigue of both brain and nerves. Moods will be changeable. There is an unusual symptom of craving for some particular food in an attempt to relieve irritation and nausea of the stomach.

A Final Warning

According to Jesse Stoff, MD (previously quoted on the topic of CFS), "The Epstein-Barr virus not only weakens the surveillance system that guards against deviant cells, but is itself oncogenic, meaning that under the right circumstances it can create deviant cells and be responsible for the creation of several different varieties of cancer." If this is so, it is a scary virus, indeed.

The research indicates that EBV acts as an initiator and must be potentiated by a "promotor". Research into what constitutes a promotor continues. The list of EBV-associated cancers grows every day.

The common denominator seems to be confusion of the immune system as to what is and what is not foreign to the body and is an invading organism or cell. In other words, the same thing that is causing such an increase in allergies may also be causing an increase in EBV-related cancers.

The first thing that comes to my mind is the immune-suppressant drugs added to "required" vaccinations and given so freely to our children, starting as day-old infants in the hospitals where they are born. The second link seems to be the vast array of chemicals that we ingest or take into our bodies in other ways every day. There are likely other links to the increased number of suppressed immune systems today.

According to some studies, EBV attacks the anti-body producing B-cells. Once inside, ***the virus causes the B-cells to reproduce the virus along with any new B-cells that are produced***. The very cells that are usually the defenders have now become a production line for the problem. As the T-cells set about destroying the virus, the B-cells are also destroyed, resulting in a severe immune deficiency as these important B-cells are destroyed. Just like soldiers in battle dying from friendly fire, some T-cells are destroyed in the battle against the virus filled B-cells. The thymus, where T-cells are produced, then goes into over-drive to make up the losses. This over-production of T-cells over an extended period of time results in thymus gland fatigue. The fatigued thymus then produces immature and atypical T-cells, thus deepening the immune system compromise and opening the body to disease, perhaps even including the EBV-related cancers as well as the susceptibility of chronic fatigue patients to other bacterial and viral illnesses.

The best defense is often a good offense. Whether or not you suffer from the Eptein-Barr virus or chronic fatigue, strengthen your immune system every day in every way that you can. Do not wait until you are fighting something nasty to get to work on your health.

COLDS

No one that I know of has yet come up with a cure for the common cold but homeopathic treatment can certainly move the symptoms along with relief coming faster than it would otherwise.

COLDS #1 (7X)

ALLIUM CEPA (red onion) Allium has more symptoms of common colds and hay fever than any other remedy. If you have cut up raw onions, you have a pretty good idea of the symptom picture. Symptoms include dull headache, lots of fluent coryza, sneezing, sinusitis, burning and itching in those poor little red eyes, and hoarseness and pain in the throat—often extending out to and including the ear.

EUPHRASIA OFFICINALIS (eyebright) This remedy is effective for hay fever with watery eyes. It does not matter, homeopathically speaking, whether the symptoms are from an allergy or from an infection; the symptom picture is what determines remedy choice. Other symptoms of Euphrasia include conjunctivitis with sticky mucus, burning and swelling of the eyelids, feeling as if there were sand in the eyes, and catarrhal headache with profuse discharges from eyes and nose. Euphrasia also effects the nose and chest, as well as the eyes. Symptoms are better from open air and worse for wind and sunlight.

ACONITUM NAPELLUS (monkshood) Aconite is for colds that come on after exposure to cold wind or cold weather. Aconite illnesses are usually acute, and are always sudden and violent with high fever being common. Some other symptoms are earache, dryness and heat in the eyes, eyelids are hard, red and swollen, and the nose is stopped up. There may be acute inflammation of the throat with high fever. Mental and emotional symptoms include many forebodings and fears.

ARSENICUM ALBUM (white oxide of arsenic) This is the first remedy to reach for in any acute ailment but is particularly useful for colds, hay fever, influenza,and food poisoning. Shortness of breath with the current illness is a keynote symptom. Mental and emotional symptoms include extreme restlessness, or anxiety and restlessness manifesting alternatively.

COLDS #2 (7X)

ECHINACEA ANGUSTIFOLIA/PURPUREA (purple coneflower) In both herbal and homeopathic form, echinacea is a blood and immune tonic and brings strength to the immune system. Echinacea is indicated for lymphatic inflammation, recurring ear infections, strep throat, full feeling in the upper part of the lungs, stuffy nose and head, dullness from headache, aching in limbs, sleepiness with confusion and weakness, and chilliness with nausea.

RANUNCULUS SCELERATUS (marsh buttercup) The keynote of Ranunculus sceleratus is the severe burning and scraping sensations in the throat. There may be fluent coryza with attacks of sneezing accompanied by headaches in which the head feels as if it were too large. The tongue is coated and mapped. There may be pain over the region of the liver with the feeling that diarrhea is about to set in as the illness progresses.

THUJA OCCIDENTALIS (arborvitae) Some of the symptoms of Thuja include constant dry, hacking coughs—usually in the evenings after lying down, chronic ear infections with purulent discharge, swelling of the inner ear with loss of hearing, and conjunctivitis with burning and stinging of the eyelids.

ZINGIBER OFFICINALE (ginger root) Some symptoms of Zingiber that apply here are smarting and burning of eyes, sensitivity to light with stinging pain, pain over the eyebrows, painful respiration, scratching sensation in the chest, dry hacking cough with morning mucus, and watery coryza in the nose and obstruction in sinuses with thick mucus.

CONGESTION #1 (6X)

EQUISETUM HYEMALE (horsetail) Equisetum is a deep acting anti-sycotic (miasmic). There will be confusion of sounds with a dull, transient pain and stiff feeling behind left mastoid. This remedy is often used in bladder infections and to support the kidney and bladder during infectious attacks. Symptoms include nocturnal bed-wetting with the bed-wetting being more common only when the child dreams.

NATRUM MURIATICUM (sodium chloride) With Nat mur there is a tendency to catch colds, have hay fever, or suffer from a wide range of allergies. The mucus membranes will be dry and then, alternatively, produce white or clear, acrid discharges. There will be buzzing, humming, ringing, and roaring in the ears, as well as great weakness and weariness with the weakness felt in the morning even before leaving the bed. Other symptoms are cold limbs and coldness along the spine, eyes sensitive to light with the light causing tears to stream down the face. Emotionally, Nat mur people are depressed with feelings of isolation, the isolation being brought on by their own reserved and introverted personalities.

VIOLA ODORATA (sweet-scented violet) Viola's most specific and wide ranging action is on the ears. Congestive type headaches hold the secondary place in the remedy picture. Physical symptoms include pain in the ears that continues into the eye balls, frequent ear infections beginning almost at birth, stitching pain beneath the ears, and roaring sounds in the ears. Mental and emotional symptoms include a description of childish behaviors including—but not limited to—weeping with no explanation, refusing to eat what was just demanded, and an ornery aversion to morning.

CONGESTION #2 (9X)

CHICORY (flower essence) Mental/emotional imbalance as it applies to caring for or controlling others is part of this flower picture. There is a martyr syndrome—constantly serving others, but with a lot of built-up resentment. Physical symptoms include congestion in the bronchial tubes with difficulty breathing in and out. The breathing difficulties are linked to holding on to this self-inflicted hurt and self-pity and the feeling of not being appreciated for all that one does. Many times the self-pity becomes a way of manipulating and controlling family members and friends.

IRIS VERSICOLOR (blue flag) Congestion and pain in the throat and bronchial tubes. The symptoms get worse in the evening and during the night. There is burning in the region of the pancreas with abdominal tenderness and vomiting of any food eaten, ringing in the ears with deafness, and chronic pain in the forehead with a headache that alternates sides of the forehead from time to time or remains over the left eye. There is profuse salivation and vomiting during the headaches and great itching of the skin at night.

MAGNESIA SULPHURICA (magnesium sulfate—Epsom salts) Epsom salts have been used for many years as a cathartic and as a homeopathic remedy it has shown itself useful for dysentery and gallstone colic. This is a remedy for panting and coughing after exercise or walking. The most marked symptoms are with the skin, urinary tract, and female reproductive system. With females, indications are thick leucorrhea, as profuse as the bleeding during menses, with pain in the back and thighs on movement. This remedy is also used for weakness of the thyroid.

THUJA OCCIDENTALIS (arborvitae) Thuja is specific to asthma and breathing difficulties in children (sometimes linked to vaccinations). Physical symptoms include rapid exhaustion and emaciation, chronic sinus infections with the unusual keynote of sweat only on the parts of the body that are uncovered. Thuja has been for many years the leading remedy for ill effects of vaccinations. Emotional and mental symptoms include feeling isolated and all alone, self-contempt, and depression. Symptoms are worse at night and, interestingly, worse when talking.

COXSACKIEVIRUS INFECTIONS—**General Information**

Coxsackieviruses are part of the enterovirus family of viruses that can live in the human digestive tract. They can spread from person to person, usually on unwashed hands and surfaces contaminated by feces. In most cases, coxsackieviruses cause mild flu-like symptoms which go away without treatment. In some cases, however, they lead to the more serious illnesses discussed below.

Coxsakievirus can produce a wide variety of symptoms. About half of the people infected with coxsackievirus have no symptoms. Others suddenly develop high fever, headache, muscle aches, and some also develop a sore throat, abdominal discomfort, or nausea. A child with a coxsackievirus infection may simply feel hot but have no other symptoms. The fever lasts about 3 days, then disappears.

This virus is responsible for different symptoms and diseases according to the part of the body affected. ***Hand, foot, and mouth disease***, in children, is a type of coxsackievirus that causes painful red blisters in the throat and on the tongue, gums, hard palate, inside of the cheeks, and the palms of hands and soles of the feet. No parent likes to see this disease in their homes. Coxsakievirus is implicated in other throat infections and in hemorrhagic conjunctivitis in both children and adults.

Occasionally, coxsakieviruses can cause more serious infections. Among these more serious situations are such things as viral meningitis, which is an infection of the meninges (the membranes that envelop the brain and spinal cord), encephalitis (another serious brain infection), childhood insulin-dependent diabetes, osteoporosis, and myocarditis (an infection of the heart muscle). Myocarditis is most prevalent among children and among men around the age of 40 (for reasons which I do not understand). As the virus enters the heart cells, the immune system reacts by attacking and damaging both infected and normal heart cells. The progress of the heart disease continues *even after the virus has been eliminated from the body because the immune system now sees the heart tissue as a danger and continues to fight to eradicate it.*

One of the harsh facts about coxsakievirus is that even when a person has recovered from an infection and has no remaining symptoms at all, they may shed infectious organisms for weeks. A fetus or newborn is a risk if the mother becomes infected near the delivery date.

COXSACKIE VIRUS REMEDY (12X)

COXSACKIEVIRUS NOSODES The coxsackie virus nosodes are placed in the remedy on the assumption that the introduction of the energy pattern of the virus into the body will stimulate the body's immune and energy systems to search out, identify, and destroy the virus and then cleanse the body of the dead viruses. Using an "exact" instead of a "similar" is not homeopathy in its pure form, but since this critter mutates quite rapidly, it is probable that the homeopathic given will be following the " law of similars" as it attacks viruses which have mutated.

FILIX MAS (male fern) The remedy picture of this remedy contains mostly abdominal and intestinal symptoms but one proving is interesting—it includes violent dyspnea (difficult, labored breathing with shortness of breath) without a cough but accompanied by stitches in region of the heart and obscure symptoms of pericarditis. The prover was described as being of lymphatic-nervous temperament and much weakened by long illness.

This remedy is used for the elimination of tapeworms and for inflammation of the lymphatic glands.

The trace mineral, selenium (found in many herbals), significantly reduces instances of the mutations which create the "master" strains which are responsible for the more severe and debilitating forms of this virus. Sufficient amounts of this mineral in the body would improve the odds against serious infection.

DECONGESTION (12X)

ERYNGIUM AQUATICUM (button snake-root) This remedy acts on the mucus membranes, particularly of the head and chest. Symptoms include thick, yellow discharges, cough, oppression of the chest with the inability to take a full breath, as well as inflammation of the left eye and the eustachian tube with thick yellow mucus discharges from the nose.

IRIS VERSICOLOR (blue flag) Symptoms include congestion with the remedy showing a particular affinity for detoxifying the digestive system. Appendicitis with sudden attacks of diarrhea are mentioned.

MYRRH (gum myrrh) Myrrh quickens the pulse, raises the body temperature with great sweating and prostration. This is a remedy for enfeebled states with excessive mucus discharges.

THYMUS SERPYLLUM (wild thyme) Thymus has an effect on the urinary organs with the elimination of uric acid as its prime function. It is useful for respiratory infections of children, dry nervous asthma, and pressure in the head that creates ringing in the ears.

DETOX #1 (6X)

ARSENICUM ALBUM (white oxide of arsenic) This is a deep-acting polycrest remedy for dealing with influenzas and poisonings and has a particular affinity for the liver. Symptoms include sudden great weakness and shortness of breath. Arsensicum is a restorative for all systems of the body (digestive, urinary, circulatory, lymphatic, glandular).

BERBERIS VULGARIS (barberry) Berberis is useful in arthritic and hepatic disorders, reduces kidney inflammation and helps with kidney and gallstone pain. It aids the body in detoxifying from chemical and metal poisoning and strengthens the body overall.

GLYCYRRHIZA GLABRA (licorice root) This is a great liver remedy, both in detoxification and protection. It is powerfully anti-inflammatory and is used as a virus fighter.

LYCOPODIUM CLAVATUM (club moss) Lycopodium is best suited to progressive chronic illnesses with great weakness. Lycopodium is also excellent for problems with digestion and for liver dysfunction.

NATRUM MURIATICUM (sodium chloride) This is a deep grief and sorrow remedy, and is for the weakening of the immune system, and damage to heart, kidneys, and spleen that these emotions engender.

NUX VOMICA (poison nut) Nux is preeminently for men who have been under stress for a long time and is useful for the stomach and bladder, for sleep disorders, irritable nerves, and for fiery tempers.

PHYTOLACCA DECANDRA (pokeweed root) Phytolacca acts on the glandular system and helps eliminate infection and inflammation. It has a special affinity for fibrous and osseous tissues and the sheaths and fascias of the muscles of the shoulders and arms.

STILLINGIA SYLVATICA (Queen's root) This remedy acts on respiratory, lymphatic, eliminative and glandular systems. It brings the "poison" to a pustular head and then eliminates it from the body.

THYROIDINUM (thyroid gland extract) Thyroidinum is useful for stimulating, strengthening, and regulating the thyroid and has a profound action on the heart, especially in cases of valvular heart disease.

TRIFOLIUM PRATENSE (red clover) Trifolium pratense is useful as a blood purifier and powerful detoxifying agent. It is indicated for anyone with predisposing factors for any type of cancer and is useful for respiratory illnesses with hoarseness, choking, chills, and cough at night—whooping cough.

DETOX #2 (9X)

This remedy is specific for mercury poisoning and detoxification.

CADMIUM BROMATUM (cadmium bromide) Cadmium bromatum is comparable to Cadmium sulphuratum. Symptoms include vomiting, burning in the stomach, esophagus, mouth, and throat.

KALI SULPHURICUM (potassium sulfate) Symptoms include colic pains, distended abdomen, mucus rattling in lungs, and nausea and vomiting. This remedy aids in the transfer of inhaled oxygen to all the cells through the mechanism of red blood cells.

NATRUM SULPHURICUM (sodium sulphate) This is the leading remedy for treating the results of head injuries. Nat sulph aids the elimination of excess fluid from the system, often producing great thirst.

TARTARICUM ACIDUM (tartaric acid) is the agent in pineapple that so many people are allergic to, making it, done homeopathically, useful for gastritis, pain at umbilicus, flatulence, thirst, and vomiting.

The above symptoms are a partial description of the symptoms of mercury poisoning. As the remedies are removing the symptoms, the underlying causation—the mercury poisoning—is being detoxed and carried from the system.

DETOX #3 (6X)

Formulated for use in MSG detoxification.

MSG ISODE (monosodium glutamate) is an isode acting to detoxify the cells of the brain, nerves, muscles, and the inter-cellular fluids which have been "clogged" and poisoned by this toxic substance.

KALI PHOSPHORICUM (potassium phosphate) Kali phos is found in the cells of the brain, nerves, muscles, blood (both corpuscles and plasma), and in the inter-cellular fluids. Taking Kali phos does not provide this nutrient—there is no material dose of a substance in a homeopathic remedy, but it does have an action on the mechanisms of the body that cause the uptake of this trace mineral. The presence, or utilization, of Kali phos strengthens the cells and allows them to detoxify. Kali phos is indicated if there is nervous prostration or brain fatigue in which any mental exertion aggravates the symptoms.

DETOX #4 (9X)

LAPPA ARCTIUM (burdock) As an herbal remedy, burdock is a liver cleanser of great ability and is known to encourage intestinal peristalsis and protect the blood against acidosis. Homeopathically, Lappa arctium affects the skin, sweat glands, liver, kidneys, joints, and the uterus (a remedy specific for uterine displacement and prolapse).

TARAXACUM OFFICINALE (dandelion) Dandelion's chief traditional use is for liver obstruction and kidney difficulties. Some symptoms of Taraxacum include headaches due to liver disturbances, frequent desire to urinate, jerkings and shooting pains in the muscles of the neck, profuse night sweats, and impatience and irritability.

TRIFOLIUM PRATENSE (red clover) The materia medicas list this remedy for blood disorders, coughs, cancers, fibroids, and whooping cough, and other coughs that are worse at night, and for sore throat with hoarseness.

YUCCA GLAUCA (Soapweed) Yucca, as an herbal remedy, is used for osteoarthritis, high blood pressure, migraine headaches, inflammation of the intestine that is present with colitis, high cholesterol, stomach disorders, diabetes, poor circulation, and liver and gallbladder disorders.

MALVA NEGLECTA (marshmallow) As an herbal remedy, marshmallow is a mild diuretic but its great strength lies in the abundance of vitamins and trace minerals that it contains. Homeopathic remedies contain no material dose of substances but theory holds that they can stimulate the body to better uptake and utilize the vitamins and minerals which the herbs contain.

RHEUM PALMATUM (turkey rhubarb) Hahnemann's proving of Rheum confirmed many of its traditional uses. Some of these uses include improving digestion and appetite, strengthening the kidneys and the bowels, and acting as a mild stimulating tonic and cleanser to the liver and the blood. Interestingly, symptoms for this remedy are mostly left-sided.

The herbs in this combination, here homeopathically potentized, are traditionally used in the removal of aberrant cells and tissues from the body. Most are commonly known homeopathics with provings and symptom pictures, Malva neglecta and Yucca glauca are not. The descriptions above are based on the traditional uses of these common herbs.

DETOX #5 (6X)

This remedy is for ridding the body of the toxic ingredients of vaccinations and other poisons.

JUNIPERIS COMMUNIS (juniper berries) Juniper has a powerful action on the kidneys and is indicated by dragging pain in the back, bladder irritation, great thirst, and stomach distension with tenderness.

NATRUM SULPHURICUM (sodium sulphate) This is the leading remedy for treating the results of head injuries. Nat sulph aids the elimination of excess fluid from the system, often producing great thirst, and is used for chronic diarrhea and debilitation.

RADON is included because of its reputation for having a normalizing effect on cellular abnormalities. Some of the literature goes so far as to use terms like squamous cell, small cell, and large cell carcinomas and lung cancers.

THUJA OCCIDENTALIS (arborvitae) Thuja has been for many years the leading remedy for ill effects of vaccinations and for situations where a person has never been well since a vaccination reaction. Emotional and mental symptoms include feeling isolated and all alone, self-contempt, and depression. Symptoms are worse at night and, interestingly, worse when talking. Some of the other things mentioned in Thuja provings are proliferating abnormal cells, distended abdomen, cysts, polyps, rapid exhaustion and emaciation, and chronic sinus infections.

CIMICIFUGA RACEMOSA (black cohosh) Cimicifuga is a polycrest remedy for women and is indicated for puerperal fever and any form of sepsis. This remedy has a wide action on the cerebrospinal and muscular systems and is used for pain in the joints and in the limbs. Emotionally there are feelings of gloom and dejection.

GELSEMIUM SEMPERVIRENS (yellow jasmine) I consider Gelsemium to be a remedy for the convalescent/recovery stage of many things. It can be especially useful whenever a cleanse or detox program has produced unwanted symptoms. A few symptoms for which Gelsemium might be useful include the limbs feeling heavy—almost paralytic, dizziness, drowsiness, headache as if there is a band around the head, and dull pains up and down spine. Gelsemium is also a treatment for chronic fatigue of liver origin.

NUX VOMICA (poison nut) Nux is a remedy for people of zealous fiery temperaments. Some symptoms include chilliness—cannot get warm no matter what, spasms and convulsions from poisoning, blurred vision, painful and ineffectual urging to urinate, and ***headache from chemical toxicity.***

CHELIDONIUM MAJUS (greater celandine) This is a major liver, respiratory, kidney, portal and venous system remedy making it of great benefit in this combination.

ISODES OF ALDICARB Aldicarb is a multi-use pesticide used in agricultural and horticultural settings. It is considered one of the most acutely toxic pesticides ever registered in the United States. Aldicarb i*nhibits the enzyme responsible for the transmission of messages to nerves.* Some of the symptoms of poisoning by this pesticide include tightness in the chest, difficulty breathing due to bronchial constriction, increased bronchial secretions, sweating, salivation, nausea, vomiting, diarrhea, abdominal cramps, and involuntary urination These isodes have been placed in this formula to aid in the detoxification from these and other harmful substances which create symptom pictures similar to aldicarb poisoning.

INFORMATION ABOUT ALDICARB AND THE FDA AND EPA

The first highly publicized outbreak of aldicarb poisoning, which sickened more than 2,000 people, occurred in California in 1985. It took a full 25 years for the *announcement* of the *phase-out* of this poison to occur. The phase-out was still ongoing (meaning aldicarb was still in nearly full use) in 1993. The EPA and FDA rely mostly on voluntary agreements, instead of on bans, to avoid lawsuits from manufacturers. The EPA assistant administrator overseeing pesticide programs said that she faced "the need to exercise due process in making sure that the company producing the chemical had a fair hearing." Apparently, a fair hearing, when you are a drug manufacturing company, takes many years.

Years later, in 2007, the EPA concluded that there were "potential human health risks" but approved aldicarb's continued use with added precautions such as larger setbacks between fields and water wells and reduced amounts applied to crops. This situation—the continued wrangling of the new *phase-out* announced in 2010—goes on and on with its use on citrus and potatoes finally being halted in 2012.

Aldicarb has been banned in Europe for several years now and a new agreement has been reached in the United States with Bayer, the sole manufacturer of this pesticide. ***Under the new agreement, Bayer will end its distribution by 2017 and all usage will stop by 2018. In other words, although the effects, especially on babies and small children, have been known since 1985, it has taken the EPA and the FDA these many years to get this chemical pulled from use on our food supply. Incredible, but typical!!***

DETOX #6 (7X)

Formulated for overcoming the effects of misuse, over-use, or allergies to penicillin.

PENICILLINUM (penicillin) The homeopathic penicillinum has been used to antidote the effects of penicillin when it has been over prescribed to patients or when there has been an allergic reaction. This isode may be helpful for those who have a family history of allergic reactions to penicillin. Some symptoms of this remedy include fatigue, diarrhea, fever that continues for a long time, kidney pains, and feelings of icy-coldness in different parts of the body. Allergic reactions may bring on anaphylactic shock and become very serious, even life threatening, very quickly. This remedy is also indicated for those who have never been well since taking this drug and is indicated for any symptoms for which this drug would have been prescribed allopathically.

NATRUM LACTICUM (sodium lactate) .Natrum lacticum is useful for gout, uric acid, unusual hunger and thirst, great weakness of lower limbs, arthritis-like pains, rapid swelling of entire body and "chalk stones" in fingers.

THUJA OCCIDENTALIS (arborvitae) Thuja has long been considered a major remedy for the after effects of vaccines and other chemical toxins. Emotional symptoms include self-contempt, feeling isolated and all alone, and depression.

DETOX #7 (6X)

For detoxification from chemical additives.

This combination is made up of three distinct parts. The first part contains the homeopathic isodes of various ***laboratory produced imitations*** of naturally occurring amino acids. The isodes are in the remedy to stimulate the body to find and dispose of the residue of these drugs. The second part of this remedy is the homeopathic isode of methanol (or wood alcohol). The third part is homeopathic remedies whose great strengths lie in the support and strengthening of the glandular system.

In order to understand this remedy and its ingredients, some explanation is necessary. I will try to keep this lesson in chemistry and anatomy as simple and as short as I can and still get the most necessary pieces of this complicated subject presented.

First: Glutamic acid, phenylalanine, and aspartic acid are *naturally occurring amino acids*—in other words, *they are found in the foods that we eat every day. We need them because they are precursors and initiators of many essential metabolic processes in the body.* ***In their natural state—they are not dangerous to our bodies.***

Second: MSG (originally) is the *naturally occurring* and very abundant sodium salt of glutamic acid. MSG is responsible for some of the flavors we enjoy most in meats and certain vegetables. MSG was first isolated as a flavor enhancer in Japan in an attempt to duplicate the taste of an edible seaweed that is used as a base for many Japanese soups. MSG's popularity as a flavor enhancer grew, worldwide, very rapidly.

There are three ways to produce MSG—hydrolysis of specific vegetable proteins, bacterial fermentation, and *chemical synthesis.* As always, chemically synthesized anything is *not natural* because man has yet to produce a *single substance* that is truly *nature identical!* Really and truly, this is a fact!

Fortunately, most MSG that is produced and marketed today is done using the bacterial fermentation method. Unfortunately, whenever safety studies are conducted on this and other products, it is rarely specified which type is being used and it is almost never reported which one was used if it is known.

Man-made, laboratory-produced, chemical imitations have at least one molecular connection that is turning the wrong way (left rotating, designated by an l in the formula name). These laboratory produced imitations of natural molecules are always toxic to one degree or another!

Third: Aspartyl-Phenylalanine (aspartame) is a combination of ***man-made, chemically produced phenylalanine and man-made, chemically produced aspartic acid.*** There have been many studies conducted that show a wide variety of results as to the safety of this product. There is also a long and sordid history of the FDA's failure to protect the public it is sworn to serve from this and other such chemicals.

Fourth: Wood alcohol (rubbing alcohol), used in Part Two, should not be ingested or placed on the skin if it is at all possible to avoid doing so. (I know, we have been taught to use it as a disinfectant!)

Fifth: The isodes that have been placed in this remedy are NOT the isodes of the *naturally occurring* amino acids. They are the isodes of the *man-made, laboratory produced, toxic imitations of the real thing.* These isodes are there to help the body recognize those poisons and eliminate them and then stimulate the body to repair whatever parts of the damage that has been done that can be repaired.

Sixth: Some of the homeopathic remedies in Part Two are polycrest remedies for supporting and strengthening the glandular system and the nerves. Others, such as Thuja, are there because they are known to help the body throw off the effects of chemical poisoning.

PART ONE:

GLUTAMIC ACID ISODE (a laboratory produced amino acid)
PHENYLALANINE ISODE
ASPARTIC ACID ISODE
MSG ISODE (monosodium glutamate the sodium salt of glutamic acid)
ASPARTYL-PHENYLALANINE ISODE (Aspartame—phenylalanine and aspartic acid combined)

PART TWO:

METHANOL ISODE (wood alcohol—rubbing alcohol is a more common name)

PART THREE:

CHAMOMILLA VULGARIS (German chamomile) This remedy is especially suited for highly emotional, temperamental, and overly sensitive children and adults. Some other relevant symptoms include profuse sweating (as the body tries to throw off toxins?), headaches that are made worse by stimulants of any kind, flatulence and colic, distended abdomen, earache, and many symptoms linked to nerve irritation.

CUPRUM METALLICUM (copper metal) Cuprum is one of the most important remedies for the reappearance of symptoms that were formerly suppressed by toxic drug treatments. This remedy affects the nerves and is used for convulsions and cramps of a violent nature especially in the fingers, toes, and calves. When this remedy is needed, there will often be a metallic (toxic drug) taste in the mouth.

MYRRH (gum myrrh) Myrrh is a stimulant and a tonic. It produces a quicker pulse, raises the body temperature, and produces vomiting and purging if that is what is necessary.

THUJA OCCIDENTALIS (arbor vitae) As already mentioned, Thuja is placed in this remedy because it is known to be of benefit in never well since a vaccination or drug program.

DETOX #8 (12X)

Aids in cleansing from environmental toxins and poisons.

CALCAREA SULPHURICA (calcium sulphate) Indicated for glandular swelling and dysfunctions, connective tissues issues, pain over the liver, cleansing and support of the liver, burning and itching of the feet, and weakness of the legs. The person is probably sleepy during the day but wakeful at night.

FERRUM PHOSPHORICUM (iron phosphate) Symptoms include debility and weakness from toxic poisoning, low iron and hemoglobin counts, a variety of blood conditions where blood volume is normal but fluids are increased out of normal proportion to solid particles (thin blood, not just iron deficiency anemia).

NATRUM NITRICUM (sodium nitrate) Natrum nitricum is used in the treatment of inflammations and hemorrhages of all kinds. The mental/emotional picture of this remedy is ill-humor and being unwilling or unable to find the energy for mental or physical exertion.

STRONTIUM NITRICUM (strontium nitrate) There have been far too few provings of this remedy but it is known to be indicated for the sort of bad taste in the mouth that is associated with drug poisoning, headache, albumin in the kidneys, intestinal irritation, arthritis, and a variety of nervous conditions.

CHERRY PLUM (flower essence) Cherry Plum is said to help those suffering from inflammation of and damage to the nervous system. This remedy is indicated for lack of impulse control, obsessive-compulsive disorders, and perfectionist or ritualistic behaviors. A very useful remedy for eliminative system disorders and for use in detoxification programs.

DETOX #9 (12X)

Aids in detoxification from industrial solvents.

DI-METHYL FORMAMIDE is also known as methylbenzene, toluene, and phenylmethane and is isolated from tolu balsam, which is certainly not a poisonous or toxic plant. Isolation of a single constituent, however, often creates a *drug* with pronounced toxicity. Such is the case here. Toulene is used in acrylic fibers, plastics, pesticides, synthetic leather, paint stripper, paint, fuel oil, as a cleaning agent, and as a solvent in many pharmaceutical drugs. It is known to cause disorientation, giddiness, dizziness, euphoria, confusion progressing to unconsciousness, convulsions, headaches, fatigue, sleep disturbances, achiness, numbness and tingling.

HYDRAZINE is found in rocket fuels and is the gas precursor in automobile air bags. It is also used as a solvent in pharmaceutical drugs. Hydrazine has been linked to depression and recent studies indicate that it is a neurological toxicant. Other studies show alarming links to the onset of lupus.

TRICHLOROETHYLENE Recent studies indicate that trichloroethylene is a neuro-toxin, although "safe" levels are still being determined. This chemical is used in cleaning products, paint and varnish, and is part of the decaffeination process. It is also used as a solvent for rubber and is a common contaminant in soil and water.

This combination is entirely made up of isodes. It may be necessary to follow it with whatever remedy most closely matches the remaining symptoms. (Isodes, like nosodes, require an intercurrent remedy.)

DETOX #10 (12X)

Aids in detoxification of industrial solvents from the body.

TEREBINTHINIAE OLEUM (oil of turpentine) Children are particularly sensitive to chemical poisoning. Fortunately, they also respond quickly to homeopathic treatment. This remedy works on the lingering effects of exposure to paint, paint thinners and removers, and many other chemicals.

THALLIUM SULPHURICUM (thallium sulphate) There are very few provings and only a short list of symptoms. These include hair loss, emaciation, tremors, paralysis, night sweats, and pulmonary distress.

IRIDIUM METALLICUM (iridium metal) Iridium is one of the heaviest metals making it, according to Scholten, a remedy for deep miasmic conditions. Symptoms include exhaustion, weakness, nervousness, restlessness, hair falling out, and partial paralysis and weakness of the muscles.

CIMICIFUGA RACEMOSA (black cohosh) Cimicifuga is a polycrest with a wide action on cerebrospinal fluid and muscles manifesting as pain in joints and limbs. There will be feelings of gloom and dejection.

GELSEMIUM SEMPERVIRENS (yellow jasmine) This is a remedy for extreme prostration, the convalescent stage of an illness, and for recovery from exposure to or ingestion of toxic chemicals. A very useful remedy for chronic fatigue that is caused by a toxic liver.

NUX VOMICA (poison nut) Nux symptoms include chilliness—cannot get warm. There are spasms and convulsions, blurred vision, painful, ineffectual urge to urinate, and headache from chemical toxicity.

CHELIDONIUM MAJUS (greater celandine) This is a major liver, respiratory, and venous remedy. It is indicated for great debility, drowsiness after eating, yellowness and biliousness from liver congestion.

BERBERIS VULGARIS (barberry) Keynote is the rapid changing of symptoms. Useful in liver disorders, venous stasis in the pelvic region, inflammation of the kidneys and kidney stones, and arthritic pains.

DETOX #11 (12X)

Aids in detoxification of asbestos and other toxins from the body.

FILIX MAS (male fern) Relevant symptoms for Filix mas are inflammation of lymphatic glands, abdominal pain and bloating with diarrhea and vomiting, parasites, pale face with blue rings around the eyes, and pain in bladder with frequent urination.

MERCURIUS SOLUBILIS (mercury vivus) The mental symptoms of Mercurius are very pronounced. They include restlessness and constantly changing one's mind (and everything else possible), poor self-confidence, and weak memory. With Mercurius there is enlargement of the lymphatic glands and destructive inflammation of bones, cellular tissues, and joints. Other symptoms include tremors, convulsions, and shortness of breath when going upstairs or walking quickly.

THIOSINAMINUM (mustard seed oil) Symptoms include enlarged lymphatic glands, adhesions, dissolving of scar tissue and keloids, a sensation of heat and burning in affected parts, stricture of the rectum, and depression with an aversion to consolation.

DETOX #12 (9X)

CONIUM MACULATUM (poison hemlock) This is an ancient poison (given to Socrates), the action of which is progressive, ascending paralysis which kills when respiratory failure sets in. For whatever reason—in this case, some sort of toxicity from which the body needs to detox—the body is stiffening, the muscles become weak, the chest becomes tight, the glands become painful, and eventually there is weakness of body and mind with trembling all over.

AESCULUS HIPPOCASTANUM (horse chestnut) The most marked action of this remedy is on the lower bowels and on the venous system of the pelvic area. Other symptoms include liver disorders, degenerative hip disease, swollen glands, sacroiliac pain, varicose veins, and waking with the mind feeling dull and confused.

MERCURIUS SOLUBILIS (mercury vivus) The symptom picture of Mercurius is listed above in the Detox #11 remedy.

BARYTA CARBONICA (barium carbonate) This is a remedy for serious destruction of the body ocurring with overwhelming debility. The symptom picture includes enlargement of the glands, problems with the outer layers of the heart muscle and the blood vessels, and progressive mental weakness.

DULCAMARA (woody nightshade) The leading indication for Dulcamara is that every symptom gets worse for getting cold and damp. An odd feature of Dulcamara is that it will antidote the unnecessary activities of Mercurius, which is also found in this remedy. Dulcamara is an excellent remedy for swollen glands, mononucleosis, and arthritis.

DETOX #13 (7X)

BAPTISIA TINCTORIA (wild indigo) One of the strengths of this remedy is its effect on sepsis that is in the blood! Descriptive phrases applied include indescribable sick feeling all over—weak and tremulous as if just recovering from an illness—muscular soreness and putrid states erupting all over the body.

CANTHARIS VESICATORIA (Spanish fly) I would assume that this particular remedy is in this combination because sometimes when the body needs to detox most, it cannot do so effectively because of inflammation in the kidneys. This remedy is indicated any time there is constant urging to urinate but the urine is scanty, cutting and burning.

SARSAPARILLA OFFICINALIS ***(wild licorice)*** Historically, this remedy as an herb acts on the urinary organs, genitals, skin, and bones and is mostly a remedy for ailments that are occurring on the right side of the body.

TEREBINTHINIAE OLEUM ***(oil of turpentine)*** The symptom picture of this remedy has been added to over the years by overdoses in allopathic practice and from accidental poisonings. As a homeopathic, it should be wonderful in detoxing the body from this chemical and from other chemicals that produce a similar symptom picture. A few of the keynote symptoms include enormous distention of the abdomen, burning pain in the region of the kidneys with the urine smelling like violets, and quickened respiration.

DIARRHEA #1 (9x)

This one is a favorite remedy of a great many people!!

PENICILLINUM ***(penicillin)*** The homeopathic penicillinum has been used to antidote the effects of penicillin when it has been over prescribed to patients or when there has been an allergic reaction. This isode may be helpful for those who have a family history of allergic reactions to penicillin. Some symptoms of this remedy include fatigue, diarrhea, fever that continues for a long time, kidney pains, and feelings of icy-coldness in different parts of the body. Allergic reactions may bring on anaphylactic shock and become very serious, even life threatening, very quickly. This remedy is also indicated for those who have never been well since taking this drug and is indicated for any symptoms for which this drug would have been prescribed allopathically.

VALIUM ***(Diazepam)*** Valium is used in the treatment of anxiety disorders and for short-term relief from anxiety and panic attacks. Side effects make a good list of the symptoms for which the remedy is indicated. Some of the side effects of this drug include mental confusion, memory loss, depression, anxiety, incontinence, nausea and vomiting, diarrhea, involuntary muscle spasms, increased sensitivity to touch and to pain, and difficulty urinating or inability to hold urine.

Whenever I type a list of drug side-effects like this, I realize once again how grateful I am to Heaven for providing us with wonderful alternatives to drug therapy—if we will avail ourselves of them—and how grateful I am for the wonderful ways we have to detox the body from drugs and other toxic poisons.

ARSENICUM ALBUM ***(white oxide of arsenic)*** Arsenicum is a leading polycrest—an absolutely amazing whole body remedy—for anything to do with the digestive and intestinal tracts and many other systems. A few (very few) keynote symptoms—besides diarrhea—include burning pain in the stomach and abdomen, rumbling and cramping pains in the bowels, violent squeezing and constriction in the umbilical region, and enlargement of the liver and the spleen.

DIARRHEA #2 (9x)

FILIX MAS ***(male fern)*** Symptoms if Filix mas include diarrhea and vomiting, abdominal pain and bloating, inflammation of lymph glands, pale face with blue circles around the eyes, and frequent but painless hiccupping. Filix is sometimes used in the treatment of tapeworms and other parasites. Symptoms are made worse from eating sweets.

KALI SILICIUM ***(potassium silicate)*** This is a deep acting remedy. Symptoms include emaciation, weakness, chilliness, pain in liver region, flatulence, nausea, stiffness of the body, and twitching of muscles.

NATRUM SULPHURICUM ***(sodium sulphate)*** Involuntary and unexpected stool when passing flatulence, yellow watery stools, and itching of the anus. Feels every change from dry to wet and always feels best in warm, dry air. This remedy balances water in cells and eliminates excess very efficiently.

DIGESTIVE #1 (9X)

This remedy is specific to Geophage, a condition in which children (occasionally adults) consume earthy things such as dirt and clay. Geophage, as well as Pica (which is a similar condition), seems to be linked to poor absorption of minerals or the lack of trace minerals in the diet. These and other eating disorders may be benefited by this remedy.

CHELIDONIUM MAJUS (greater celandine) Chelidonium is a poppy and allied to Opium and Sanguinaria. This is an outstanding organ remedy with particular affinity for the liver and gallbladder and the relief of pain and congestion in those locations.

NATRUM SULPHURICUM (sodium sulphate) Common symptoms of Nat sulph relating to digestion include nausea, gas, bloating, and headache with constipation. A great many foods produce uncomfortable diarrhea. There is a strong desire for ice and ice cold water.

CALCAREA CARBONICA (calcium carbonate) The first indication for this remedy is malnutrition from lack of, or slow absorption of, vitamins and minerals. Other symptoms include glandular swellings, lack of appetite when tired or working too hard, ***cravings for eggs and for indigestible things,*** vomiting of bile, frequent sour belchings, sour vomiting, pain in the liver and gallbladder regions, and a tendency to form gallstones. Unrelated to digestive issues (unless being caused by digestive malfunctions) are joint disorders, weak ankles, and cramps in the legs at night.

DIGESTIVE #2 (7X)

Specific to flu-like symptoms caused by one of the Norwalk viruses.

Homeopathic Ingredients: NORWALK VIRUS NOSODE (norovirus)

This family of viruses is the most common cause of intestinal disturbances in the United States. They can be ingested in contaminated food or water or can be passed from an infected person to someone else. Symptoms include intense nausea and vomiting usually lasting only a day or two, diarrhea, stomach cramps, headache, and low grade fever. The most serious effect is dehydration if a person is unable to keep liquids down for too long a period of time. *Please remember that with homeopathic treatment, it is not necessary to have ingested a particular strain of virus or bacteria to benefit from the remedy made from it. You need only have a similar symptom picture.*

ARSENICUM ALBUM (white oxide of arsenicum) This is the first remedy to reach for in any stomach and intestinal upset because it has the widest range of digestive symptoms in its picture.

IPECACUANHA (Ipecac root) Ipec symptoms include cramps with nausea and vomiting, nausea from smell of food with violent hunger when nausea is over, violent cramping pains, gastroenteritis, and nausea not better for vomiting. The most outstanding keynote of Ipecacuanha is *continual persistent nausea.*

NUX VOMICA (poison nut) A remedy for intense, driven people who cannot bear noises, odors, light, or touch and who are easily offended by the careless words of others. Keynote digestive symptoms include cravings for stimulants, but worse for them, feeling of weight and pain in the stomach, region of stomach sensitive to pressure, constant sour taste in the mouth, nausea and vomiting in the morning, and the ***stomach and abdomen are very sensitive to touch***.

PODOPHYLLUM PELTATUM (May apple) Indian tribes used the root to expel worms. This remedy acts on the duodenum, which is an unusual and important function. Symptoms include rumbling and shifting of flatus, heartburn, gagging, empty retching, nausea, diarrhea, and weakness after stool.

VERATRUM ALBUM (white hellebore) Veratrum album is an important remedy for many body systems. The symptoms, taken together, add up to a profound prostration and collapsed state with extreme coldness. All symptoms indicative of veratrum are violent and sudden. With digestive issues, there will be copious evacuation—vomiting, diarrhea, salivation, sweat, and urine. The nausea and vomiting will be aggravated by the least motion.

KALMIA LATIFOLIA (mountain laurel) Kalmia has only a few symptoms that are digestive in nature. Among them, however, is pain in the stomach that is *worse for bending over.* This type of pain is sometimes indicative of heart issues, of which there are many in the Kalmia picture. One heart symptom is palpitations that are *worse for bending over,* linking the heart and the stomach symptoms together. The symptoms of nausea and diarrhea, with dizziness, may have a possible link to the heart.

DIGESTIVE #3 (9X)

KALI NITRICUM (potassium nitrate) Symptoms related to digestion include loud rumbling in abdomen, burning in the stomach, severe pain after every meal, usually on the right side, burning in urethra with diminished urine or frequent, profuse clear urine.

THIOSINAMINUM (mustard seed oil) Some digestive system symptoms of Thiosinaminum are flatulence of stomach and bowels that is worse after eating., pyloric stenosis, and stricture of the esophagus. This remedy aids in dissolving scar tissue, keloids, and removing intestinal obstructions. Useful for strictures of the urethra indicated, in part, by increased urination during the night.

DIGESTIVE #4 (7X)

HYDRASTIS CANADENSIS (golden seal) Some symptoms of Hydrastis are burning pain in the umbiiical region, flatulent colic with faintness, sharp pain in the spleen region, gurgling in ileocecal region, weak digestion with debility, stomach ulcers with emaciation, and vomiting nearly everything eaten. The materia medicas also list this remedy for use against stomach and colon cancer.

ANACARDIUM ORIENTALE (marking nut) Digestive symptoms include great emptiness in the stomach with weakness and irritability, gnawing hunger, desire to nibble, hypoglycemia—worse from fasting or missing a meal, indigestion and pain that is worse when the digestion of the last meal is complete and lasts until the next meal is taken, eating temporarily relieves all discomfort, constipation, headache worse by mental exertion and is made better by eating. The headache comes with optical illusions, flashing lights and halos.

CONDURANGO (condor plant) Condurango is a fairly recent treatment for stomach ailments with symptoms such as ulceration, vomiting of food, constant burning pain, and stricture of the esophagus with burning pains behind the sternum where food seems to stick. Condurango is also a treatment for skin ailments and for relationship issues.

PULSATILLA NIGRICANS (windflower) This remedy has a very clear emotional picture. Symptoms in the digestive realm include painful distended abdomen with loud rumblings and abdominal colic from eating ices, fruits, pastries, fat and greasy things. Other symptoms include a bitter taste that diminishes the enjoyment of all foods, heavy feeling in the stomach, and vomiting of food that was eaten long before.

IPECACUANHA (ipecac root) Cramps with nausea and vomiting, nausea from smell of food with violent hunger when nausea is over, violent cramping pains, gastroenteritis, and nausea not better for vomiting. The most outstanding keynote of Ipecacuanha is continual, persistent nausea.

DIOXINS (12X)

ISODE OF TATRACHLORODIBENZO-P-DIOXIN (Agent Orange) AND SIMILAR CHEMICALS re chemical compounds which are very poisonous. Today, it is claimed that dioxins are no longer deliberately made (see next paragraph), but are the by-products of some industrial processes such as the production of PVC pipes, the bleaching of paper, and the burning or fossil fuels. Dioxins occur naturally as the result of forest fires, volcanoes and the incomplete incineration of waste. Any person living in an industrialized nation has dioxins in his or her body and could probably benefit by having the body recognize and remove as much of them as possible, while rebuilding and repairing body organs and tissues from the damage that has been brought about.

It is unclear how harmful low doses are. Some animals begin to show symptoms of poisoning when they are given doses only 2 or 3 times the level of dioxins in the average person's body. Past research indicated that dioxins increase the risk of certain kinds of cancer but lower the risk of others according to the amount of exposure. More recently it is being claimed that epidemiological evidence does not indicate that TCDD is carcinogenic at even low doses. Perhaps it is just my paranoia showing, but I do not trust revised information that allows chemicals previously deemed harmful to continue to be marketed. Add to this the fact that removal of Agent Orange as a carcinogenic allowed the government to avoid responsibility for many sick and suffering Vietnam war vets, and I become very sceptical indeed. Glyophosate, a major ingredient of Agent Orange is, according to some sources, an ingredient of *Roundup*. Of course there are those, mostly the usual people who defend Monsanto, who claim that glyphosates are harmless to humans and certainly not carcinogenic.

There are many scientists that believe that dioxin poisoning can cause organ disease, an increased risk of cancer and heart attacks, a suppressed immune system, hormonal imbalances, diabetes, menstrual problems, increased hair growth, weight loss, and the facial cysts known as chloracne. It takes a long time for symptoms to show up, often making it difficult to determine where the poisoning took place.

DICHLOROPHENOXYACETIC ACID—2,4-D (chlorinated pesticides), TRICHLORPHENOL, PENTACHLOROPHENOL—PCP (chlorinated phenols)

Chlorinated phenols and chlorinated pesticides are used in agricultural pesticides worldwide. Scholarly articles indicate that children with even low levels of these phenols (laboratory produced) have a higher risk of parent-reported ADHD compared to children with levels below the limit of detection.

Animal studies have also reported hair loss, decreasing body weight, and a weakened immune system from oral exposure to these chemicals. Other animal studies indicate possible effects such as skeletal deformities, kidney defects, altered levels of sex hormones, reduced production of sperm, increased risks of miscarriages, and weakened immune responses ***in the offspring*** of many of the animals exposed and tested. ***Of course, none of these tests meet the standards of the FDA and the EPA for actionable risk factors in humans because they were done on animals!***

Since this remedy is comprised of isodes, it may be advisable to take a follow-up remedy according to symptoms when a regimen of this combination is finished.

ENERGY ALIGNMENT

BERBERIS VULGARIS (barberry) Berberis is useful in arthritic and hepatic disorders, reduces kidney inflammation and helps with kidney and gallstone pain. It aids the body in detoxifying from chemical and metal poisoning and strengthens the body overall. The mental picture of Berberis vulgaris is one of indifference and apathy. The person is mentally and physically tired and does not want to do much of anything. There is a dislike of the dark that is quite pronounced.

CIMICIFUGA RACEMOSA (black cohosh) Cimicifuga is a polycrest remedy for women. It is most suited for women who suffer from rather extreme mood swings and who tend to become easily overexcited. Other symptoms include sadness, anxiety, and irritability where these emotional symptoms may be tied to hormonal imbalances. Black cohosh is considered to be a remedy for the darkest states of depression—a brooding state of dark hopelessness, often tied to a history of sexual abuse, alcoholism, or drug abuse. The dark moods of Cimicifuga are usually worse just before the menstrual cycle.

SULPHUR (brimstone) Sulphur is one of the great polycrest remedies for the things that are common to the human condition and is a major anti-psoric remedy. Sulphur is frequently needed after an acute illness which did not completely clear up, relapsed, or is failing to respond to a remedy that was working well even though the symptom picture has not changed. Sulphur also has a reputation for moving a case along when the vital/immune response of the patient is deficient.

COLOCYNTHIS (bitter cucumber) Colocynthis is especially suitable for irritable persons who are easily angered, for ailments in people resulting from anger, ailments as the result of silent grief, and emotional and energetic upsets from being too much affected by the misfortunes of others. The picture of colocynthis includes depression, joylessness, a disposition to weep and cry, offended by everything and everybody, wants to be left alone, and becomes angry when questioned.

LEDUM PALUSTRE (wild rosemary) One of the major indications of Ledum is cold all the time due to the general lack of heat being generated in the core of the body. Interestingly, although cold nearly all the time and cold when first getting into bed, the heat of the bed soon becomes intolerable. An interesting emotional note that indicates serious energy issues in the body is aversion to friends and company to the point that sometimes the person has such a desire for solitude that they avoid even the sight of people.

PICRICUM ACIDUM (picric acid) Picricum is a remedy for people who are worn out both physically and mentally. Anemia that fails to respond to treatment, pins and needles sensation in the limbs, and burning in many parts but especially along the spine and in the legs are also seen. The mind is weary, weak, and forgetful, and mental exertion makes things even worse—even just a little bit of reading is too much to be handled.

AMMONIUM MURIATICUM (Sal ammoinic) Ammonium symptoms include irregular circulation with the blood seeming to be in constant turmoil with many pulsations. The emotional patterns include a desire to cry, but cannot do so, melancholy with unfounded apprehension from internal grief, and involuntary and usually unfounded aversion to certain persons.

ARGENTUM METALLICUM (silver metal) One of the keynotes of this remedy is an insatiable desire for sugar. A keynote of Argenticum that is more than intriguing is that the tissues of the body, especially the cartilages, thicken resulting in problems with the joints and bones. The cartilage of the ribs becomes particularly painful, especially on the left side.

ER911 (3X) *(please see Rescue Remedy)*

ER911 is the Bach flower essence formula known as Rescue Remedy or Five-Flower Formula but with Arnica montana added. Just like Rescue Remedy, ER911 is most effective when used during any trauma or emergency, by helping the person cope with extreme pain and shock. This remedy is also effective for extreme fatigue of physical or emotional cause. Like Rescue Remedy, ER911 is useful in hysteria, such as that of a small child who has been stung by a bee or a person who has suffered a severe trauma. The addition of Arnica makes it even more effective and a specific for blunt force trauma and bruising as well as being helpful for the confusion that is so much a part of the Arnica symptom picture.

ARNICA MONTANA (leopard's bane) Arnica is the #1 remedy for trauma and all of its effects, recent or remote. Other conditions for which Arnica is indicated in the materia medicas are tumors in many parts following injuries, compound fractures, influenza with sore bruised muscles, mental or emotional shocks, never the same since a trauma, fright or grief, head injury or strokes that affect mental functions, hematoma, strain on the heart from violent running, and palpitations after shock or injury.

The mental and emotional symptoms include fear of the approach of anyone, many fears, and mental issues from head injury or strokes.

ESSIAC

The plants in this remedy have reputations as herbs as either blood purifiers, cancer fighters, or as outstanding nutritional herbs. Each ingredient has a listing in the materia medicas, although some of them have very few provings and very little is known about them except their herbal uses.

LAPPA ARCTIUM (burdock) Herbally, burdock is a serious blood and liver cleanser and is often employed in fights against cancer. Homeopathically, Lappa arctium is considered to affect the skin, liver, joints, kidneys, stomach, intestines, and uterus. Indicated for vertigo with nausea and vomiting.

RUMEX ACETOSA (sheep sorrel) Herbally, sheep sorrel is a very strong blood and liver cleanser. Symptoms from homeopathic provings include convulsions with staring and sunken eyes, exhaustion, pain in the esophagus that is worse when swallowing, lack of appetite but intense thirst, violent pains in the intestines, rapid but weak pulse, and sweating so severe it soaks the blankets.

ULMUS FULVA (slippery elm bark) Indicated for malnutrition, boils and ulcers, and herpes/syphilitic eruptions. This remedy is known mostly in herbal form, where it is used extensively to soothe irritated internal organs and tissues.

RHEUM PALMATUM (turkey rhubarb) This is a remedy for persistently acidic people. (Cancers grow best in an acidic environment.) Other symptoms include fear of death, colicky pain in abdomen rising up to the chest, cool sweat on the face, loss of appetite with food having a bitter taste, burning when urinating, disordered liver with jaundice, sour smelling sweat even right after bathing. The sweat leaves a yellow stain on clothing and bedding. This remedy is often indicated in nursing babies when they get sores in their mouth accompanied by sour smelling diarrhea.

TRIFOLIUM PRATENSE (red clover) Herbal remedies have a reputation for retarding the growth of cancerous tumors and improving the overall health of the patient. Trifolium pratense is listed in homeopathic materia medicas for blood disorders, cancer, and for those with a predisposition to the emotional patterns associated with increased risk for cancer. Trifolium is often a part of remedies suggested for cancer. Other symptoms include confusion and headaches on waking, cold hands and feet, increased flow of saliva, hay fever, and irritation of pharynx and trachea with hoarseness and choking.

NASTURTIUM AQUATICUM (watercress) Nasturtium homeopathic remedy is used for conditions relating to malnutrition or malabsorption of nutrients. The American Journal of Clinical Nutrition claims that watercress helps to reduce free radical damage to cells. Research published in this journal indicates that watercress (whole food form) turns off the signal that tells the body to create the new blood vessels needed to sustain tumor growth. Amazing, if true! It isn't known if the homeopathic remedy reduces free radical damage or blocks the blood supplies needed by tumors but the connection between herbal and homeopathic remedies is always very close and fascinating. It is known that Nasturtium aquaticum aids with cirrhosis of the liver and edema (dropsy is the term used for edema in homeopathic texts).

CARDUUS BENEDICTUS (blessed thistle) The plant is said to have obtained the name "benedictus" because of its reputation as a heal-all plant. Homeopathic symptoms include cutting pains in the abdomen, bitter burnings in the stomach, vomiting, diarrhea, pain and constriction in the trachea, swelling of the veins, twitchings and disturbance of vision, and blackness before the eyes for a short time.

FUCUS VESICULOSUS (bladderwrack) Fucus is a potent remedy that strengthens and heals tissues. Indications are obstinate constipation, thyroid enlargement, yellow tinge to skin—especially of the face, intolerable headache with the forehead feeling as if compressed by a ring, nausea, vertigo, difficulty breathing, nosebleeds, and vomiting of bright red blood. This remedy is renowned for use with goiter.

EXHAUSTION #1 (7X)

FERRUM PHOSPHORICUM (iron phosphate) Ferrum phos is considered useful for anemia and debilitating weakness. According to Robin Murphy's materia medica Ferrum phos stimulates the blood to increase hemoglobin. This remedy is also useful for the first stages of all inflammatory disorders, for those who take cold easily, and is useful for fresh wounds, contusions, sprains, and bruised soreness on the chest, shoulders, and muscles.

HOMERIA COLLINA (cape tulip) The picture of Homeria is a state of total collapse with severe weakness and near insensibility. The pulse is irregular and the pupils are dilated. There is great coldness with severe nausea and vomiting.

RANUNCULUS BULBOSUS (buttercup) Some of the symptoms are weakness, fainting, trembling and heat in the head with coldness in hands and feet. The symptoms are made worse by atmospheric changes, sudden exposure to cold or heat, and much worse in wet and stormy weather.

EXHAUSTION #2 (9X)

EQUISETUM HYEMALE (horsetail) Horsetail, in any form, is considered a remedy for the urinary tract. Symptoms that apply here include urine retention, constant desire to urinate, passing large quantities of clear, light-colored urine which brings no relief, irritability, poor uptake of calcium, easily fatigued mentally, cystitis, and diabetes.

KALI PHOSPHORICUM (potassium phosphate) Phosphorus remedies always include a picture of exhaustion and fatigue, anemia, nervous sensitivity, weakness, a tendency to tire easily, and brain fatigue. The slightest labor seems a heavy task and there is anxiety with nervous dread.

RHUS AROMATICA (fragrant sumac) Rhus aromatica is a remedy for diabetes and kidney disorders. Other symptoms include emaciation, weakness, trembling. This remedy is especially indicated following uterine hemorrhage or bleeding in the kidneys.

EXHAUSTION #3

FORMICA RUFA (red ant) Formica rufa symptoms include unusual and unaccountable weakness of the lower limbs with pain in the hips, depression, remarkable mental acuity during the day but forgetful and often apprehensive and morose in the evenings.

PSORINUM (scabies nosode) Two unusual keynotes of this remedy are great debility without any identifiable disease or cause and great prostration after acute disease. People who need this remedy suffer extreme sensitiveness to cold—sensitivity is so severe that there is great dread of the least cold air or drafts.

EYE IRRITATION #1 (4X)

***EUPHRASIA OFFICINALIS* (*eyebright*)** Euphrasia affects the mucus membranes of the eyes, nose, and chest with the eye and nose symptoms extending to the skin around them. Eye symptoms include conjunctivitis with acrid discharge, the effects of allergies and hay fever on the eyes, eyes sensitive to light and watering all the time, and burning and swelling of eye lids as if there is sand in the eyes.

***NATRUM MURIATICUM* (*sodium chloride*)** Symptoms if Nat mur include light sensitivity with photophobia worse for bright light or sunlight, tears stream down face when coughing, eyestrain, muscles around eyes become weak and stiff, pain in eyes when looking down, styes, and swollen lids with a heavy feeling.

***RANUNCULUS BULBOSUS* (*buttercup*)** Symptoms include day blindness with occasional night blindness, photophobia, a mist before the eyes, pressure and smarting in eyes, pain over right eye which is better standing or walking. None of these symptoms are keynotes for this remedy.

EYE IRRITATION #2 (6X)

***FERRUM PHOSPHORICUM* (*iron phosphate*)** Among Ferrum phos's other symptoms and uses (besides anemia and exhaustion) are some very distinctive eye issues. These include conjunctivitis without mucus, red eyes, inflamed burning sensation in eyes, feeling of sand under eyelids, suffused eyes with pressure on bending over and vision becomes blurred, and stye on lower eyelid.

***MANCINELLA VENENATA* (*manganeel apple*)** One of the major uses of Mancinella is for problems with the eyes and with vision. Specific to Mancinella symptoms include burning eyes, smarting on closing the eyes, light sensitivity, dull ache behind the eyes, eyelids heavy and sore, intense inflammation with loss of vision for several days at a time. Mental keynote is sudden vanishing of thoughts.

***RESERPINUM* (*alkaloid of Rauwolfia serpentina*)** The only eye issue I can find for Reserpinum is myosis (contraction of the pupil of the eye). Perhaps this remedy is added here because of the headaches for which it is indicated. These headaches include migraines and headaches on waking in the morning that is better for food and worse again just before lunchtime (these symptoms indicate problems balancing and maintaining blood sugar levels more than they point toward eye strain, however).

***THUJA OCCIDENTALIS* (*arbor vitae*)** Thuja acts chiefly on the mucus membranes and stimulates the body to deal with bacterial invasions. Symptoms applicable to this combination are blood-red eyes that tear up a lot, conjunctivitis after vaccination, styes and tumors, constant ache in the eye made worse by bright light, and eye infections—both mild varieties and more dangerous types.

***URTICA URENS* (*stinging nettle*)** Urtica urens is indicated for anything that burns. Eyes feel weak and sore, pain in eyes as if from a blow, feels like sand in the eyes, and the eyes burn and sting a lot.

***WYETHIA HELENOIDES* (*poison weed*)** The major symptoms of Wyethia include itching at the inner canthus of the eye—usually of the *left eye*, and hay fever symptoms with swollen and sore glands—usually on *right side of neck*.

FATIGUE #1 (6X)

***SCUTELLARIA LATERIFOLIA* (*skullcap*)** A man named Hale, who introduced Scutellaria to the homeopathic world, said that "Its calming effects on the nervous system have been known ever since the settlement of New England." This remedy is excellent for tiredness and weakness of whatever cause, cardiac irritability, inability to concentrate on study or work, dull frontal headache, migraine that is worse over the right eye, explosive headaches, and restless and unrefreshing sleep.

ARSENICUM ALBUM (white oxide of arsenic) Arsenicum is a very deep-acting remedy, affecting every organ and tissue in some way. Arsenicum also acts on the nerves. A keynote of Arsenicum is sudden great weakness from trivial causes, shortness of breath, and being extremely nervous and restless. Arsenicum is particularly strengthening to the muscles, nerves, lungs, and digestive systems and is a polycrest for influenza, food poisoning, and many other things. This is a remedy with which everyone should be familiar as it will be needed by every person more than once in their lives.

GELSEMIUM SEMPERVIRENS (yellow jasamine) Gelsemium is a remedy with a strong affinity for the recovery stages of illnesses and for fatigue and illness that is brought on by anxiety, anticipation, fear, or bad news. Some keynote symptoms are muscular weakness and paralysis, aching all over, poor circulation, dizziness, drowsiness, trembling, apathy, and one pupil dilated and the other contracted (may indicate something amiss in the brain).

The symptoms of Gelsemium may go as deep as complete prostration both mentally and physically. Gelsemium is a polycrest remedy. There are pages and pages of symptom descriptions other than the ones reported here having to do with fatigue.

PHOSPHORICUM ACIDUM (phosphoric acid) Phosphoricum acidum is specific for conditions from a weakened immune system brought on by an acute illness, loss of vital fluids, or by grief and loss. Symptoms include debility, exhaustion, emaciation, fatigue of a chronic and continual nature, hair loss, mental debility followed by physical debility, wants nothing and likes nothing, and very sleepy during day with the weakness being a little bit better for a short nap.

FERRUM PHOSPHORICUM (iron phosphate) Ferrum phos is a remedy for anemia, recovery from hemorrhage (I have seen this impressive thing personally), venous disorders, debility, weakness, and the early stages of any inflammatory disorder. Ferrum phos is said to increase hemoglobin production and the absorption of iron.

ECHINACEA ANGUSTIFOLIA/PURPUREA (purple coneflower) Echincea treats blood poisoning and septicemia from a cut, wound, surgery, or childbirth. Listless feeling that is worse in the evening, with weakness felt in stomach, bowels, heart, and knees. Vertigo accompanies the symptoms and there is slowness in every action and even in the speech. Echinacea, in both herbal and homeopathic form is considered a support to the immune system and is said to bring relief from the effects of vaccinations and chemical toxins.

MEDICAGO SATIVA (alfalfa) *(For some strange reason this is NOT listed by Latin name in Murphy's Materia Medica but rather is listed as Alfalfa).* Favorably influences nutrition and the uptake of vitamins and minerals which results in improved mental and physical vigor. Alfalfa is also listed as a remedy to help with hypoglycemia—weak and shaky if food is not taken about every 3 hours, as well as weak kidneys with frequent urge to urinate.

FATIGUE #2 (6X)

KALI TARTARICUM (potassium tartrate) There are only a few symptoms known for this remedy and most of them refer to emaciation, weakness that is so severe they can scarcely walk, thighs and legs feel paralyzed, great thirst, and often with diarrhea and vomiting.

RESERPINUM (alkaloid of Rauwolfia serpentina) Symptoms include sleepiness especially after meals, slowing down of mind and body, general weakness, trembling, anxiety, difficulty working, violent attacks of vertigo, and melancholy. Although very tired there are periods of hyperactivity and aggressiveness at times in most sufferers.

TRIGONELLA FOENUM GRAECUM (fenugreek) Fenugreek, in herbal form, causes sugars to be absorbed from foods more slowly and blood sugar levels to remain more stable. This herb also has an effect on the release of blood sugars stored in the liver. I can find very little information on this plant in homeopathic form. I hope there are some provings done soon and that I hear about them as soon as they happen.

WYETHIA HELENOIDES (poison weed) The symptoms—few as are known to us—include nervousness, uneasiness, apprehensive feelings, depression, inability to accomplish mental work, averse to company, impatient, and quarrelsome.

FATIGUE #3 (8X)

CANTHARIS VESICATORIA (Spanish fly) Spanish fly has an effect on digestive, liver, and abdominal complaints, inflammation of brain tissue, with paleness and anxious restlessness seen in all situations. A keynote is sudden loss of consciousness with the face becoming abnormally red.

GINSENG (wild ginseng) A major symptom of ginseng is general coldness with especially cold hands. Ginseng *strengthens the ability of the body and the mind to withstand stress,* calms the mind, and promotes feelings of courage.

KALI IODATUM (potassium iodide) All Kali based remedies have to do with despondency and the trivial details of life seeming like too much to cope with. Kali iodatum has a regulating influence over the functions of the organs having to do with nutrition, growth, and development and also works on neuralgia and inflamed nerves.

MYRTUS COMMUNIS (myrtle) This remedy has mostly to do with heart and lungs but there is a clear symptomatic indication for this remedy that includes extreme tiredness in the afternoon that is worse from atmospheric changes.

FATIGUE #4 (9X)

EPHEDRA VULGARIS (ma huang) This wonderful herb is no longer available to us in anything but homeopathic form. Since it was a wonderful convalescent herb (in herbal form and not made in to a white powder drug that causes a lot of side-effects), this is a tragedy. I miss this herb in the convalescent stages of serious illnesses such as pneumonia. Some homeopathic symptoms include fatigue and weakness that begins early in the morning and lasts all day long, apathy toward nearly everything, stiff neck, and insomnia with great longing for sleep.

GINSENG (wild ginseng) A major symptom of ginseng is general coldness with especially cold hands. Ginseng *strengthens the ability of the body and the mind to withstand stress*, calms the mind, and promotes feelings of courage.

LONICERA XYLOSTEUM (fly woodbine) Keynote symptoms are trembling of the whole body, sleepiness, constant deep sleep with half-open eyes (scary to look out, especially with children), coldness of limbs, and profuse cold perspiration.

ZINCUM PHOSPHORICUM (zinc phosphate) According to homeopathic tradition, Zinc phos removes the mental depression and weakness following cerebral congestion and strokes. Other symptoms include nervousness, brain exhaustion, nervous vertigo, hands cold with perspiring feet, and nervous headache. The fatigue of Zinc phos is very great with total or near total disinclination to do any mental exertion at all. The person may be in a happy and enthusiastic mood followed by gloom and discontent.

FATIGUE #5 (9X)

LEDUM PALUSTRE (wild rosemary) Ledum affects the fibrous tissues of joints, especially the tendons of the ankles and heels. Symptoms include confusion of the mind, difficulty thinking, cold all the time with the limbs being particularly cold. This combination is often indicated as a treatment for Lyme disease and other "spirochete" caused illnesses with the symptoms having begun at the time of insect stings or bites. There is pain gradually rising from the feet to the head.

ELAPS CORALLINUS (Brazil coral snake) Like other snake remedies, Elaps includes issues of the blood with destruction of blood cells causing hemorrhages which are dark in color all over. This remedy is also indicated for parasites moving through the blood to other locations in the body. There is a cold feeling in stomach and often terrible coldness all over the body.

FEVER (6X)

SAMBUCUS NIGRA (Elder) Symptoms of Sambucus nigra include dry burning fever while asleep with copious sweating on waking, a constant state of fretfulness, spasms in the respiratory area, shortness of breath, snuffles in infants which prevents nursing, deep dry cough, fever without thirst, constant state of fretfulness, and colic with nausea, and earache.

MENTHA PIPERITA (peppermint) Peppermint, as an herb, has always been good for fevers. Homeopathic symptoms include colds, dry coughs, sore throat, a dry and painful throat, and headache with tension toward the ears. Symptoms are worse on rising but better returning to bed.

FIVE FLOWER FORMULA (SEE RESCUE REMEDY)

FLU SYMPTOMS #1 (9X)

This symptom is a favorite of many people because it works!

CHERRY PLUM (flower essence) Dr. Bach placed this remedy, and the Red Chestnut that is also in this combination, under the category of *For Those Who Have Fear.* The mind is overstrained and out of balance after prolonged mental effort. The mental exhaustion leads to digestive disturbances, prostration, flu-like symptoms, stage fright and performance anxiety with nausea.

RED CHESTNUT (flower essence) Extreme physical nervousness and anxious weakness, tightening in the stomach and abdominal region from fear, along with grief and fearful worry about family members. With the fear there are sometimes feelings of helplessness and self-blame for things that she feels that she might have done differently or things that she failed to do.

FERRUM MURIATICUM (iron chloride) Symptoms include cramping, chronic diarrhea, passage of blood and mucus, face pale and anemic, vertigo, sleeplessness, and a sensation of coldness alternating with heat with this pattern possibly lasting for several hours.

KALI SULPHURICUM (potassium sulphate) Symptoms include colicky pains, an abdomen that is cold and distended, headaches that are worse in a warm room and in the evening (worse for warmth and in the evenings is true of most Kali sulphuricum symptoms), pressure and feeling of fullness in the stomach, nausea, vomiting, and vertigo.

FLU SYMPTOMS #2 (6X)

ACONITE NAPELLUS (monkshood) The symptoms of Aconite that apply to the flu are pressure in the stomach, burning from stomach to esophagus, painful hiccups, and vomiting of clear water every time one sits up. Aconite is indicated for any acute, sudden, violent illness that comes with a high fever.

FERRUM PHOSPHORICUM (iron phosphate) Ferrum phos aids in lowering fevers, especially in infants and children and is suited to those who catch colds and sore throats easily. There are coughs made worse from going outside. This remedy is excellent for the first stage of ear infection. The symptom picture includes sour belchings, chill while eating, pain in stomach that gets worse after eating, vomiting of undigested food and bright red blood. Ferrum prevents suppuration from earaches and conjunctivitis.

BRYONIA ALBA (wild hops) Bryonia is less rapid in its action than Aconite, but it goes deeper in its effects and ***often takes up the healing work where Aconite leaves off.*** Symptoms include splitting headache, aching bones and muscles, sharp pain when swallowing, pleurisy with sharp pains, hacking cough, fever, nausea, and vomiting. All symptoms are worse from the slightest motion.

EUPATORIUM PERFOLIATUM (boneset) Eupatorium symptoms include severe chills with terrible aching in bones, vomiting preceded by thirst, vomiting everything eaten, weak pulse, and great weakness and prostration. Sweating relieves all the symptoms but the headache and the cough is worse at night.

GELSEMIUM SEMPERVIRENS (yellow jasmine) Gelsemium is a remedy with a strong affinity for the recovery stages of illnesses and for fatigue and illness that is brought on by anxiety, anticipation, fear, or bad news. Gelsemium is keynoted by either the failure of energy levels to return to normal after an illness or complete exhaustion that just will not go away. Other symptoms include drowsiness, trembling, aching muscles, headache, chilliness and pain up and down the spine, fever with thirstlessness.

FUNGUS #1

ASPERGILLUS NIGER (the fungus that causes black mold on fruits, etc) I can find no information on this fungus as a homeopathic remedy so I will list the symptoms of the fungus as it lodges in the lungs and creates a fungal ball there. These include non-productive cough, fever, pleuritic chest pains, shortness of breath, nasal congestion and pain, sinusitis, weakened immune system, and fungal ear infections that may degenerate into hearing loss.

CANDIDA ALBICANS (thrush fungus) Candida albicans is a naturally occurring yeast-like fungus that lives in various mucus membranes of the body and in the intestinal tract. Under certain conditions natural balance is upset and the candida multiply and travel through the bloodstream to many parts of the body where they do not belong and cause a variety of nasty symptoms. Nevertheless, the root cause of all of the symptoms is the out-of-balance state in the intestinal mucosa. This fungus is the same fungus as the one that causes thrush in babies and candida symptoms in grown people.

MEZEREUM This remedy is listed for use against such things as Herpes zoster and shingles. Symptoms include enlarged glands, eruptions, bruised and weary feeling in the joints, violent neuralgia around the face and teeth, eruptions that have thick leathery crusts under which pus collects, vanishing of thoughts while speaking, and irresolution about decisions.

SULPHUR (brimstone) Sulphur is listed for boils, herpes, skin disorders, difficult respiration with much rattling of mucus, unhealthy skin which breaks out and suppurates, soles of the feet burning and needing to be uncovered, and many other symptoms that might be related to a fungal infection in the body. Sulphur is a remedy that is indicated when the immune system/vital energy is deficient and the healing reaction to closely matching remedies is not sufficient to produce a cure.

ARSENICUM ALBUM (white oxide of arsenic) Arsenicum is a polycrest remedy for many things but among them are symptoms related to flu symptoms created by bacterial infections, food poisoning, intermittent fever, malaria, glandular swellings, ringworm, ulcers, worms, colitis, and anorexia.

PIX LIQUIDA (pine tar) This remedy is known as a stimulating expectorant in chronic bronchitis and tuberculosis and as a stimulant to healing of the skin in psoriasis and scaly eczema. A keynote of this remedy, when things have progressed to an extreme state, is constant vomiting of black fluid with pain in the stomach, pain at a spot at about the third left costal cartilage, and skin that itches intolerably with eruptions on the back of the hands.

FUNGUS #2 (7X)

Isodes of Cryptococcus neoformans, C. laurentii, C. albidus **Cryptococcus is a genus of fungi found in soil worldwide, especially where there are a lot of bird droppings. Cryptococcus infrection may cause pneumonia-like illness, with shortness of breath, cough and fever. Some strains may cause central nervous system infection or inflammation with fever, headache, changes in mental state or memory loss.**

GALLBLADDER DISTRESS (7X)

CHINA OFFICINALIS (Peruvian bark) This is a polycrest remedy with many pages of symptoms in the materia medicas. Those symptoms that apply to this remedy are gas and bloating of the abdomen, indigestion, severe diarrhea, intestinal candida overgrowth, gallstone colic, and a hot face with cold hands and body.

FILIX MAS (male fern) The symptom picture of felix mas includes many abdominal and stomach disorders, some of which are an absolute match for a gallbladder attack—things such as great pain in the abdomen with diarrhea and constant vomiting and becoming ill after taking food and particularly worse after eating sweets and sweets mixed with milk products. Other symptoms include nausea, bloated abdomen with boring pains, and torpid inflammation of the lymph glands. Used for the destruction of worms, parasites, and intestinal bacterial infestations that create cramping, nausea, and vomiting.

NATRUM SULPHURICUM (sodium sulphate) Common symptoms of Nat sulph relating to digestion include nausea, gas, bloating, and headache with constipation, a great many foods producing uncomfortable diarrhea, burning pain in the abdomen, cramps with flatulence, acid indigestion with heartburn, sour vomiting of green bilious vomit, and there is a strong desire for ice and cold water.

GLADULAR/LYMPH #1 (8X)

BELLADONNA (deadly nightshade) Belladonnas acts on the brain, nerve centers, glandular and lymphatic systems. The symptoms are notable because of their sudden onset and include loss of appetite, glands that are red, swollen and tender, vision difficulties, nausea and vomiting, ear pain, and tinnitus.

CALCAREA IODATA (calcium iodide) Calcarea iodata is indicated for many symptoms that are glandular in nature such as enlarged tonsils, croup, varicose veins, breast tumors, thyroid tumors, and cysts. Other symptoms include weariness of the whole body, constant severe but dull headache at the forehead and temples, tired feeling in the calves of the legs, and light-headedness.

CONIUM MACULATUM (poison hemlock) Applicable symptoms include breasts that enlarge and become painful before and during menses, breast cancer with hard tumors, tumors that appear at the site of old injuries, stitches in breasts and in nipples, prostate issues, prostate cancer, ovarian issues, aching in lumbar and sacral areas, and progressive debility of body and mind.

ECHINACEA ANGUSTIFOLIA/PURPUREA (purple cone-flower) In both herbal and homeopathic form, Echinacea is a blood and immune stimulant and tonic. It is indicated for lymphatic inflammation, recurring ear infections, strep throat, full feeling in the upper part of the lungs, stuffy nose and head, dullness from headache, aching limbs, sleepiness with confusion and weakness, and chilliness with nausea.

HEPAR SULPHURIS CALCAREUM (calcium sulphide) This is an excellent glandular remedy and is indicated by a tendency for mucus membranes to suppurate. The lesions spread by the formation of small papules around the sides of the old lesions. Being a glandular remedy, there are symptoms that apply to every gland and to every system that the glandular system affects (in other words, all of them).

SULPHUR IODATUM (sulphur iodide) This remedy is useful for painless enlargement of glands and for tissues that are thickening after inflammation. It is also useful for many other obstinate skin afflictions such as pustular eruptions and suppurating acne.

KALI IODATUM (potassium iodide) Applicable symptoms are glandular swellings with glands enlarged and indurated, diffused sensitiveness of glands and of the scalp, glands that have begun to atrophy, pains long after an injury, small boils, and itching eruptions—worse in the heat.

KALI MURIATICUM (potassium chloride) Kali mur is indicated for the ill effects of vaccinations giving it a very long list of symptoms, many of them obviously applying to the glandular system.

MERCURIUS SOLUBILIS (mercury vivus) People needing this remedy are often described as human thermometers (that's mercury!)—up and down and constantly changing, especially in moods and energy levels. There will be dejection and discouragement offset by periods of euphoric happiness.

Mercurius also has a strong action on the lymphatic system. Mercurius increases glandular activity, with enlarged glands and glandular problems making up a large part of the remedy picture. Excessive saliva with a metallic taste in the mouth (possibly indicating that Mercurius is a remedy useful in the treatment of toxic poisoning). Symptoms are worse from any change in temperature or weather.

PHYTOLACCA DECANDRA (pokeweed root) Phytolacca acts on the glandular system, helping to eliminate infection and inflammation. It has a special affinity for fibrous and osseous tissues with symptoms such as mastitis in the breasts, hardness of the glands in right side of the neck, and swelling of the axillary glands. Phytolacca also acts on the sheaths and fascias of muscles of the shoulders and arms. Many phytolacca problems manifest with high fever alternating with chilliness and great fatigue.

PULSATILLA NIGRICANS (windflower) Pulsatilla affects many glandular and hormonal issues. All symptoms are worse from warmth or stuffiness of a room. Symptoms include food lodging in the throat, anemia, varicose veins, and a person experiencing "never the same since puberty or childbirth" symptoms. This is a remedy for people with mild, yielding dispositions whose symptom picture is constantly changing.

SOLIDAGO VIRGAUREA (goldenrod) The common use of this remedy as an herb and as a homeopathic is as a diuretic and for chronic kidney inflammation. Murphy's Materia Medica calls this remedy the "homeopathic replacement for the catheter".

GLANDULAR/LYMPH #2 (8X)

EUPHRASIA OFFICINALIS (eyebright) The symptom picture of Euphrasia includes glandular swellings, prostate gland disorders, clogged lymph glands, amenorrhea and other female hormone disorders, and catarrh in the chest, and allergies. A full range of eye disorders are this remedies specialty.

HEPAR SULPHURIS CALCAREUM (calcium sulphide) This is an excellent glandular remedy and is indicated by a tendency for mucus membranes to suppurate. The lesions spread by the formation of small papules around the sides of the old lesions. Skin eruptions are almost always an indication that the internal lymph and the lymph system just below the skin is clogged. There are symptoms here that apply to every gland and to every system that the glandular system affects (in other words, all of them).

VIBURNUM OPULUS (cramp bark) Pelvic problems that include a "sick" feeling all over that can be indicative of glandular and lymphatic issues. Another keynote symptom is involuntary bladder release when coughing or walking and bladder irritation. This remedy is indicated for cramps in the abdomen and legs of pregnant women and has strong hormonal and glandular components.

GLANDULAR SUPPORT #1 (9X)

Specific to pineal gland support.

CHAMOMILLA VULGARIS (German chamomile) Chamomilla is particularly suited for children and pregnant women. The picture includes profuse sweating (in adults), tender breasts from lymph gland swelling, and menstrual cramps with a lot of pain and irritability. Most of the symptoms of Chamomilla are linked to either glandular/hormone issues or nerve irritation.

CUPRUM METALLICUM (copper metal) Symptoms include spasms, convulsions, and cramps in toes, fingers, and calves. A few symptoms, such as a metallic taste in the mouth and grinding of teeth, may be indicative of a liver burdened with toxins or poor absorption of minerals—glandular issues.

MYRRH (myrrh gum) Myrrh is a tonic and stimulant herb. Homeopathic symptoms include enlarged tonsils, lymph nodes, and glands, with general overproduction of mucus.

THUJA OCCIDENTALIS (arbor vitae) The native habitat of a plant is considered by many herbalists to be indicative of that plant's strengths as a healing catalyst. Thuja loves swamps and is indicated for enlarged glands, soft and spongy warts, and skin eruptions that appear only on covered parts of the body Thuja is the #1 remedy for "never the same since vaccination" glandular repair.

GLANDULAR SUPPORT #2 (6X)

The first four ingredients of this remedy are the same as the one above—Glandular Support #1—and are specific to the pineal gland. Listed below are descriptions of the other homeopathics that have been added to the combination above to create this combination. Note the inclusion of 4 more mineral/metal remedies, in addition to the Cuprum that is among the 4 remedies discussed above in Glandular Support #1 and a part of this remedy also. Remedies from this grouping (sometimes called *elements)* have the emotional characteristics of problems with structure and organization (either too much or too little), disconnected thinking—considering each body part separately instead of understanding how each system relates to other systems—when it comes to health matters, disconnection in relationships, and money issues.

ALUMINUM SILICATA (aluminum silicate) This is a deep acting remedy for croup in the lower portion of the larynx and the upper part of the trachea, lung problems with coughing of much mucus, and chronic complaints of brain, spinal cord, and nerves.

NICCOLUM CARBONICUM (nickel metal) Niccolum carb is for periodic headaches of very severe and intense nature, swollen glands with the glands in the throat sore to external touch, and coughs which bring on dizziness or convulsion—the person must be held sitting up to avoid this. Mental/emotional symptoms include becoming angry if contradicted and just plain quarrelsome most of the time.

PLUMBUM METALLICUM (lead metal) Plumbum affects the muscles, nerves, spinal cord, glandular system, kidneys, and the blood and blood vessels—quite a comprehensive list. Mental/emotional symptoms include mental exhaustion following physical labor, slow perception, increasing slowness and apathy, and the inability to find the right word when speaking.

KALI PHOSPHORICUM (potassium phosphate) Schuessler used this remedy for conditions of depleted nerves, among other things. Kali remedies have to do with the fulfilling of one's duties and Phosphoricum remedies always indicate great fatigue. This remedy is a polycrest for mental and physical prostration brought about by a combination of overworking and psychological factors like excitement, worry, and frustration.

A malfunctioning glandular system is inevitable, eventually, in the symptoms picture of this remedy. Perhaps it is the result of other problems in the body or maybe struggling glands were part of the cause of the collapsed state that eventually occurred.

RANUNCULUS BULBOSUS (buttercup) This is a remedy for liver dysfunction related to toxins of any kind (those found in everyday life and those, such as alcohol and prescription drugs, that are deliberately put into the body). As always, when the nerves and glandular system have been disturbed, the person becomes quarrelsome, irritable, and anxious.

VALERIANA OFFICINALIS (valerian) Valeriana is a remedy for oversensitivity of the nervous system with the unusual characteristic of being worse from rest but also worse from standing. The mood and emotions are changeable (constantly) with emotions ranging from the highest joy to the deepest grief and back again, often very quickly. Impatience and irritability will also be seen.

The irritation of the nerves will become so pronounced as to trigger hysterical spasms of muscles and an inability of the person to hold still when supposedly sitting still. They wiggle and squirm all over the place. There will be terrible insomnia from nightly nervous itching and muscular spasms from the excitement of the day.

I am not sure why this remedy is included in a glandular support combination except that when the glandular system is out of balance nerve issues will not be far behind as illustrated by the next remedy (Glandular Support #3).

GLANDULAR SUPPORT #3 (9x)

Emphasis on nervous disruption from glandular malfunction.

CHELIDONIUM MAJUS (greater celandine) Chelidonium is a ***major liver and gallbladder remedy.*** Symptoms include gallbladder pains, liver-related headaches—frontal and sometimes centered over the right eye, nausea, vomiting, and jaundice due to hepatic and gallbladder obstruction.

CRATAEGUS OXYACANTHA (hawthorn berries) Crataegus is placed in this combination because it is a great heart tonic and blood pressure stabilizer. It is useful for insomnia and certain types of nausea.

AVENA SATIVA (oatstraw) Avena improves the uptake of the nutrients needed by the brain and nervous system and is one of the best tonics for recovery from a debilitating illness. Sleeplessness with nervous exhaustion is a keynote and mental exertion always aggravates the symptoms until recovery is complete.

LOBELIA INFLATA (indian tobacco) Lobelia, as an herb, has a long and interesting history. (See the story of Samuel Thompson in Butterfly Miracles with Herbal Remedies for the whole story.) This great herbalist described Lobelia (the herb) as the greatest remedy of which he made use in his practice.

Homeopathically, Lobelia is a vasomotor stimulant and increases the activity of all body processes with a particular emphasis on the pneumogastric nerve.

Some issues and symptoms (only a few of the many) include prickling and itching all over body with nausea, issues from clogged mucus—such as occur in the sinuses, ears, heart and lungs, headache with vertigo, and great chilliness. Lobelia is specific for conditions that "drag on"—never quite allowing the person to return to full health and vigor.

EQUISETUM HYEMALE (horse-tail) The major focus of this remedy is for support of the urinary tract. Symptoms include profuse urination of clear and watery urine or the opposite, less common, situation of urine that is cloudy and filled with mucus and albumin.

GLANDULAR SUPPORT #4 (6X)

Specific to support of the pineal and pituitary glands.

The pineal gland, located in the center of the brain, was considered the "seat of the soul" in ancient times. Along with the pituitary gland, the pineal gland regulates many endocrine functions and plays a starring role in degenerative disease and aging.

The pituitary regulates blood pressure, body temperature, growth, motor function, the reproductive system, sleep habits, the passage of calcium into and out of all cells, the metabolism of carbohydrates, cellular respiration, the regulation of temperature, the creation and health of collagen in cells, the regulation of DNA, enzyme activity, and lymphocyte production. That is quite an impressive list!

The pineal gland has an integral role in body cycles and behavior patterns. Because the pineal gland has a regulatory and inhibitory function on the thymus and thyroid, it directly impacts hormones, circulation and cardiovascular health.

The blood/brain barrier does not protect the pineal gland and even large toxic molecules can enter and become a threat to it. The pineal gland is stimulated by sunlight and the geomagnetic fields of the earth.

One interesting note on the pineal gland is that, when healthy, it gives "the power to endure prolonged physical exertion without taking food and without feeling fatigued. "

With the exception of Vespa crabro and the Pituitary glandular isode, these are little known remedies with little or no information given in the materia medicas. Taken together, however, they stimulate these two glands and have a direct impact on the body functions mentioned above.

GYMNOCLADUS CANADENSIS (American coffee-tree) One thing that is listed for this remedy is "pain in the front part of the head following influenza." Frontal headaches are often caused by liver issues. Other symptoms include swelling of the face and head, and hives.

STERCULIA ACUMINATA (kola nut The first symptoms that I found listed for this remedy was fatigue and weakness of no known origin that was being blamed on psychosomatic causes (Neurasthenia). What little information that is available indicates that this is a remedy for circulation and the correction of cardiac rhythms and that it acts as a diuretic.

PELARGONIUM RENIFORME (African geranium) This is a remedy that is completely unfamiliar to me. The only information I can find, having to do with healing, is that it was used by soldiers for dysentery and as a purgative for their horses.

PITUITARIA ANTERIOR LOBE ISODE (pituitary gland isode) The homeopathic symptoms of this remedy are based on 5 years of clinical observation by Dr. David Flores Toledo of Mexico. Dr. Toledo believes that this remedy deserves to become one of the great polycrest remedies of our generation. The symptom picture includes hormonal disorders of many types and descriptions, flatulence and rumbling after eating, low backaches and pain in the sacral region before menses, involuntary urination, palpitations while lying on the back, brown spots on the face, constipation, and hemorrhoids (among others).

VESPA CRABRO (wasp) This remedy is much like Apis and is an excellent remedy for bee stings and allergic reactions to bee stings. A keynote is stinging, burning pains that pierce deeply. There may be nerve and muscular excitement, itching over the whole body, trembling, burning pain with urination, inflammation of the right eye, and problems with the left ovary and with the cervix.

HAIR & NAILS (8X)

The hair and nails are a direct reflection of the overall health of the body. Whenever the body is suffering a deficiency of nutrients it will be reflected first in the hair and the nails as the body considers them less essential than internal organs. It does not matter whether the body is nutrient deficient because of poor eating habits or because of poor assimilation. The ingredients of this combination address both issues.

PHOSPHORICUM ACIDUM (phosphoric acid) Phosphoricum acidum is helpful in improving the absorption of vitamins and minerals and is specific for hair loss and brittle nails, especially when the nutritional deficiency is associated with grief. Other symptoms are mental debility followed by physical weakness, blue rings around the eyes, diabetes, frequent urination at night, and vertigo in the evening.

ANTIMONIUM CRUDUM (native sulphide of antimony) Besides crusts on the scalp, brittle nails, and nail fungus Antimonium is noted for food allergies, gastrointestinal disorders, lack of appetite, and arthritic pains of joints and fingers.

ARSENICUM ALBUM (white oxide of arsenic) This is a great polycrest for a multitude of things. Among them are stomach, intestinal, and nutrient absorption difficulties. Circular bare patches where there is no hair, scalp very sensitive and cannot be brushed, hair becoming grey very early, falling out of hair, and chronic eruptions on the head that are filled with pus. The fingernails are blue and discolored.

SILICA TERRA (pure flint) Although Silica should be remembered for its ability to expel foreign objects from the body, Silica is also noted for improving defective nutrition that is due to poor assimilation of nutrients. Silica is the first remedy I think of if my hair becomes dry or my nails become brittle. Some symptoms applicable to this remedy are a tendency to easy exhaustion, arrested development, unhealthy skin, and pus formation—particularly abscesses around fingernails and whitlows (thickening of the skin around the fingernails.

THUJA OCCIDENTALIS (arbor vitae) Thuja is noted for symptoms arising after vaccinations and exposure to chemical toxins. (For interesting reading on early acknowledgement of the toxic side-effects of vaccines, see the "comments" section in Thuja occidentalis in Robin Murphy's Materia Medica—very disturbing, but educational). Symptoms that apply to use in this remedy include white scaly dandruff, dry hair that splits and falls out, and nails that are brittle, ribbed, soft, distorted, discolored and crumbling.

HEADACHES #1 (6X)

ACONITUM NAPELLUS (monkshood) There are several varieties of Aconite headaches. These include congestive headaches, headaches with a very hot sensation inside the head, pulsations in the forehead, violent squeezing or bursting pain in the forehead, scalp being sensitive to touch during the headache, and scalp sensitive to cold air and strong winds.

Nearly all Aconte symptoms come on suddenly and there is a tendency to phobias and panic attacks.

BELLADONNA (deadly nightshade) The headaches of Belladonna include congestive headache with a red face, throbbing headache of great proportions often felt in the forehead, throbbing and hammering headache, headaches that are worse for light and noise, headaches worse for or brought on by lying down in the afternoon. The keynote of Belladonna is the violence and suddenness of the attacks and the congestion of the blood, often in the head.

BRYONIA ALBA (wild hops) Some symptoms of Bryonia include migraine headaches which are worse for any motion, pressure headaches, bursting and splitting headaches, vertigo on rising, and head feeling as if it has been hit from the inside with a hammer. The headaches are worse from motion, from stooping, and from opening the eyes. A couple of keynotes are that the hair is very greasy, dandruff is rough and uneven, cold sweat on the head , and the person is exceedingly irritable—just wants to be left alone.

IRIS VERSICOLOR (blue flag) Symptoms include gastric or hepatic headaches, headaches that begin with blurring of the eyes, chronic pains in forehead, dull throbbing on right side of the forehead, frontal headache over left eye with nausea, and neuralgic pains beginning over one eye then changing sides. What an interesting variety of headaches is found in this remedy!

NUX VOMICA (poison nut) Nux headache symptoms include a variety of migraines, headaches brought on by sunlight, toxic headaches from the effects of drugs and alcohol, congestive headaches associated with hemorrhoids, and a scalp that is very sensitive to touch. People who respond to Nux are highly strung and fast moving. They are often angry and impatient when spoken to and suddenly angry with very little provocation.

HEADACHES #2 (6X)

ACETALDEHYDE ISODE (weed sprays) This is common ingredient of weed sprays. Symptoms listed are coughs, respiratory distress, diarrhea, nausea, vomiting, and possibly/probably being carcinogenic. Even if you choose not to use these weed sprays personally, acetaldehyde is a common soil and water contaminant. This is probably a good thing to make a point of detoxing from.

IRIS VERSICOLOR (blue flag) The symptoms of Iris versicolor are listed under Headaches #1 remedy.

MILLEFOLIUM ACHILLEA (yarrow) The headache symptoms of yarrow include piercing thrusts of pain in the head—worse stooping or bending over, throbbing in the arteries of the head and face, confused dull headache in the evening, and vertigo with nausea. Uses other than with kidney ailments are many and varied. This is a remedy with whom everyone should be familiar as a homeopathic, as an herb, and as an essential oil. Yarrow was one of fiver herbs that Brigham Young said every person would have need of.

HORMONE BALANCER (6X)

GINSENG (wild ginseng) Ginseng, as an herb, is an amazing and world-renowned remedy with emphasis on balancing hormones and on building vigor and stamina. Ginseng alleviates fatigue and weakness and helps a person endure under prolonged stress or heavy physical labor more easily. Ginseng is more than specific for the malfunction of reproductive organs and systems; it is absolutely amazing in this sphere.

DAMIANA APHRODISIACA (Turnera) Damiana is another great invigorator of the system—with a particular affinity for sexual weakness, hormonal imbalances, and glandular dysfunction. Is said to dispel fatigue and restore clearness of mind.

INCONTINENCE (6X)

Urinary tract inflammation and leaking of urine.

KALI PHOSPHORICUM (potassium phosphate) This is a remedy for fatigue brought on by too much striving to leave no duty or responsibility undone and done in the best possible way—no matter the cost in personal energy.

The kidneys are always about fear and the kidney symptoms associated with this remedy reflect the fear of not having done or been enough. There is nocturnal bed-wetting in children and in the elderly, urine that is very yellow in color, and urine coming in stops and starts.

APIS MELLIFICA (honey bee) The kidney symptoms of Apis include acute kidney infection, a sore or bruised feeling over the region of the kidneys, burning when urinating, frequent and involuntary urine, and dragging pain in lumbar region.

CAUSTICUM (caustic potash) Involuntary passage of urine when coughing or sneezing, urine dribbles or passes slowly, involuntary retention of urine after labor or after surgical procedures, and burning in the urethra. Causticum people cannot bear to see injustice and are obsessive motivated by causes. When kidney symptoms appear, there must be some sort of underlying fear in the emotions somewhere.

FERRUM PHOSPHORICUM (iron phosphate) Ferrum is usually thought of because it increases hemoglobin and is specific for the early stages of inflammatory disorders. Nevertheless, it has a special affinity for the kidneys. Symptoms include bladder paralysis, bed-wetting, need to urinate immediately after every drink of water, and a frequent need to urinate due to irritation at the neck of the bladder.

NATRUM MURIATICUM (sodium chloride) Nat mur has the unusual symptom of difficulty urinating in the presence of others (bashful bladder). There is also pain just after urination, and a need to urinate that comes on very suddenly—can't control the flow, and the urine is clear with red sediment.

The ailments of Nat mur are usually accompanied by depression and feelings of isolation and/or were brought on by grief—either acute or chronic. There is backache with a keynote of bends over easily but hurts or has great difficulty straightening back up. The spine is sensitive to touch or pressure.

INDIGESTION #1 (7X)

EUPHORBIUM OFFICINARUM (gum EUPHORBIUM) Indications for this remedy are intense burning pains as if something hot is in pit of the stomach. Burning pains are part of the picture all over the body with this remedy. There is also heartburn, hiccups, nausea with shuddering, and ulcers.

CAFEINE (coffee alkaloid) Abdominal pulsation is a keynote of this remedy as far as stomach symptoms go. Another symptoms is anxiety with constriction of the neck and throat at periodic intervals of about 15 minutes. Vomiting relieves this and most other symptoms. It is odd to me that there are so few symptoms listed in the materia medicas for this remedy. Practical experience alone has provided us with a list of common negative reactions to caffeine to serve as symptoms for which this remedy might be useful.

PULSATILLA NIGRICANS (windflower) Emotional symptoms include mild temperament, being emotional and tearful, craving affection and sympathy, and being filled with quiet resentment. There is a bitter taste in the mouth that interferes with the enjoyment of food, a painfully distended abdomen, indigestion from rich, greasy, fatty foods, flatulence, and vomiting after fruits, pastry or ice cold things.

INDIGESTION #2 (6X)

EPIGEA REPENS (gravel weed) Symptoms of Epigea include uric acid building up throughout the body, kidney stones, cystitis, and great rumbling in bowels.

HOMERIA COLLINA (cape tulip) Symptoms include obstinate, chronic constipation, toxic poisoning from whatever source, severe nausea and vomiting, collapse with cold limbs, irregular pulse, dilated pupils, and near insensibility.

KALI MURIATICUM (potassium chloride) Symptoms of Kali mur include abdominal tenderness, uncomfortable fullness after eating anything, colic with diarrhea, pressure in liver region, peritonitis, itching in urethra, indigestion with whitish gray tongue, and stomach pain with constipation. Fatty or rich foods almost always cause indigestion.

MANCINELLA VENENATA (manganeel apple) Symptoms related to this remedy are rumbling in the abdomen, burning stomach pains, continual choking sensation rising from the stomach, vomiting followed by severe colic and profuse diarrhea, and such severe heartburn that it feels as if there are flames rising from the stomach. Cold aggravates the symptoms but the person craves cold water.

RANUNCULUS SCELERATUS (marsh buttercup) Burning in mouth, throat, or stomach, burning and rawness of the tongue with patches peeling off, nausea worse after midnight, sore burning behind the xiphoid cartilage, and the sensation of impending diarrhea are some symptoms of Ranunculus.

VIBURNUM OPULUS (cramp bark) The symptom picture includes sudden cramps and colicky pains in pelvis with the pain worse by pressure around the umbilicus. There is no appetite or desire for food but, alternatively, there may be constant nausea that is relieved by eating.

INFECTION FIGHTER #1 (9X)

Anti-microbial, useful for a variety of infections, but is especially indicated for strep and staph infections.

This is an herbal preparation potentized according to homeopathic principles. Only Echinacea has a symptom picture based on homeopathic provings listed in the materia medicas. Lomatium and usnea are listed with herbal information only—usnea only as a headache remedy. Oregon grape, pau d'arco, and usnea are effective against a wide variety of bacteria (including strep and staph), fungal infections, yeasts, and the new strains of molds that are occasionally found in the lungs with osha being renowned as an immune stimulant. This combination is especially good for children.

ECHINACEA ANGUSTIFOLIA/PURPUREA (purple coneflower) Echinacea is a blood and immune tonic and is indicated for lymphatic inflammation, recurring ear infections, strep throat, upper lung congestion, stuffy nose and head, and even for such things as insect bites and stings and snakebites.

LIGUSTICUM PORTERI (osha) There are no homeopathic provings or remedies for sale that I can find record of; the formulator of this remedy must have created it for use here. The herb, however, is wonderful and has a particular affinity for respiratory problems of any nature. It is used for cardiovascular ailments and for the parasympathetic and sympathetic nervous systems. Osha stimulates circulation and promotes eliminative sweats. This herb is considered an immune stimulant and a regulator of white blood cells.

LOMATIUM DISSECTUM (lomatium) The area of expertise of Lomatium is the stomach and digestive problems, particularly if they are connected to bacterial issues.

MAHONIA AQUIFOLIUM (Oregon grape) This is one of the most fascinating herbs that I know of. It can be used as a substitute for goldenseal but does not have goldenseal's tendency to cause trouble for those who have blood sugar issues. Oregon grape is renowned in the herbal world for its ability to cleanse the liver, increase the production of bile, and cleanse the blood. This wonderful herb is also used for infectious conditions in the stomach and intestinal tract. There are no homeopathic provings that I know of for Oregon grape but with its herbal uses, it should make a wonderful homeoapthic.

USNEA BARBATA (a lichen) Usnea has very few homeopathic provings but as an herb it has unique properties which make it particularly effective against staph and strep strains and their various mutations. Usnea is also a great anti-fungal herb and is listed for headaches in Murphy's Materia Medica.

Each of these plants has a long history of use against infections.

INFECTION FIGHTER #2 (12X)

FILIX MAS (male fern) Symptoms for Filix mas include diarrhea and vomiting, abdominal pain and bloating, inflammation of lymph glands, pale face with blue circles around the eyes, and frequent but painless hiccupping. Filix is sometimes used in the treatment of tapeworms and other parasites, as well as for intestinal bacterial infestations. All symptoms are made worse from eating sweets.

MYRRH (myrrh gum) Myrrh is prized and respected for its antiseptic properties and for its abilities to cause the discharge of mucus from the body. Myrrh raises the body temperature and creates sweating (a good way to kill nasty bacteria and viruses). Myrrh is listed in homeopathic literature for stomach disorders, thrush, tonsillitis, sore throat, gum and mouth disorders, respiratory weakness with difficult expectoration, and to relieve infected or abscessed glands.

PENICILLINUM (penicillin) The homeopathic uses of this remedy would be much the same as those achieved by the drug itself with the additional benefit of detoxing and repairing the body from any side-effects or allergic reactions connected to the drug if it had ever been taken. One of these symptoms is a fever that continues for a long time and is worse in the evening.

INFECTION FIGHTER #3 (12X)

This remedy is specific to viral infection.

CETRARIA ISLANDICA (Iceland moss) The herb is antiseptic and expectorant and the homeopathic remedy is used for respiratory infections and chronic digestive problems.

ERYNGIUM AQUATICUM (button snake-root) This is a remedy for urinary disorders, congested mucus membranes, thick yellow mucus discharges from anywhere in the body, and is useful for inflammation of the eustachian tube.

IRIS VERSICOLOR (blue flag) This remedy is specific for viral infections with painful burning sensations, clogged liver, and kidneys stressed by the overload of dead and dying bacteria. An unusual keynote symptom is pain beginning over one eye and then moving to the other eye.

TARAXACUM OFFICINALE (dandelion) Some of the symptoms listed in the medicas are congestion and pain in the ears, bladder congestion, liver congestion and weakness, gallstones, irresistible drowsiness after meals, heat without thirst, tongue coated with a white film and raw red patches, and copious urine.

INFECTION FIGHTER #4 (9X)

This is an all-purpose anti-microbial remedy.

This remedy is made from a tincture combination that we have used in my home and business for many years. Some of the ingredients have no known (to me) homeopathic provings. There are many instances in the medicas where the provings were done using tinctures of the plant or animal material instead of using the homeopathic form. The symptoms produced are then listed as the symptom picture of the remedy. That is what I have done here.

MAHONIA AQUIFOLIUM (Oregon grape) This is one of the most fascinating herbs in use. Oregon grape can be substituted for goldenseal but does not have goldenseal's tendency to negatively affect blood sugar in sensitive persons. This herb is renowned for cleansing the liver and blood and increasing the production of bile. It is also used for infectious conditions in the stomach and intestinal tract. There are no homeopathic provings that I know of for Oregon grape.

USNEA BARBATA (a lichen) Usnea has very few homeopathic provings but as an herb is has unique properties which make it particularly effective against staph and strep strains and their various mutations. Usnea is also a great anti-fungal herb. Usnea is listed for headaches in Murphy's Materia Medica.

ECHINACEA ANGUSTIFOLIA/PURPUREA (purpleconeflower) Echinacea is a blood and immune tonic and is indicated for lymphatic inflammation, recurring ear infections, strep throat, upper lung congestion, stuffy nose and head, and even for such things as insect bites and stings and snakebites.

PHYTOLACCA AMERICANA (pokeweed root) Phytolacca is a polycrest remedy for glandular and lymphatic issues. It is indicated for glands that are swollen with heat and inflammation—particularly breasts and tonsils. Phytolacca acts on scar tissue, is useful for sore throats, and for muscular soreness all over. Keynote symptoms are high fever alternating with chilliness and great debility and prostration.

TRIFOLIUM PRATENSE (red clover) Red clover is primarily a blood cleanser and a rebuilder of cartilage. The materia medicas list this remedy for blood disorders, coughs, cancers, fibroids, and whooping cough and other coughs that are worse at night, and for sore throat with hoarseness. Some other symptoms and issues are lungs that are full with chills and cough at night, confusion and headaches on awakening, and cold hands and feet. Robin Murphy's materia medica lists this remedy as a preventive for mumps and cancer and as a retardant for cancerous growths.

MILLEFOLIUM ACHILLEA (yarrow) Yarrow acts on capillaries, arteries, veins, and mucus membranes as a tonic and astringent. This remedy is useful for ulcerations of the throat with pain on swallowing and for wounds which bleed profusely. Yarrow aids with injuries, falls and sprains, and bruises.

INFECTION FIGHTER #5 (9X)

Aids in the relief of inflammation and fever associated with the flu, viral colds, and minor infections.

ECHINACEA ANGUSTIFOLIA/PURPUREA (purple cone-flower) Echinacea is a blood and immune tonic and is indicated for lymphatic inflammation, recurring ear infections, strep throat, tonsillitis, upper lung congestion, stuffy nose and head, and even for such things as insect bites and stings and snakebites.

ACONITUM NAPELLUS (monkshood) Aconite illnesses are usually acute, and are always sudden and violent with high fever being common. Some other symptoms are earache with pain, dryness and heat in the eyes, croup, influenza, bronchitis, pneumonia, chills, and is useful any time the nose is stopped up. There may be acute inflammation of the throat with high fever. Mental and emotional symptoms include many forebodings and fears.

ARNICA MONTANA (leopard's bane) While Arnica is usually considered a remedy for injuries and traumas, it also has symptoms that make it useful in this infection fighting remedy. Some of these symptoms are influenza with fever, aching pains that accompany illness, violent, spasmodic cough and burning or a feeling of rawness in the chest. The person is usually sleepless and restless when overtired and all symptoms are better from lying down. The nose feels sore and cold.

BAPTISIA TINCTORIA (wild indigo) This remedy has a history of effective use with epidemic influenza. Other symptoms for which this remedy is considered useful come with high fever and include such things as septicemia, toxemia, blood poisoning, headache with fever and delirium, extreme diarrhea, and lungs feeling tight and compressed with a feeling of suffocation. Prostration comes on rapidly, the brain feels sore and there is confusion, as if the person is intoxicated.

RHUS TOXICODENDRON (poison oak) Rhus toxicodendron is indicated for a great many things that have nothing to do with infections and it is important to remember one of the basic rules of homeopathy—that it is the symptom picture, and not the cause of the ailment, that matters. Symptoms include fevers with blisters, appendicitis, influenza, hoarseness, rashes, swollen glands, headache in occiput, and the mind and the senses become cloudy. There is pain and stiffness in the small of back and no appetite for any kind of food. Symptoms are better from heat and from a hot bath and worse from overexertion.

SANGUINARIA CANADENSIS (bloodroot) Sanguinaria is useful for blood disorders, croup, burning sensations, distended veins and temples, pneumonia, cough of gastric origin, dry cough, tickling in throat, and chill with nausea. This is a right-sided remedy.

BRYONIA ALBA (wild hops) The symptoms of Bryonia include coughs, headaches, influenza, nosebleeds, sharp pain when swallowing, pleurisy, whooping cough, and mucus membranes are all dry with excessive thirst. Modalities include better for rest and aggravated by motion. Mental/emotional symptoms include being exceedingly irritable and wanting to be left alone.

STREPTOCOCCINUM (streptococcus nosode) This is a nosode made from the streptoccus virus and is used for chronic sore throats and streptococcal infections, for people who are susceptible to catching colds and sore throats, for many types of infections, tonsillitis., otitis and mastoiditis, pleurisy, acute sinusitis, and severe bronchitis.

GELSEMIUM SEMPERVIRENS (yellow jasmine) Gelsemium is a remedy with a strong affinity for the recovery stages of illnesses and for fatigue and illness that is brought on by anxiety, anticipation, fear, or bad news. Gelsemium is keynoted by either the failure of energy levels to return to normal after an illness or complete exhaustion that just will not go away. Other symptoms include drowsiness, trembling, aching muscles, headache, chilliness and pain up and down the spine, and fever with thirstlessness.

INJURIES (9X)

HYPERICUM PERFORATUM (St. Johns' wort) Hypericum is one of the most important polycrest remedies of all time! Hypericum is indicated for wounds to nerve-rich areas of the body such as fingers and toes. Hypericum injuries are distinguished by several unique traits. Two of these traits are that wounds are more tender than appearance would indicate they should be and the pain from the wound is shooting or coming in spasms. Hypericum is useful for any type of infected wound, the bites of animals and insects, injuries to the tailbone, neuralgia, pinched nerves in back, sciatic pain, and pain from puncture wounds.

CALENDULA OFFICINALIS (pot marigold) Calendula is a remarkable healing agent, applied locally or given internally in homeopathic potency. Calendula promotes the rapid healing of wounds, cuts, abrasions, lacerations, and broken skin surfaces. Calendula prevents scar tissue formation, stops bleeding—especially from the scalp or mouth, and is excellent before or after surgery.

INSOMNIA #1 (6X)

FERRUM PHOSPHORICUM (iron phosphate) Ferrum phos is said to increase hemoglobin production and the absorption of iron. This remedy is useful for inflammation and for the first stages of inflammatory disorders. Part of the picture is issues which create insomnia where there is restless sleep with anxious dreams, slight fever causing wakefulness, and the night sweats common to anemia. The bad night is usually followed by great depression in the morning.

KALI PHOSPHORICUM (potassium phosphate) Kali phos is considered "the nerve nutrient" in tissue salt theory. There is sleeplessness from worry, over study, or business troubles, sleeplessness from over-active mind, and sleepwalking when sleep is finally achieved. Kali phos people are sensitive, nervous and easily tired out completely by worry or mental fatigue. The exhaustion often comes with pains and weight at back of head.

MAGNESIUM PHOSPHORICA (magnesium phosphate) Some insomnia keynotes of Mag phos include sleepiness when attempting to study or read, insomnia from exhaustion, waking due to leg or foot cramps, sleep disturbed by troubled dreams, and drowsiness in the morning hours. There is such severe yawning that it feels as if the jaws will be dislocated—painful and uncontrollable enough to cause tears and there are spasmodic twitchings of facial muscles. The neuralgic pains are relieved by warmth.

INSOMNIA #2 (6X)

VALERIANA OFFICINALIS (valerian) Valerian is always about over-sensitiveness of the nerves. This is reflected in sleeplessness and insomnia. The person cannot sleep before midnight, their sleep is disturbed with tossing and anxious confused dreams, sleeplessness from nightly itching, muscular spasms from excitement, profuse sweats at night, and cramping of hands and feet that prevents sleep.

COFFEA CRUDA (unroasted coffee) With Coffea, the mind and memory are active until midnight preventing sleep but then the person awakes at 3 a. m. and only dozes the remainder of night. There is great nervous agitation and restlessness, spending the night tossing about in anguish. The person is sensitive to noises—sleepless as long as there is any sound or light and wakes again at the slightest sounds.

PULSATILLA NIGRICANS (windflower) Pulsatilla is for people of basic mild temperament who are emotional, tearful, and like consolation. A person with Pulsatilla characteristics is sleepy in the afternoon, wide awake in the evening even until very late, restless at first sleep and takes a long time to fall asleep. She then wakes unrefreshed, confused, and grumpy in the morning. A person in the Pulsatilla pattern generally sleeps on their back and prefers to have their hands above their head.

BELLADONNA (deadly nightshade) Everything about Belladonna is extreme and throbbing. The person is kept awake by pulsation of blood vessels—throbbing in carotid and temporal arteries—and jerks during sleep, waking during the night full of fear with dreams of falling, and there is often a tickling, dry cough that is worse at night. The person will be wakeful because they are oversensitive to light, noise and even minor movements of other people in the bed or the room.

ARSENICUM ALBUM (white oxide of arsenic) The insomnia symptoms of this polycrest remedy include sleeplessness from anxiety and nervous exhaustion, violent startling with twitching and trembling of limbs during sleep, and being kept awake by heartburn and shortness of breath.

ACONITE NAPELLUS (monkshood) Aconite is indicated by sleeplessness caused by fear, fright or anxiety. There are anxious dreams, physical and mental restlessness, and vertigo that is worse on first rising. Children of this pattern cry and complain, and are very restless.

LEPTANDRA VIRGINICA (Culver's root) Insomniac symptoms of Leptandra are restless sleep after midnight and then feels very ill the next day. Other symptoms include weakness, gloominess, irritability, dull frontal headache, and aching eyes.

PENTHORUM SEDOIDES (Virginia stonecrop) There is no mention of sleep disorders with Penthorum but there are many symptoms that indicate nervous issues that would very likely create insomnia that should probably be listed. These nerve symptoms include headaches, lack of focus in life, vertigo, and dull aching in the kidneys.

ZINCUM BROMATUM (zinc bromide) With Zincum bromatum there is alternating wakefulness and a sleep so deep that it is stuporous. There is pain in the nerves of the head and face. Zincum bromatum is predominantly a remedy for teething children but is occasionally used for other people.

INTESTINAL CLEANSE (9X)

QUASSIA AMARA (Quassia wood) Quassia is listed in the medicas as a digestive remedy and as a treatment for worms . Certainly the symptoms upon which it acts indicate parasite infestations.

Among these symptoms are pressure and pain in the liver and, sympathetically, in the spleen, very acute sticking in the hepatic region followed by dull pain, fatty liver, pain in the muscles above the liver, dyspepsia with flatus, acidity, and heartburn. Symptoms outside the digestive area, but understandable as connected to serious trouble there, include copious urination day and night—the child wakes up with the bed drenched, fatigue and weakness with great hunger, drawing pains in calves, severe drawing pains in cervical muscles, and cold limbs with a sensation of coldness running over the back.

JUGLANS NIGRA (black walnut) Juglans nigra is similar to Julans regia and is another remedy, in both herbal and homeopathic form, that is noted for the expulsion of parasites. Juglans nigra is especially noteworthy because it affects the spleen even more acutely than it does the liver—an usual traint among homeopathic remedies. Symptoms includes bloating, flatulence, nausea, and emaciation—certainly all symptoms consistent with parasites.

ABSINTHIUM ARTEMISIA/ARTEMISIA ABSINTHIUM (common wormwood) This is a far more deep acting remedy than any of the others in this combination. It has all of the usual symptoms associated with parasites and other serious intestinal problems, but also has actions on the liver, spleen, and intestinal tract with a special emphasis on the gallbladder.

Absinthium also has in its symptom picture indications for parasite infestations that have been acting on the body for a very long time, causing serious nutritional and nerve deficiencies. These symptoms include convulsions preceded by trembling, marked tremors of nerves, tongue, and heart, spasmodic facial twitching, headaches, nervousness, vertigo, and loss of memory.

FILIX MAS (male fern) The symptoms of FIlix mas include great pain in the abdomen with diarrhea and constant vomiting, gnawing and boring in the bowels, bloating, inflammation of lymph glands, pale face with blue circles around the eyes, frequent but painless hiccupping, and worms and worm colic. Filix mas is used in the treatment of tapeworms and other parasites, as well as for intestinal bacterial infestations. All symptoms, as would be expected with parasites, are made worse from eating sweets.

SYZYGIUM AROMATICUM (clove) I can find no provings for clove as a homeopathic remedy but clove essential oil is considered anti-fungal and anti-parasitic as well as an excellent antibiotic, antiseptic, expectorant, and antispasmodic.

There are many instances in the medicas where the provings were done using tinctures of the plant or animal material instead of using the homeopathic form. The symptoms produced are then listed as the symptom picture of the remedy.

INTESTINAL/STOMACH DISTRESS #1 (10X)

VINCA MINOR (lesser periwinkle) When Vinca minor is indicated the person's abdomen will be full, tense and painful. The intestinal tract will rumble and gurgle and then pass offensive flatus. Keynotes are that the stool will be first very hard then overly soft, indicating a problem with moisture levels in the last part of the colon. Passing the stool is exhausting with burning in the anus. When vomiting occurs, it will be copious and be very bitter and yellowish-green in color.

PSORINUM (scabies nosode) Psorinum is a remedy with many allergies, including food allergies, in its picture. The result of these allergies in the intestinal tract is constipation with pain in the lumbar region, chronic diarrhea in the early morning, involuntary stools while sleeping (a nasty pattern), burning hemorrhoids, and stools that are bloody and excessively fetid.

LOBELIA PURPURASCENS (purple lobelia is very similar to Lobelia inflata but is grown in Australia) Lobelia, both as an herb and as a homeopathic remedy, is useful in neutralizing ***poisons in the blood*** from a congested colon. SarsaparillA is another herb with this characteristic. Lobelia is excellent for the repair of diverticula inflamed or infected pouches in the intestinal wall) in a septic colon.

Interestingly (and exactly what you would expect in the homeopathic world), an overdose of this herb brings on chills—which is one of the outstanding aspects for which Lobelia as a homeopathic remedy bring relief. These chills, along with the accompanying slowing of the heart rhythm, have given this herb an undeserved bad reputation. I say undeserved because the action is exactly what the body needs, both to heal and to alert you that it is time to let the body make use of what you have provided and get on with healing without any more of the remedy.

PLATINUM METALLICUM (platina metal) A symptom which sets this remedy apart, and indicates the need for this remedy, is the alternating of the physical and mental symptoms. If they are not feeling sad, arrogant, contemptuous, or wounded in their pride, which seems to keep them stuck somehow, the physical indications for this remedy will come online. Then, as the physical ailments are treated, the unpleasant mental/emotional patterns emerge. ***This requires treatment to a very deep level to eradicate this pattern completely!***

Physical symptoms include colic from toxic poisoning, pain in the umbilical region extending through into the back, a lot of flatulence and abdominal pain, and sensations of constriction of the stomach and abdomen.

VESPA CRABRO (wasp) Vespa is usually thought of as a remedy for bee stings but is also indicated for boils. Skin conditions of the magnitude of boils almost always indicatE a congested colon. Because the colon is not able to eliminate things that would be very harmful to the body, they are brought to the surface, encapsulated into a boil, and expelled—eventually, after much pain and suffering. There will be heat in the stomach, with indigestion and nausea during the evening hours.

INTESTINAL/STOMACH DISTRESS #2 (15X)

KALI CYANATUM (potassium cyanide) Kaly cyanatum is a deadly poison, but readily available because of its use in photography. Cyanide (material dose not homeopathic) is a favorite method of suicide and attempted suicide. I don't understand this as it would be such a painful way to go! The symptom picture of this remedy is actually drawn from the symptoms observed in suicide attempts and from a small number of homeopathic provings.

Symptoms include pains in abdomen and groin, severe burning in the stomach, sharp gastric pains, and such copious and horrendous vomiting that it brings on momentary bouts of unconsciousness. There can be, in later stages, vertigo. Headache, convulsions, and agonizing neuralgia are experienced in the facial area and involve the trigeminal nerve.

VERBASCUM THAPSUS (mullein oil) Mullein, in herbal form, is soothing and healing to mucus membranes and this effect carries into the homeopathic form. Symptoms include incessant gurgling and rumbling with inflation of the abdomen, violent and painful pressure in the abdomen, sensation of emptiness in the pit of the stomach which disappears with a rumbling noise, frequent hiccups, hemorrhoids, and empty or bitter risings into the esophagus with nausea, constipation, diarrhea.

PARIS QUADRIFOLIA (one berry) This is an anti-psoric remedy with the psora keynotes of being hungry soon after a meal and a "sinking" feeling in the stomach. Other digestive symptoms include weak digestion (many things irritate and absorption of nutrients is impaired), stomach often feels heavy as if it contains a stone, there is rumbling and rolling in the abdomen, and a lot of abdominal pain.

LOBELIA INFLATA (Indian tobacco) Lobelia, both as an herb and as a homeopathic remedy, is useful in neutralizing ***poisons in the blood*** from a congested colon. Symptoms include a distended abdomen with shortness of breath, extreme nausea and vomiting, nausea with prickling and itching of the skin, and diarrhea. Lobelia is excellent for the repair of diverticula (inflamed or infected pouches in the intestinal wall) often found in a septic colon and creating painful bloating and a foul odor.

Interestingly (and exactly what you would expect in the homeopathic world), an overdose of this herb brings on chills—chills being one of the aspects of Lobelia as a homeopathic remedy. These chills, along with the accompanying slowing of the heart rhythm, have given Lobelia an undeserved bad reputation. I say undeserved because the action is exactly what the body needs, both to heal and to alert you that it is time to let the body take over the healing process. (I know that this information was just presented a moment ago but I felt that it was important enough to mention in each remedy's description.)

INTESTINAL/STOMACH DISTRESS #3 (6X)

NEPETA CATARIA (catnip) Nepeta is a diaphoretic, tonic, antispasmodic, diuretic, and carminative. Because it produces free perspiration it is useful for many types of toxic and infectious situations. Symptoms include abdominal pain, colic, diarrhea, flatulence, cramps, and indigestion. Children become fretful and irritable from the pain of indigestion.

MENTHA PIPERITA (peppermint) With Mentha piperita indigestion is most often seen in the evening two hours after dinner. There is weight in the stomach that extends into the ears, flatulence, and a lot of stomach pains. Mental symptoms include mental dullness when rising early with the opposite, more balanced pattern of waking up eager for work and being extraordinarily productive and effective.

FOENICULUM SATIVUM (fennel) This is another remedy whose information in the medicas is based on the herbal uses of the plant. T he action of this remedy is milder on the stomach than cumin or dill but is more relaxing to the digestive tract overall. Foeniculum sativum is useful for stomach cramps, flatulence, and many types of diarrhea.

INTESTINAL/STOMACH DISTRESS #4 (7X)

Created for use against the cryptosporidium parvum protozoa (Crypto).

CRYPTOSPORIDIUM PARASITIC PROTOZOAN (protozoa) that exists in rivers and lakes. This parasite can cause intestinal illnesses. Infestations are commonly seen in people suffering from auto-immune disorders, chronic fatigue, and allergies. Overuse of antibiotics allows the parasite to grow unchecked. There are some studies that indicate that chlorine in drinking water actually alters the protozoa's walls, making them better able to multiply faster than normal in the human intestinal tract.

Symptoms of Cryptosporidium infestation in humans include diarrhea, abdominal pain, nausea, vomiting, and low-grade fever. The symptoms often come and go, lasting less than 30 days. Immune deficient patients are more susceptible, making this critter quite deadly to cancer patients undergoing chemotherapy and to anyone who has a suppressed immune system or has just suppressed it on purpose (with a vaccine, for example). Occasionally, dehydration from a severe case has caused death.

ARSENICUM ALBUM (white oxide of arsenic) Arsenicum is a leading polycrests and is a restorative for all systems of the body (digestive, urinary, circulatory, lymphatic, and glandular) but has a particular affinity for the liver and the intestinal tract. A few (very few) keynote symptoms include burning pain in the stomach and abdomen, rumbling and cramping pains in the bowels, violent squeezing and constriction in umbilical region, diarrhea, and enlargement of the liver and the spleen Great deep-acting polycrest remedy for dealing with influenzas, stomach flu, intestinal distress of any description, poisonings, and parasites. Remedy picture also includes sudden great weakness and shortness of breath.

INTESTINAL/STOMACH DISTRESS #5 (10X)

GUARANA (Brazilian coco) Symptoms of Guarana include debility after a debilitating disease, chronic diarrhea, and spasms of the bladder. This is a remedy for nervous exhaustion. Nerve symptoms include reduced vitality, congestive or throbbing headache, headache followed by vomiting, loss of appetite, restless nervousness, and neuralgias.

PLUMBAGO LITTORALIS (plumbago) I can find very little information about plumbago as a homeopathic and none at all about it as an herbal remedy. Symptoms that are listed include profuse milky saliva, vertigo after eating, and an aversion to every food presented or suggested.

CROTALUS HORRIDUS (timber rattlesnake) Crotalus, being a snake remedy, as action on the blood, heart and liver and is a remedy for septic conditions. Symptoms include intestinal hemorrhage, heat and tenderness of abdomen, liquid stools, involuntary stools, aching in liver region, and vomiting.

INTESTINAL/STOMACH DISTRESS #6 (6X)

This remedy is for use with food poisoning situations.

SALMONELLA TYPHI (nosode) This nosode is one of several Salmonella bacterium and is the one responsible for typhoid fever. It would seem to me that Salmonella enterica would be a closer match if looking for a nosode for Salmonella infestation. However, "like cures like" is the homeopathic principle and S. enterica, as a nosode, would be "exact acting on exact", which is a very different treatment pattern .

This remedy is meant to help with the sudden onset of symptoms such as nausea, abdominal cramping, bloody diarrhea with mucus, dehydration, chronic infection and inflammation of the gallbladder and bile ducts, chronic pancreatitis, and high fever. There may be mental confusion and vagueness.

ARSENICUM ALBUM (white oxide of arsenic) Please see the description of Arsenicum album under the Intestinal/Stomach Distress #4 remedy discussed previously.

KIDNEY #1 (6X)

ASPARAGUS OFFICINALIS (asparagus) Symptoms of this remedy having to do with the kidneys include cystitis, frequent urination with stinging and a peculiar smell, thirst, and kidney stones and crystals. Restlessness increased by motion. Pain near shoulders. There may be pain in forehead and root of nose, shooting pains in the heart region after a meal, belching, flatulence, vertigo and dizziness.

PENTHORUM SEDOIDES (Virginia stonecrop) Symptoms include a dull ache in kidneys, the bladder being sore to touch, a burning sensation when urinating although the urine tests as alkaline, and a scaled sensation in the tongue.

URTICA URENS (stinging nettle) Many symptoms of this remedy have "burning" included in their description. Symptoms related to the kidneys include bleeding from the bladder, uric acid toxemia, kidney/ bladder disease, gravel in the kidneys, and acid urine with itching.

KIDNEY #2 (7X)

JUNIPERUS COMMUNIS (juniper berries) This is one of my favorite herbs although I only use it in combinations and a bit sparingly. The homeopathic symptoms picture includes scanty urine with blood and the smell of violets, and a feeling as though there is a weight in kidney region.

POLYGONUM SAGITTATUM (arrow-leaved tearthumb) This homeopathic remedy has only a few lines in Murphy's Materia Medica and all of those are for something kidney related. They include pains of nephritic colic, suppurative nephritis—inflammation of the kidneys and sharp pains along the spine.

KIDNEY #3 (7X)

CYPRIPEDIUM PUBESCENS (yellow lady's slipper) Lady's slipper was a herb of great renown in former years as a nervine. Unfortunately, it has been on endangered species lists for years and we can no longer purchase it. The homeopathic remedy is the best that we can do. Symptoms for this remedy, homeopathically, include neuralgia, nervousness, intestinal trouble, debility after gout (uric acid crystals and cellular waste in the tissues of the extremities, sleeplessness, indifference, and vertigo.

LYCOPODIUM CLAVATUM (club moss) Symptoms pertaining to the kidneys include hot urine with red sand, aching the kidneys that is better for urinating, backache before urinating that is better after urine passes, gallstones or kidney stones or gravel, eczema, nasal troubles since childhood, low blood sugar, and a great desire for sweets, and oozing behind ears. The emotional pattern linked to kidneys is fear; anxiety and suspiciousness are simply the manifestation of the problem in the kidneys.

EUPHORBIUM OFFICINALIS (eyebright) The most marked keynote of this remedy is terrible burning pains as if a live coal were on or in that body part whether it be bones or internal organs.

MANCINELLA VENENATA (manganeel apple) This is a remedy with *serious* mental and skin issues in its symptom picture. Hair loss after illness. These include skin problems with excessive blisters, herpes, and severe sore throat. There is sudden vanishing of thoughts and a fear of going completely insane.

PENICILLINUM (penicillin) This remedy is indicated for those who have had kidney issues and have never been well since taking this drug. It is also indicated for many of those symptoms for which the drug might be prescribed allopathically.

RADIUM BROMATUM (radium bromide) Pure radium is a white powder that has the property of adhering to ferrum (iron). This property illustrates the close relationship of radium and ferrum and gives us clues as to the homeopathic uses of radium. One of the uses for this remedy is for x-ray burns. This remedy is also indicated for kidney irritation, albuminuria, and the increased elimination of sediment, bedwetting, itching all over the body, and skin disorders. Radium bromide was used historically for epithelioma, which is an abnormal growth of the layer of tissues that covers the surfaces of organs and other structures of the body.

THIOSINAMINUM (mustard seed) Thiosinaminum is used in cases of scar tissue formation, strictures of the urethra and painful urination, and urine that is increased in quantity but has no increased sediment or albumen.

KIDNEY #4 (7X)

EUPHRASIA OFFICINALIS (eyebright) Symptoms include frequent, copious urination, bladder being very irritable at night, dribbling urine, conjunctivitis, watering eyes, and burning and swelling of eyelids.

IPOMOEA PURPUREA (morning glory) Although Ipomoea is used solely as a drastic purgative in allopathic medicine, it has many uses in the homeopathic world. (As an herbalist, I often remarked that there had to be some use for this stubborn weed. I finally found some in homeopathy!)

The ipomoea picture includes many symptoms for the kidneys. These include severe pain in the left kidney with nausea, kidney stones and gravel, kidney disorders with pain in the back (this seems to occur predominantly on the left side), chilliness alternating with flashes of heat and copious sweat. Emotional symptoms include a strong desire for solitude, loss of memory, hypersensitivity to noise, and anxiety with palpitations. This remedy is specific to night terrors in children who have worms.

NATRUM SULPHURICUM (sodium sulphate) Nat sulph symptoms include kidney and bladder irritation and distress, frequent urination, diabetes, burning pain in urethra, urine loaded with bile, scanty dark urine with the need to get up several times in the night, bruised pain in lumbar region, severe pain at the back of the neck and base of the brain with soreness up and down spine and neck.

TEREBINTHINIAE OLEUM (oil of turpentine) Some symptoms of Terebinthiniae are burning and drawing pain in the region of the kidneys and running along the ureters, cystitis, irritable bladder and kidneys, bleeding from the bladder, scanty suppressed urine with the odor of violets, and pains that alternate between navel and bladder that is better for walking, and stiff muscles. There will be feelings of lethargy, agitated sleep with frequent waking, and anxiety and confusion related to uric acid deposits—mental symptoms set up by renal (urinary) failure.

KIDNEY #5 (7X)

FICUS RELIGIOSA (ashwathya) With Ficus there is a frequent desire to urinate and the urine contains blood. The emotional mood is quiet, sad, melancholic. Mental exertion causes sweat on the feet, and vertigo while sitting or stooping.

KALI SILICIUM (potassium silicate) The symptom picture of Kali silicium includes stiffness over body and limbs, twitching of muscles, gouty, small bumps under the skin, offensive sweat on the feet, and vertigo while sitting or stooping.

NATRUM SILICICUM (sodium silicate) Natrum silicicum is a very deep-acting remedy whose symptom picture includes headaches, chronic gout, chilliness, dryness of mouth and throat, and nervous headache from mental exertion.

THUJA OCCIDENTALIS (arbor vitae) Kidney symptoms of this remedy include paralysis of the bladder sphincter, burning pain on urination, urine that is dark red in the morning with a strong smell, and there is complete inability to focus and concentrate.

KIDNEY #6 (7X)

Aids in decreasing inflammation of the urogenital tract.

HEPAR SULPHURIS CALCAREUM This remedy is specific for the bladder difficulties of elderly men. Symptoms include slow voiding without force, weak bladder, seems as if some urine always remains, putrid odor of urine, itching. Emotions include overly sensitive to impressions, extreme irritability, peevishness, and impulsive behavior.

SABAL SERRULATA This remedy also includes prostate enlargement and weakness along with the kidney symptoms. (Incidentally, this remedy is also good for undeveloped breast glands.) Other symptoms are bed wetting, cystitis, impotency, urine incontinence, pain in the region of the kidneys, and fear of going to sleep.

CHIMAPHILA UMBELLATA One of the main focuses of this remedy i suppressed urine in infants and acute inflammation of the urinary tract in adults. This remedy includes many types of kidney and bladder disorders, as well as prostate enlargement, scanty urine loaded with ropes of mucus with sediment, nephritis, straining before flow comes, burning during urination, and clots of blood passing with urine. Modalities include better from walking and worse in damp weather.

Meridian Balancing Combinations

Over 5,000 years ago, the ancient Chinese discovered an entire system of subtle energy in the body that is only now able to be "read" by our modern diagnostic and imaging tools. Energy disturbances in these subtle systems precede the manifestation of abnormal patterns of cellular organization and growth.

There is a primary energetic substance of which everything in the universe is composed. Physical matter and energy are two different manifestations of this primary substance. Matter, which vibrates at a very slow frequency, relatively speaking, is referred to as physical matter. Matter which vibrates at speeds exceeding the velocity of light is know as subtle matter. Subtle matter is just as real as the more dense form of matter.

The Chinese have mapped out twelve meridians, or pathways, along which this energy travels in the human body. These meridians were named for the life function associated with them. To the majority of scientists in the western hemisphere, these meridians seem like imaginary structures because there are no published anatomical studies of them in orthodox medical journals to substantiate their existence. The medical community does admit, however, that there is much about "energy" in the human body that cannot be explained in terms of circulation, nerves, or by the electrical impulses that they can trace.

Meridians are the pathways of communication between the various parts of the human body/mind/soul complex. Through these meridians pass an invisible nutritive energy known to the Chinese as ch'i. The ch'i energy enters the body through specific points and flows to deeper organ structures, bringing life-giving nourishment of a subtle energetic nature.

The meridians, and specific acupuncture points along them, have been mapped by modern technological methods—electronically, thematically, and radioactively. Normal energy over one of these points, when healthy and vibrant, is approximately 100,000 ohms. With practice and awareness this energy can be felt and located by the human hand, with micro-electrical voltage meters, and with muscle testing. It is often easier to feel a point with your hand when the point is not functioning correctly.

A strong and balanced flow of energy through the body's meridians is important to optimal health. Blocked meridians create imbalanced energy flow to organs which contributes to disease states within the body. There are emotional and mental characteristics associated with each pair of meridians. In fact, some of what we call personality is dictated by the way the energy is flowing through our meridians.

Energy flow through the meridians can be slowed or entirely blocked by a number of factors, including traumatic injury, emotional trauma, chronic illnesses, parasite infestations, and chemical toxicity. Impaired flow in a meridian is often responsible for slow healing of wounds and injuries, as well as slow response to herbal, chiropractic, or homeopathic treatment.

The idea of using a homeopathic combination to improve flow along a meridian is a good one. There is one homeopathic combination for each meridian listed on the next few pages. The basic symptom picture of each single remedy within the combination is explained separately. This will enable you to choose for yourself whether to take a low-potency combination remedy, or zero in on a particular remedy contained in the blend and take just that one in a higher potency.

A very brief description of the emotional pattern of each meridian is given. You should be able to draw a fairly accurate picture of the meridian's out-of-balance state by the descriptions of the single remedies.

GOVERNING VESSEL MERIDIAN BALANCE (6X)

Moving forward on life's path with faith and confidence—or—Embarrassment and reluctance to move forward at all

The governing vessels controls the peripheral nervous system which collects information and controls certain bodily functions such as the heartbeat, the kidneys, and hormone levels.

ARSENICUM ALBUM (white oxide of arsenic) Arsenicum is a leading polycrest—absolutely amazing restorative for all systems of the body (digestive, urinary, circulatory, lymphatic, and glandular). A few (very few) keynote symptoms include burning pain in the stomach and abdomen, vomiting, diarrhea, and enlargement of the liver and the spleen. Arsenicum is a great deep-acting polycrest remedy for dealing with stomach and intestinal distress, poisonings, and parasites. Remedy picture also includes sudden great weakness and shortness of breath, constricted air passages, asthma, and pulmonary edema.

AURUM METALLICUM (gold metal) This is a remedy that is indicated for acute mental depression—the kind of hopelessness that can lead to suicide! The person will be oversensitive to pain and to noise. There are many physical symptoms. A few of the keynotes include high blood pressure, rapid pulse that is feeble and irregular, carotids and temporal arteries throb visibly, and angina pectoris.

BARYTA CARBONICA (barium carbonate) The mentals of this remedy that indicate the governing meridian include increasing mental weakness and some learning disabilities in children. There is a wide range of physical symptoms listed.

CACTUS GRANDIFLORUS (night-blooming cereus) Desire to be alone, sadness and melancholy, fears that something bad is about to happen, and an irresistible inclination to weep are some of the emotional symptoms of this remedy. Physical symptoms include constriction as from an iron band around the head, very acute pains and stitches in heart with the pulse being feeble and irregular, endocarditis with mitral valve insufficiency together with violent and rapid action, heart murmurs, low blood pressure, aneurysm of large arteries and heart, and arteriosclerosis.

There are many symptoms unrelated to the heart but the heart symptoms are very pronounced and are a primary focus of this remedy as is typical of remedies that affect the governing meridian.

CALCAREA CARBONICA (calcium carbonate) This remedy is one of 3 remedies that are considered the standard around which all anti-psoric remedies are grouped. Symptoms include digestive difficulties and improper absorption of nutrients, glandular issues, many heart and kidney issues.

LITHIUM CARBONICUM (lithium carbonate) The mental patterns of this remedy includes manic depression and obsessive compulsive disorders. The heart symptoms include the odd keynote of eye symptoms showing up with the heart trembling, fluttering of the heart, and heart pain.

LYCOPODIUM CLAVATUM (club moss) Mentals include panic attacks and many fears, anger and irritability. There seems to be a connection to being the child of domineering or abusive parents. Indigestion with pain and distress in gastric region. Once again, as with all things to do with the governing meridian, there are issues such as hypoglycemia, diabetes, and food allergies.

MERCURIUS SOLUBILIS (mercury vivus) The keynote of this remedy is the changeableness of the symptoms, mental and physical—in other words, stress, confusion, and the interruption of energy flow in the central and governing meridians.

NATRUM SULPHURICUM (sodium sulfate) This number is particularly indicated after a head injury has interrupted the flow of the governing meridian up over the back of the head and over the face.

SPIGELIA ANTHELMINTICA (pinkroot) Neuralgia of the fifth cranial nerve with heart disorders and neuralgias.

TARENTULA HISPANICA (Spanish tarentula) When the governing meridian is struggling there will be twitching, involuntary movements, restlessness of lower limbs, migraine headaches, hysteria, burning and painful boils. Mental and emotional symptoms will include destructive impulses and erratic behaviors. The person will find being still extremely difficult. All symptoms and pains of Tarentula will be violent and painful.

This remedy is indicated for multiple sclerosis and Parkinson's disease and is known to palliate the agony and pains of the dying process.

CENTRAL VESSEL MERIDIAN BALANCE (6X)

Firmness, balance between logic and emotion, considerate of—without being unduly influenced by—other people's energies or opinions—or—
An unrealistic sense of shame, guilt, shyness, and discomfort around people

The central vessel is affiliated with the central nervous system and, when depleted, makes a person vulnerable to the negative energies around them.

APIS MELLIFICA (honey bee) There is a great deal of swelling or puffing up in various parts of the body found throughout this remedy. The edema usually come with burning sensations. Some symptoms include congested ovaries with fluid buildup, burning in the kidneys with dark urine, and allergic reactions. A person benefited by this remedy will show anxious restlessness and fidgeting, be constantly busy, and worse from heat of any kind.

ARSENICUM ALBUM (white oxide of arsenic) A keynote of Arsenicum that applies very specifically to the central vessel is ***sudden great weakness from trivial causes.*** Arsenicum acts on the nerves producing neuralgias, anxiety, fastidiousness, anger, mania and depression. Physical symptoms include nerve pain all over the body and the malfunctioning of organs and systems.

BELLADONNA (deadly nightshade) The first thing listed in the materia medicas for Belladonna is that it acts upon t he brain and nervous system centers. A keynote of this symptom is the suddenness and violence of any attack on the body. This suddenness and depth of pathology is because the weakened central meridian is unable to protect the body as it is meant to.

CONIUM MACULATUM (poison hemlock) The effect on the nervous system of this remedy is a spreading paralysis that begins in the lower extremities and moves upward. The legs and the gait are often the first things affected, as is seen in chronic ailments like Parkinson's disease, but the debility is progressive until all nerve and brain functions—and, therefore, all bodily functions—are affected. The eyes, fed by this meridian, often show distress when the energy here is either too agitated or to low.

FERRUM METALLICUM (iron metal) The affinity of this remedy for the central vessel is seen in the intense restlessness or the opposing symptom of too worn out to move. The sensitivity to pain, irritation at even slight noises, anger when contradicted, and changeable moods are also symptoms of weakness in this meridian.

LACHESIS MUTA (bushmaster snake) More than most snake remedies, Lachesis shows the great weakness and prostration of nerve disorders. There is also the telltale erratic aspects found in the pains often alternating sides of the body very rapidly, wandering arthritis pains, and the mind and conversational topics jumping from place to place with great rapidity. Nervous headaches are common.

MERCURIUS SOLUBLIS (mercury vivus) Once again, weakening of the central vessel is seen in the lightning fast changeableness of this remedy and in the list of things that make symptoms worse—there is nothing mentioned that makes the symptoms better. Emotional symptoms include restlessness that is especially pronounced at night, poor self- confidence, irresolute when a decision needs to be made, and homesickness.

PULSATILLA NIGRICANS (windflower) The dependent, affection- and sympathy-craving patterns of Pulsatilla are driven by such weakness in the central vessel that the boundaries between self and others are very blurred. Moods come and go, the person is emotional and tearful, feels forsaken and abandoned or put upon by others. Even pain in the body is indecisive, moving about and going to the part being pressed against or lain on. A Pulsatilla personality requires time alone when no other person's energy is invading their weakened personal space and can get very annoyed if they feel that someone is pushing them into something against their will. Being hugged (energy fed into the weakened central meridian) improves all symptoms.

SEPIA SUCCUS (cuttlefish ink) Sepia is a remedy for those, usually women, who are mentally and physically worn out. There are weak veins, fluctuating hormones, a weak bladder, poor circulation, ***sagging tissues and organ***s, vision difficulties, and oversensitive to noise. The woman often feels as though the responsibilities of family life and the things required of her as a wife and mother are toomuch to bear.

THUJA OCCIDENTALIS (arbor vitae) This remedy is a great polycrest for coping with the damage done to the nervous system by vaccinations and other toxic chemicals. The list of symptoms under "mind" in the materia medicas is the longest, and most depressing to read, of any remedy that I know of. A few of the mental/emotional symptoms include dullness of mind, uses wrong words or omits words and syllables, depression with a feeling of being isolated and alone, self-contempt, mistrustful and fearful of strangers.

Incidentally, Thuja is a remedy for polyps and warts.

GALLBLADDER MERIDIAN BALANCE (6X)

Feeling of love, adoration and compassion for other people—or—Deep rage, more intense and longer lasting than mere anger

The gallbladder is the only yang organ in the body that is a storage receptacle and that influences both the emotional and physical aspects of the unhealthy patterns associated with it.

ARSENICUM ALBUM (white oxide of arsenic) Arsenicum is a very deep acting remedy that affects every organ and body system, with a special emphasis on the liver and the gallbladder. The compassion for other people that is key to this meridian often becomes anguish and anxiety about everything and everybody. The anger at the unfairness of the world and at "man's inhumanity to man" may manifest as being intensely domineering and demanding, seeking to control the environment and people around him so as not to have anything to trigger his anger.

BELLADONNA (deadly nightshade) The intensity of this meridian is seen in the suddenness of the onset and the violence of all symptoms and ailments to which people needed Belladona are prone. There are a lot of symptoms having to do with the glands and the lymphatic system.

CALCAREA CARBONICA (calcium carbonate) Calcarea carb is foremost among the calcarea remedies and is one of 3 remedies that are considered the standard around which all anti-psoric remedies are grouped. Symptoms include a specific listing for use with gallstones and many descriptions of digestive difficulties and improper absorption of nutrients. There is a whole list glandular issues other than the gallbladder, and many symptoms related to the heart and kidneys.

CARDUUS MARIANUS (St. Mary's thistle) The action of this remedy is centered on the liver, the gallbladder and the ducts of those systems. General symptoms in these areas include the gallbladder being swollen and painful, gallstones, liver and spleen disorders including cirrhosis, hepatitis and liver related headaches, and a characteristic bitter taste in the back of the mouth.

COLOCYNTHIS (bitter cucumber) Colocynth was used as a purgative in allopathic practice and is useful homeopathically in acute disorders of the digestive and intestinal tract. The pains found in various locations in the body are described as radiating, agonizing, cutting, tearing, sudden, and atrocious, to name just a few descriptions. There is sudden horrible cramping with tearing pains. There are also a great many types of neuralgia with chilliness and the person is greatly affected by the misfortunes of others, as is typical with gallbladder meridian issues.

LYCOPODIUM CLACATUM (club moss) Lycopodium is the third member of the triumvirate of remedies that are used together for so many ailments common to all of mankind (the psora miasm displaying itself). A few of these symptoms include bloated abdomen, food allergies, diabetes, hypoglycemia, hernias, stiffness and weakness in the joints, aneurysms, hair loss, and great weakness of the digestive system. As you can see from the physical symptoms, this is truly a much needed remedy by most people (the definition of a polycrest) remedy.

Mental/emotional symptoms include weak memory, dyslexia, indecisiveness, poor self-esteem, and panic attacks. There is a strong desire for sweets but sweet make all symptoms worse.

NATRUM SULPHURICUM (sodium sulphate) As always, this remedy is particularly indicated after head injury. Nat sulph captures excess fluid in cells and guarantees its elimination from the body. Pain through lower left chest. Gallbladder and digestive disorders are clearly a part of this picture but are not keynote to it. All symptoms are worse for any type of cold and damp.

NUX VOMICA (poison nut) The keynote of Nux is the fiery temperament which cannot bear noises, odors, light, or music. There are many abdominal and stomach symptoms listed, gallbladder problems being among them, although Nux is very much a remedy for nerves.

PHOSPHORUS (the element) The Phosphorus personality is oversensitive to outside opinions and environmental signals. Phosphorus, alone or in other natural mineral combinations always indicates a certain level of prostration and nervousness. The stomach symptoms are described as and "empty and all gone" feeling. There is ravenous hunger during a fever with cravings for cold food and drink. The cold drink makes the person feel better for a moment but it is vomited as soon as it becomes warn in the stomach.

SEPIA SUCCUS (cuttlefish ink) The materia medicas do not mention the gallbladder in connection with this remedy but there are many symptoms associated with weak digestion and the liver is sore and painful. Sepia is a remedy for those who are mentally and physically worn out from either real or perceived overwork and stress. There are disorders of the venous system, prolapsing of organs, and many issues having to do with hormones.

LIVER MERIDIAN BALANCE (6X)

Happy and cheerful, full of joy—or—Feelings of anger and annoyance all the time toward everyone and everything

ARSENICUM ALBUM (white oxide of arsenic) As expressed previously with the gallbladder meridian, Arsenicum is a very deep acting remedy that affects every organ and body system, with a special emphasis on the liver and the gallbladder. The compassion for other people that is key to this meridian often becomes anguish and anxiety about everything and everybody. The anger may manifest as being intensely domineering and demanding, seeking to control the environment and people around him so as not to have anything to trigger his anger. Arsenicum is a polycrest remedy for absolutely everything having to do with digestive issues. It includes flu, food poisoning, bacterial infections and everything in between and along the way.

BERBERIS VULGARIS (barberry) Berberis is often useful in arthritic, hepatic (liver) disorders, and gallbladder disorders but its most important range of action is with the kidneys and upon the many and varied symptoms that arise when the kidneys are not functioning properly.

BRYONIA ALBA (wild hops) A true polycrest remedy in that it works on disorders of the blood. Symptoms will show up everywhere as a result. There are symptoms in nearly every part of the body that this remedy is listed for including, unexpectedly to my mind, slipped disks in the back with sharp pain, pleurisy with sharp pains, and dryness of mouth, tongue and throat with excessive thirst.

CARDUUS MARIANUS (St. Mary's thistle) The action of this remedy is centered on the liver, the gallbladder, and the various ducts of those systems with terrible attacks of gallstone colic, gallstones and many liver disorders. Headache shortly before meals which disappears after eating may indicate further glandular issues involving the pancreas. The digestive disorders which are associated with Carduus are accompanied by lung issues. A keynote symptom is never the same since mononucleosis or hepatitis.

CINCHONA OFFICINALIS/ CHINA OFFICINALIS (Peruvian bark) China bark was the first remedy that Hahnemann proved and even way back then it was considered a treatment for hepatitis and other liver disorders. China bark is also considered a treatment for parasites and for dysentery and diarrhea with dehydration and weakness. An enlarged and swollen liver is one of the early signs of disruption in this meridian with further trouble on the way.

KALI CARBONICUM (potassium carbonate) While there are liver issues and jaundice included in the symptom picture of Kali carb, they are by no means heavy keynotes of this remedy. The potassium salts (the Kali group) have an affinity for both solid tissues and blood corpuscles.

LYCOPODIUM CLAVATUM (club moss) Lycopodium is the third member of the triumvirate of remedies that are used together for so many ailments common to all of mankind (the psora miasm displaying itself). One thing that is common to mankind is fears of one thing and another. The kidney/bladder meridian is about fear—and about symptoms that are driven by fear. A few of the symptoms associated with this remedy include bloated abdomen, food allergies, diabetes, hypoglycemia, hernias, stiffness and weakness in the joints, aneurysms, hair loss, and great weakness of the digestive system. As you can see from the physical symptoms, this is truly a much needed by most people (the definition of a poylcrest) remedy.

NUX VOMICA (poison nut) The keynote of Nux is the fiery temperament which cannot bear noises, odors, light, or music. There are many abdominal and stomach symptoms listed, liver and gallbladder problems being among them, although Nux is very much a remedy for nerves. Even liver things as deep as hepatitis are mentioned in the decades-old literature.

KIDNEY MERIDIAN BALANCE (6X)

Full of faith and trust in the future—or—Full of fear, lack of self- confidence

APIS MELLIFICA (honey bee) The kidney symptoms of Apis include acute kidney infection, sore or bruised feeling over region of kidneys, burning when urinating, frequent and involuntary urine, difficult or slow urine, swelling or puffing up of various parts, edema, allergic dermatitis, burning and soreness when urinating, and dragging pain in lumbar region.

BERBERIS VULGARIS (barberry) Berberis is often useful in arthritic, hepatic (liver) disorders, and gallbladder disorders but its most important range of action is with the kidneys and bladder and upon the many and varied symptoms that arise when the kidneys are not functioning properly. Pimples with dry rough scaly skin.

CANTHARIS VESICATORIA (Spanish fly) The action of this remedy has to do with inflammations and swelling that burn and are violently acute. There is an almost constant urging to urinate, acute severe cystitis, and occasions when the urine is passed drop by drop, dribbling. There may be difficulty swallowing liquids.

EQUISETUM HYEMALE (horsetail) A keynote among remedies for anything to do with the bladder and the kidneys. Symptoms include nocturnal bed-wetting of children, a constant desire to urinate, the passage of large quantities of clear or light-colored urine without relief, severe pain at the close of urination. The person for whom this remedy is indicated is inclined to show a frown—the corners of the mouth at 4 and 8 on the clockface, when facial muscles are at rest.

LYCOPODIUM CLAVATUM (club moss) Lycopodium is the third member of the triumvirate of remedies that are used together for so many ailments common to all of mankind (the psora miasm displaying itself). One thing that is common to mankind is fears of one thing and another. The kidney/bladder meridian is about fear—and about symptoms that are driven by fear. A few of the symptoms associated with this remedy include bloated abdomen, food allergies, diabetes, hypoglycemia, hernias, stiffness and weakness in the joints, aneurysms, hair loss, and great weakness of the digestive system. As you can see from the physical symptoms, this is truly a much needed by most people (the definition of a polycrest remedy).

NATRUM MURIATICUM (sodium chloride) This remedy affects the emotions, heart, kidney and spleen and is suited to patients that are very thirsty all the time. A keynote of this remedy is difficulty urinating in the presence of others and pain just after urinating.

PHOSPHORUS (the element) The phosphorus personality is oversensitive to outside opinions and environmental signals. Phosphorus, alone or in other natural mineral combinations, always indicates a certain level of prostration and nervousness. The bladder is full without any urging and there may be blood in the urine.

RHUS TOXICODENDRON (poison oak) Rhus tox is generally thought of as a skin and muscle remedy. The only indications in the symptom picture that this remedy might be useful for the kidneys. These symptoms include extreme apprehension—especially at night, low back pain with the pain and stiffness being better for motion, and stiffness of muscles and joints that may be connected to uric acid crystals lying under the muscles. This type of pain is better for warmth, motion, or massage. Incontinences is also listed.

SEPIA SUCCUS (cuttlesfish ink) Sepia is a remedy for those who are mentally and physically worn out from either real or perceived overwork and stress. There are disorders of the venous system, prolapsing of organs, and many issues having to do with hormones, vein issues, and weakened or overstressed kidneys. There may be frequent urination, urine that is milky in color, and bed-wetting.

URINARY BLADDER MERIDIAN BALANCE (6X)

In tune with Spirit, authoritative, sure—or—Lack of self-confidence, impressionable, meek and compliant

ARGENTUM NITRICUM (silver nitrate) Keynotes are a great desire for sweets even though sweets aggravate, irritating the kidneys and resulting in the sugar in the urine that indicates hypoglycemia. There are a lot of fears—performance anxiety and apprehension of many types. The person wants to do things in a hurry, perhaps to get it over with. Emotional upsets bring on migraines or diarrhea.

BERBERIS VULGARIS (barberry) Berberis is often useful in arthritic, hepatic (liver) disorders, and gallbladder disorders but its most important range of action is with the kidneys and bladder and upon the many and varied symptoms that arise when the kidneys are not functioning properly. Symptoms included inflammation of the kidneys and bladder disorders including the strange symptom of pain in the thighs while urinating.

CANTHARIS VESICATORIA (Spanish fly) Cantharis is keynoted by inflammatory conditions that are violently acute and is useful for any condition in which the urine is scanty. There is a severe cystitis with a constant urging to urinate but urine is passed drop by drop, dribbling.

KALI BICHROMICUM (potassium bichromate) There is a small list of kidney symptoms listed but they are quite general and not keynotes. Care should be taken to insure that the keynote symptoms of this remedy also match along with the kidney symptoms. Among these keynote symptoms are pains that migrate from place to place, sinus headaches centered over the eyebrows, and very weak limbs. Emotionally, there is sadness which is better after eating.

MERCURIUS SOLUBLIS (mercury vivus) Mercurius is a very changeable remedy and the person is affected for the worse by any change in temperature or weather and by nearly everything else. Kidney/bladder complaints include greenish discharge from urethra, burning sensations both before and after urination, frequent urging to urinate both night and day, and urine flows in thin stream or only drop by drop.

RHUS TOXICODENDRON (poison oak) Rhus tox is generally thought of as a skin and muscle remedy. The only indications that I can find that this might be useful for the kidney and bladder is the presence of extreme apprehension—especially at night, low back pain with the pain and stiffness being better for motion, and stiffness of muscles and joints that may be connected to uric acid crystals lying under the muscles. Other symptoms relating to the urinary tract include incontinence, restless tossing ab out in sleep, and intense itching of the skin.

TEREBINTHINIAE OLEUM (oil of turpentine) Burning and drawing pain in region of the kidneys and running along the ureters, cystitis, irritable bladder and kidneys, bleeding from the bladder, scanty suppressed urine with the odor of violets, and pains that alternate between navel and bladder that is better for walking, and stiff muscles. There will be feelings of lethargy, agitated sleep with frequent waking, and anxiety and confusion. These last three symptoms are related to uric acid deposits—mental symptoms set up by renal (urinary) failure Inflammation of kidneys.

THUJA OCCIDENTALIS (arbor vitae) The emotional keynote of feeling isolated and alone is very much a kidney/bladder symptom. Other such symptoms include bladder feels paralyzed, desire to urinate is sudden and uncontrollable, kidney issues with swollen feet, and involuntary urination when coughing. Mercurius has long been considered an effective remedy for never the same since vaccinations.

LARGE INTESTINE MERIDIAN BALANCE (6X)

Confidence, feeling of self-worth—or—Guilt, low self-esteem, discouragement

ALOE SOCOTRINA (common aloes) Emotional symptoms include being dissatisfied and angry about himself and sadness in the morning that is less intense in the. Some intestine related symptoms are the abdomen feels heavy and bloated with the bloating being more pronounced on the left side, abdominal pains are better from passing burning offensive flatus, colitis, and hemorrhoids that bleed often and profusely. This is also a remedy for prostate enlargement and kidney issues in elderly gentlemen.

ALUMINUM OXYDATA (aluminun oxide) The keynote of Aluminum oxydata is memory loss and dementia with confusion as to personal identity (as is indicated by the more than casual connection between aluminum poisoning and Alzheimer's) Symptoms having to do with the large intestine include severe constipation, abdominal pain that is mostly right-sided, colic whenever the body is exposed to a chill, and an interesting note of potatoes disagreeing with digestion.

ARSENICUM ALBUM (white oxide of arsenic) Arsenicum is a great polycrest remedy suitable to many people for many things including sudden very great weakness. The liver and spleen become enlarged and painful, there is coldness and chilliness in the abdomen, gastroenteritis, and violent pains in the abdomen with anguish, and vomiting with diarrhea.

BARYTA CARBONICA (barium carbonate) This is a remedy specific to the habitual colic of children who are not thriving. The child has an unusually large abdomen and is hungry but refuses food. There is always swollen tonsils and as they grown they seem to grasp things, mentally, more slowing than normal.

BRYONIA ALBA (wild hops) The mental picture of Bryonia is irritable and very difficult to please. The abdomen displays sharp burning pains that are worse from any touch or pressure and worse from coughing or even breathing.

CARBO VEGETABILIS (vegetable charcoal) This remedy is for sick and exhausted persons who have never fully recovered from some previous illness. The abdomen is greatly distended with pains extending into the chest. There is frequent flatulent colic and constipation with nearly all foods causing distress. The person is often icy cold.

PLUMBUM METALLICUM (lead metal) Emotional keynote is mental exhaustion and depression. The navel feels retracted and tense and the abdomen feels as if it is being drawn towards the back. There is mention of this remedy helping when a young child is unable to assimilate proteins and fats properly—to the point of dying of malnutrition. A keynote symptom is distinct blue lines along margins of gums.

PYROGENIUM (rotten meat pus) Intestinal symptoms of Pyrogenium include colitis, horribly offensive brown-black diarrhea, painless involuntary stools, diarrhea with fever, septic conditions, constipation, and pain in umbilical region with the passage of sticky yellow stool.

LUNG MERIDIAN BALANCE (6X)

Humility, tolerance, teachable—or—Pride, intolerance, already-knows-it-all attitude

APIS MELLIFICA (honey bee) This remedy is much like Vespa crabro and is an excellent remedy for bee stings and allergic reactions to bee stings. A keynote is stinging, burning pains that pierce deeply. Lung symptoms include breathing with panting, edema and swelling of larynx, feelings of suffocation, short dry breathing—the person feels as if they may not be able to draw another breath. Apis is a slow-acting remedy; it should not be given up on or discontinued too soon.

ARSENICUM ALBUM (white oxide of arsenic) Arsenicum is a great polycrest remedy suitable to many people for many things. Lung symptoms include constricted air passages, hay fever, wheezing, asthma, and pulmonary edema. Arsenicum is keynoted by sudden very great weakness.

CARBO VEGITABILIS (vegetable charcoal) Carbo vegetabilis is indicated for persons who have never fully recovered from some previous illness. Their breathing is laborious, quick, and short, with burning in the chest, cough with itching of larynx, spasmodic coughing with gagging and vomiting of mucus, and if things continue to worsen there will be hemorrhage from lungs.

CHAMOMILLA VULGARIS (German chamomile) Chamomilla is a remedy for temperamental and oversensitive persons and for peevish children who demand and seem to be better for being carried about all day. Chamomilla people demand and expect someone to provide instant relief from their suffering, large a small. Lung issues include asthma that was brought on by anger, spells of dry tickling cough, hoarseness, rattling of mucus in a child's chest, and cough that is much worse between 9 p.m. and midnight but does not wake the child (only the parents).

KALI BICHROMICUM (potassium bichromate) Kali bichromicum has an affinity for the mucus membranes if the air passages, the nose, and the pharnyx. The outstanding keynote is mucus that is thick, sticky, ropy, string, touch and yellow-green in color. This mucus sticks to the throat and can only be drawn out in strings. (This is a pretty good description of whooping cough!) Other lung symptoms include asthma, a dry and annoying cough, cough with pain in sternum that extends to the shoulders, and wheezing and panting on first waking up.

PHOSPHORUS (the element) The symptoms of Phosphorus that relate to the lungs include oppressive breathing, congestion of the lungs, pneumonia of left lower lung (in the space that is hard to clear where the lung conforms around the heart), asthma with congestion, sore throats that tend to drop into the lungs, and cough which makes the whole body tremble. Phosphorus is a remedy for the tired and weak who are overly sensitive the environment and to the opinions of people around them.

SULPHUR (brimstone) The sulphur personality is absent-minded and indifferent to personal appearance—"ragged philosophers". Lung symptoms include pneumonia, a loose cough, tickling in larynx, asthmatic conditions, difficult respiration of any kind, especially when the person insists they must have the window open if they are going to be able to breathe. A very strong keynote for this remedy, and any other anti-psoric remedy, is that all ailments and complaints seem to be getting better and then relapse or linger. Sulphur should be considered when a carefully chosen, well-matched homeopathic remedy fails to act, especially in acute diseases.

STOMACH MERIDIAN BALANCE (6X)

Contentment, appreciation for what is in one's life—or—Disappointment, greed, attitude of "there is never enough"

ARSENICUM ALBUM (white oxide of arsenic) Arsenicum is a leading polycrest—an absolutely amazing whole body remedy—useful for anything to do with the digestive and intestinal tracts and many other systems. A few (very few) keynote symptoms include burning pain in the stomach and abdomen, rumbling and cramping pains in the bowels, violent squeezing and constriction in umbilical region, diarrhea, and enlargement of the liver and the spleen Great deep-acting polycrest remedy for dealing with influenza, stomach flu, intestinal distress of any description, poisonings, and parasites.

The remedy picture also includes sudden great weakness and shortness of breath. Arsenicum is a restorative for all systems of the body (digestive, urinary, circulatory, lymphatic, and glandular) but has a particular affinity for the liver.

CALCAREA CARBONICA (calcium carbonate) This remedy is one of 3 remedies that are considered the standard around which all anti-psoric remedies are grouped. Symptoms related to the stomach meridian include digestive difficulties, with malnutrition from lack of or slow absorption of vitamins and minerals, glandular swellings, lack of appetite when tired or working too hard, ***cravings for eggs and for indigestible things,*** vomiting of bile, frequent sour belchings, sour vomiting, pain in the liver and gallbladder regions, and a tendency to form gallstones.

Unrelated to digestive issues (unless being caused by digestive malfunctions) are joint disorders, weak ankles, cramps in the legs at night, glandular troubles, and many heart and kidney issues.

DIGITALIS PURPUREA (foxglove) Although a well recognized heart remedy, the action of Digitalis is on the lungs and stomach as well as the heart. The liver becomes enlarged and painful, there is shortness of breath, neuralgic pain in stomach, excessive nausea that is not better for vomiting, and heartburn. Outstanding keynotes include great guilt, but feels better for crying because weeping improves nearly all symptoms, anxiety about the future, and great weakness with the illness. The person becomes so weak they can barely communicate.

IGNATIA AMARA (St. Ignatius bean) Ignatia symptoms are always tied to an emotional state of grief, loss, and worry. There will be hiccups, belching, a great deal of flatulence—especially at night, distension of the abdomen causing inability to breathe.

LYCOPODIUM CLAVATUM (club moss) With Lycopodium there is great general weakness of the digestive system. Even eating a very small amount of food creates feelings of fullness and triggers bloating and belching. Other symptoms include many food allergies with an allergy to wheat being common with the food allergies associated with this remedy are often the underlying cause of learning disabilities such as dyslexia. Hypoglycemia and diabetes are common but there is also a great craving for sweets.

PHOSPHORUS (the element) Phosphorus is a remedy for the tired and weak who are overly sensitive to the environment and to the opinions of people around them. There are many food cravings. Among them are cravings for cold drinks, ice cream, salt, acids, spicy foods, and the person desires chocolate and sweets to an almost uncontrollable level. Most of the things they crave further upset the digestive system bringing on pain and burning in stomach, nausea, vomiting, and very fetid stools and flatus from undigested food. A strange keynote is ravenous hunger during fever which, of course, upsets the digestion even further.

***PULSATILLA NIGRICANS* (windflower)** A remedy for persons of generally mild temperament but with very changeable moods. The Pulsatilla personality is emotional and often tearful with consolation improving all symptoms. There is abdominal colic from fruits, pastries, icy drinks, and fat or greasy things. There will be belchings after eating these foods and the taste of the foods remains a long time in the mouth and with the belching.

***VERATRUM VIRIDE* (American hellebore)** This remedy picture is of hiccups that are excessive and painful with spasms of the esophagus, burning in the stomach and esophagus, nausea and vomiting but sometimes there is vomiting that is violent but without any degree of nausea. A definite keynote is that the tongue is red with a deeper red streak down the center. Another keynote is the beating of the pulse being felt throughout the body.

SPLEEN MERIDIAN BALANCE (6X)

Confidence, faith in the future—or—Anxiety about the future, lack of faith and hope, feelings of grief and loss

***ARSENICUM ALBUM* (white oxide of arsenic)** Arsenicum is a great polycrest remedy with a keynote of sudden very great weakness. The liver and spleen become enlarged and painful and there is coldness and chilliness in the abdomen with great pain.

***CARDUUS MARIANUS* (St. Mary's thistle)** The action of this remedy is centered on the liver, the gallbladder, the spleen and the various ducts of those systems. Headache shortly before meals which disappears after eating may indicate further glandular issues involving the pancreas. The digestive disorders which are associated with Carduus are accompanied by lung issues. A keynote is never the same since mononucleosis or hepatitis.

***CEANOTHUS AMERICANUS* (red root)** Enlargement of the spleen with deep-seated cutting pains and feelings of fullness and sharp pains in the area of the spleen. There is headache on the right side with the spleen pain. The emotional keynote of this remedy, when the person is ill, is discouragement and fear that they will become unfit for work.

***CINCHONA/CHINA OFFICINALIS* (Peruvian bark)** One very clear mental keynote is that the is abundant ideas and clearness of mind late in the evening. Physically, the liver and spleen are swollen and enlarged, the digestion is weak and slow, there is belching of bitter fluid, regurgitation of fluids, there may be extreme diarrhea with dehydration and weakness and intolerable pain in the lumbar region.

***KALI BICHROMICUM* (potassium bichromate)** Kali bichromicum displays painful stitches in the region of both the liver and the spleen. The pains cut through to the spine and migrate from place to place, including the loins, but after wandering about they eventually settle in the stomach.

***LYCOPODIUM CLAVATUM* (club moss)** With Lycopodium there is great general weakness of the digestive system. Even eating a very small amount of food creates feelings of fullness and triggers bloating and belching. Other symptoms include many food allergies with an allergy to wheat being common. The food allergies are often the underlying cause of learning disabilities such as dyslexia.

***PHOSPHORUS* (the element)** Phosphorus is a remedy for the tired and weak who are overly-sensitive the environment and to the opinions of people around them. There is pain in the abdomen, not always over the spleen, pain and burning in the stomach, nausea, vomiting, and very fetid stools and flatus.

PLUMBUM METALLICUM (lead metal) The most outstanding mental symptom is mental exhaustion and depression brought on by physical labor. The navel feels retracted and tense and the abdominal wall feels as if it is drawn toward the spine by a string. Hernias are common.

RANUNCULUS BULBOSUS (buttercup) The abdomen is tender to pressure, particularly over the spleen area. There is a keynote spleen symptom of muscular pain along the lower margin of the shoulder.

TRIPLE WARMER MERIDIAN BALANCE (6X)

Protection of the physical body, lightness, hope—or—Auto-immune disorders, allergies, heaviness, and depression

The triple warmer meridian is closely associated with the immune system and protects the entire body from external threats. Triple warmer gauges everything from the temperature of the room to the safety of the building we are entering or standing in and tells us if the emotional environment is safe. This meridian is responsible for the distribution of water in the cells and tissues. Triple warmer governs those feelings or inspirations that we receive that we do not mentally understand the source of.

BARYTA CARBONICA (barium carbonate) Baryta carb is a remedy that is especially indicated for infants and old age with a particular emphasis on the glandular system and auto-immune disorders. Kidney symptoms include frequent urination with the frequency increasing even more during the night. This remedy is sometimes called for in Down syndrome and delayed developmental issues of children.

CALCAREA CARBONICA (calcium carbonate) The triple warmer meridian is a necessary part of the protective apparatus of the body. Calcarea carb is one of the three polycrest anti-psoric—and therefore, triple warmer meridian remedies—that are useful to many people for many things. The psora miasm is basic to the human condition and is especially noted for chronic ailments, auto-immune disorders and any condition which seems to be getting better but then either relapses or just hangs on and on.

IODUM PURUM (iodine) Iodum purum acts prominently on the connective tissue where the energy of the meridians run. Since the connective tissue covers every organ of the body and runs through every muscle and connects muscle to bone, inflammation in the connective tissue can create a wide variety of symptoms. If the triple warmer meridian is low and there is no energetic defense for the body, the immune system compromise can be very deep.

KALI IODATUM (potassium iodide) Kali iodatum is a deeper acting remedy and is for the more desperate syphilitic miasm rather than the milder psoric miasm. All Kali-based remedies have to do with despondency with the trivial details of life being altogether too much to cope with.

Kali iodatum has a regulating influence over the functions of the organs that have to do with nutrition, growth, and development. It works on neuralgia and inflamed nerves, and has many symptoms having to do with water balance in the cells and in the tissues. Symptoms of Kali iodatum include enlarged lymph glands, liver dysfunction, arthritis, arteriosclerosis, headaches with intense pain over the eyes and at the root of the nose, tinnitus in the ears, and the skin will develop boils rather than the rashes of the psora miasm. There may be sciatica, frequent urination, nocturnal bed-wetting, pneumonia and pleural effusions being common.

LACHESIS MUTA (bushmaster snake) More than most snake remedies, Lachesis shows the great weakness and prostration of nerve disorders. There is also the telltale erratic aspects of a weakened triple warmer meridian that is illustrated by the pains of arthritis alternating sides of the body very rapidly and wandering all about. The mind and conversational topics jump from place to place with great rapidity and are most often a bit (more than a bit) sarcastic. Nervous and liver headaches are common with the liver and digestive regions being so sensitive that the person can't bear anything around the waist. This is an excellent remedy for malignant or septic states with the urine being very dark and foamy with a strong odor.

PHOSPHORICUM ACIDUM (phosphoric acid) Phosphoricum acidum is specific for conditions incident to a weakened immune system brought on by an acute illness, loss of vital fluids, or by grief and loss. Symptoms include weakness, debility, exhaustion, emaciation, fatigue of a chronic and continual nature, hair loss, heart palpitations, mental debility followed by physical debility, wants nothing and likes nothing, sleepy during day with the weakness being a little bit better for a short nap.

SEPIA SUCCUS (cuttlefish ink) Sepia is a remedy for those, usually women, who are mentally and physically worn out. There are weak veins, fluctuating hormones, a weak bladder, poor circulation, ***sagging tissues and organs***, vision difficulties, and over sensitivity to noise as the weakened triple warmer meridian fails to protect the person from stimulus and the nervous system goes into hyper drive.

SPONGIA TOSTA (roasted sponge) According to Hahnemann, spongia tosta was first mentioned as a specific for thyroid issues (goiter) by the alchemist Arnold Von Vollanova in the thirteenth century. The benefits of spongia have been attributed to the iodine contained in it and partially liberated by roasting.

The triple warmer meridian protects the physical body and is paired with the pericardium meridian whose task it is to protect the heart. There are a lot of heart symptoms in the remedy picture of Spongia tosta. Whenever the heart is compromised, there will eventually be problems in the pulmonary system (cardio-pulmonary symptoms) Some of these symptoms include asthma, bronchitis, dryness of mucus membranes, and a dry, chronic, sympathetic cough. Exhaustion and heaviness of the body with anxiety and difficult breathing are present.

THYROIDINUM (thyroid gland extract) This remedy is a sarcode made from thyroid tissue. It is meant to be used whenever the thyroid is struggling, being either low or high. A symptom that is sometimes overlooked is vomiting during pregnancy that is the result of thyroid problems. Anemia is often the result of thyroid dysfunction.

PERICARDIUM MERIDIAN BALANCE (6X)

Protector of heart and emotions, openness and peacefulness in relationships—or— Manic depressive tendencies, withdrawal and anger at perceived hurts

Because the heart, energetically, must be open and able to feel both joy and sorrow, the body has provided a strong defense and alarm system for it. In far eastern philosophy, this is referred to as the pericardium meridian. There are several other names but I prefer pericardium because the physical pericardium is the sac that surrounds and protects the heart and I like the connection between the physical and the energetic that the name implies. The job of the pericardium meridian is to protect the heart from unexpected hurt and from emotional violation. An important part of the function of this meridian is to provide us by providing an evaluation about the trustworthiness of the people around us.

ARSENICUM ALBUM (white oxide of arsenic) Arsenicum is a leading polycrest—absolutely amazing restorative for all systems of the body (digestive, urinary, circulatory, lymphatic, and glandular). A few (very few) keynote symptoms related to the heart include angina, shortness of breath, palpitations when lying on the back and becoming worse at night, heartbeats that are audible in the ears, valvular disease with intermittent pulse, and pulse more rapid in the morning. A keynote is very great weakness.

Emotional/mental patterns include extremely nervous and anxious, restlessness, weeps and whines but speaks very little, wants to be comforted and coddled, anxiety about health, and upset by any disorder.

AURUM METALLICUM (gold metal) This is a remedy that is indicated for acute mental depression—the kind of hopelessness that can lead to suicide! Aurum depression is the deepest and the most acute depression of any remedy. If it tests up for a person I am always VERY concerned. The person simply sees no way out of the pain except death. One person described it this way, "I would have killed myself if I believed that death would mean complete annihilation, but I believe that the soul goes on so death wouldn't have helped, really."

CALCAREA CARBONICA (calcium carbonate) Calcarea carb is one of the three polycrest remedies that are useful to many people for many things. It is a basic anti-psoric and very helpful for blocks in this meridian. Symptomns include food cravings, gallstones, colic, heartburn, pains in liver region, belching, cramps and increased susceptibility to cold.

GLONOINUM (nitroglycerine) This remedy is used in allopathic medicine for heart issues and as a homeopathic remedy for such things as sudden vascular congestion with violent pulsations of the carotids, throbbing bursting headache, high blood pressure, and threatened stroke. Any exertion brings a rush of blood to the heart and fainting spells. Mental symptoms include confusion with dizziness, fear from the sensation of swelling in the throat, fear of imminent death, and feelings of aversion and dislike towards her own husband and children. This last symptom is frightening to me because it would be the result—the side effect—of taking nitroglycerine, as is done in allopathic medicine, for a heart condition.

LITHIUM CARBONICUM (lithium carbonate) The mental patterns of this remedy includes manic depression and obsessive compulsive disorders. The heart symptoms include the odd keynote of eye symptoms showing up with the trembling of the heart, fluttering of the heart, constriction of the chest, and heart pain. The heart pain is worse from bending over. The entire body feels sore and heavy.

LOBELIA INFLATA (Indian tobacco) Interestingly (and exactly what you would expect in the homeopathic world), an overdose of this herb brings on chills—which is one of the outstanding symptoms of Lobelia as a homeopathic remedy. These chills, along with the accompanying slowing of the heart rhythm, have given this herb an undeserved bad reputation. I say undeserved because the action is exactly what the body needs, either to heal or to alert you that it is time to let the body make use of what you have already provided and allow it to move forward with healing.

MERCURIUS SOLUBILIS (mercury vivus) Mercurius is a very changeable remedy. Persona needing this remedy are affected for the worse by any change in temperature or weather and by nearly everything else! The keynote of this remedy is the changeableness of the symptoms, mental and physical—in other words, stress, confusion, and the interruption of energy flow. Mercurius has long been considered an effective remedy for never the same since vaccinations symptoms and situations.

NAJA TRIPUDIANS (cobra venom) Unlike most snake remedies, Naja is not a remedy for hemorrhages or septic conditions. Its primary focus is on the circulation, the heart, and the edema in tissues resulting from cardiac insufficiency. Useful for valvular disorder, heart lesion, heart damage after infectious diseases, low blood pressure, chronic nervous palpitations that prevent speaking, heart symptoms with pain in the forehead, and vertigo followed by astounding pain in right side of head. The person who would be benefited by Naja feels great anguish for any pain that others are experiencing.

PHOSPHORUS (the element) Phosphorus is a remedy for the tired and weak who are overly sensitive tto the environment and to the opinions of people around them. The heart protector is simply not protecting them or discerning between what is *themselves* and *their own decisions* and what in the environment is *harmful* and what *is in their best interest.* Interestingly, phosphorus people are often a bit clairvoyant and have a closer connection to the "other side" than is usual.

SMALL INTESTINE MERIDIAN BALANCE (6X)

Great joy, intense happiness—or—Sorrow, melancholy, depression

ARSENICUM ALBUM (white oxide of arsenic) Arsenicum, as has been stressed before in this book, is a leading polycrest and an absolutely amazing restorative for all systems of the body (digestive, urinary, circulatory, lymphatic, and glandular). A few (very few) keynote symptoms include burning pain in the stomach and abdomen, rumbling and cramping pains in the bowels, violent squeezing and constriction in umbilical region, diarrhea, and enlargement of the liver and the spleen. This is a great deep-acting polycrest remedy for dealing with influenza, stomach flu, intestinal distress of any description, poisoning, and parasites. The remedy picture also includes sudden great weakness and shortness of breath.

BELLADONNA (deadly nightshade) Everything about Belladonna is extreme and throbbing. The person is kept awake by pulsation of blood vessels—throbbing in carotid and temporal arteries. Symptoms include the abdomen being swollen and extremely sensitive to touch with cramps and colic. The symptoms come on quickly and go away just as quickly. The delusions of the mind are many and very acute and intense with Belladonna.

CINCHONA/CHINA OFFICINALIS (Peruvian bark) This is a polycrest remedy with many pages of symptoms in the materia medicas. The symptoms that apply to this remedy are gas and bloating of the abdomen, indigestion, severe diarrhea, intestinal candida overgrowth, gallstone colic, hot face with cold hands and body. Cinchona is considered a treatment for parasites and for dysentery and diarrheas with dehydration and weakness.

KALI CARBONICUM (potassium carbonate) The Kali carb emotional picture is full of fears and imaginations with hypersensitivity to pain and an obstinate and dogmatic temperament. Symptoms include throbbing at the navel, cutting pain in the intestines as if they are being torn, and liver troubles that include jaundice.

LYCOPODIUM CLAVATUM (club moss) This is a very important remedy. Murphy lists it with Sulphur and Calcarea carbonica as one of three remedy categories into which the entire materia medica can be classified. Malnutrition due to weakness of the digestion and lack of absorption of minerals from the small intestine are the primary keynotes. Nearly every symptom of this remedy flows from this lack of nutrition. Lycopodium is keynoted by hypoglycemia, diabetes, food allergies and a desire for sweets.

NUX VOMICA (poison nut) A remedy for intense, driven people who cannot bear noises, odors, light, or touch and who are easily offended by the careless words of others. Keynote digestive symptoms include cravings for stimulants, but worse for them, feeling of weight and pain in the stomach, there is a constant sour taste in the mouth, nausea and vomiting in the morning, and the ***stomach and abdomen are very sensitive to pressure and to touch.***

PHOSPHORUS (the element) Phosphorus is a remedy for the tired and weak who are overly sensitive the environment and to the opinions of people around them. Diarrhea can become so severe that it brings the person to a state of absolute exhaustion. A chronic pattern of first constipation and then diarrhea is also seen in the phosphorus picture.

PYROGENIUM (rotten meat pus) Pyrogen is the great remedy for septic states when the blood has become involved and is carrying contagion throughout the body. Bodily discharges have an offensive carrion-like odor. There will be severe diarrhea, with fever, as the body attempts to cope. The abdomen may become so bloated as to make breathing difficult. Because of the septic condition of the intestinal tract and the blood, even small cuts or injuries become infected and inflamed.

HEART MERIDIAN BALANCE (6X)

Love, forgiveness, compassion—or—Anger, judgement

AURUM METALLICUM (gold metal) This is a remedy that is indicated for acute mental depression—the kind of hopelessness that can lead to suicide! Aurum depression is the most acute depression of any remedy and if it tests up for a person I am always VERY concerned. The person simply sees no way out of the pain except for death. The person will be oversensitive to pain and to noise.

Mental symptoms become worse during cloudy weather, in winter, and worse from sunset to sunrise. Physical symptoms include high blood pressure, rapid pulse, carotids and the temporal arteries throb visibly, valvular lesions of arteriosclerosis, irregular heartbeat with the sensation that the heart has stopped beating, and angina pectoris.

CACTUS GRANDIFLORUS (night-bloooming cereus) Desire to be alone, sadness and melancholy, fears that something bad is about to happen, and an irresistible inclination to weep are some of the emotional symptoms of this remedy. The heart feels as though it is being clutched and released alternately by an iron band. There are palpitations that are worse when lying on the left side, aneurysms in the large arteries and in the heart, low blood pressure, mitral valve insufficiency with violent and rapid heart action to compensate for the valvular insufficiency.

DIGITALIS PURPUREA (foxglove) There is sudden constant pain in region of the heart, the pulse is weak and very slow, but becomes rapid with the slightest movement, there is shortness of breath and the sudden sensation that the heart is standing still. This remedy should usually be given while seeking immediate medical assistance unless the response is very immediate and very effective.

Digitalis is specific for non-closure of foramen ovale at birth. This is one of the shunts that is designed to close at birth as the baby's circulatory system moves from appropriate to in the womb to appropriate for the world in which he will be breathing air and on his own, separate from the mother. The only other solution for this problem is surgery. Certainly, the homeopathic would be worth a try before subjecting the baby to the trauma of surgery but the results of the remedy would have to be immediate. Now, isn't that the kind of results for which homeopathy is famous?

LITHIUM CARBONICUM (lithium carbonate) The mental patterns of this remedy include manic depression and obsessive compulsive disorders. The heart symptoms include the odd keynote of eye symptoms showing up with the trembling of the heart. There are flutterings of the heart muscle, constriction in the chest, and heart pain which is worse from bending over. The body feels sore and heavy.

MERCURIUS SOLUBILIS (mercury vivus) Mercurius is a very changeable remedy, mentally and physically, and the person needing Mercurius is affected for the worse by any change in temperature or weather and by nearly everything else. The keynotes of this remedy include feeling stressed, confused, and the energy flow in the body being interrupted. Poor self-confidence is a keynote of the emotional symptoms. Heart symptoms, while not heavy keynotes, include aching pain at the apex and the base of the heart, awakening with cardiac tremors, palpitations on slight exertion, shortness of breath when going up stairs, and pulse with violent beating in the arteries. Mercurius is often an effective remedy for never the same since vaccinations symptoms.

NAJA TRIPUDIANS (cobra venum) The predominant effect of snake remedies on the circulation and the heart is especially pronounced with this remedy. Symptoms include valvular disease, septic endocarditis, low blood pressure, sharp pains in the chest made worse by breathing deeply, and nervousness with excitement—so excited that they are trembling. The keynote emotional symptom is that the heart symptoms are tied to the anguish that they feel for the suffering of others.

PHOSPHORUS (the element) Phosphorus is a remedy for the tired and weak who are overly sensitive to the environment and to the opinions of people around them. The heart is literally damaged by the attempt to do everything the way everyone else wants them to. Symptoms include palpitations with anxiety while lying on the left side, breathing that is quickened and oppressed, feeling of tightness across the chest, pressure in the middle of the sternum and around the heart with the pain moving into the *right* arm and palpitation that come with numbness stiffness and coldness spreading down the *left* arm.

PULSATILLA NUTTALIANA (American pulsatilla) This remedy seems to be quite similar to Pulsatilla nigricans but is not nearly as well known. The only heart symptom listed in Murphy's Materia Medica is audible pulsation of the heart with the pulse accelerated.

MIASMS (9X)

Each miasm, and each remedy that matches it, has a long list of symptoms—too long to describe here. Please see Butterfly Miracles with Homeopathc Remedies, Book One for more detailed descriptions of miasms and miasmic theory. To my mind, understanding miasms is absolutely essential to the understanding of human nature and will help immensely with understanding and using homeopathic remedies. The descriptions below are *very* brief.

PSORINUM (Scabies nosode) Symptoms include allergies and hay fever, hopelessness that is not very deep or constant, debility, prominent unhealthy skin symptoms with itching, offensive discharges, headaches, hungry and feels unusually well just before becoming ill, and the keynote psora symptom of looking unkempt no matter how much effort is put into looking nicer.

MEDORRHINUM (Gonorrhea nosode) Medorrhinum is noted for a state of collapse and trembling, panic attacks, weakness of memory, manic depression, impulsive behavior and decision making, violent pain in the region of the kidneys, insomnia, and a sensation of a tight band across the forehead.

SYPHILINUM (Syphilis nosode) Syphilinum is of great benefit for crying infants who began crying shortly after birth and never seem to stop. There is nightly—from darkness until daylight—aggravation of all complaints with prostration and debility in the morning, sleeplessness and great restlessness at night. This is a deep and desperate remedy for deep and desperate situations, many of which center around relationship issues.

NATRUM MURIATICUM (sodium chloride) Symptoms, randomly chosen, include hay fever, dry mucus membranes, great weakness and weariness with coldness, severe depression and feelings of isolation, acute and chronic grief, holds grudges for years, photophobia, tears stream down face when coughing, fever blisters and cold sores, migraine headaches, and vertigo and vomiting during pregnancy. Consolation aggravates all symptoms with Nat mur.

VACCININUM (cowpox vaccine) The vaccinosis miasms includes all of those symptoms brought on by exposure to drugs and chemicals. A comprehensive list of those symptoms is not possible to create. A few of those symptoms include skin eruptions, strange growths, restlessness, irritability, impatience, nervousness, aching in the pit of the stomach with shortness of breath, convulsions, seizures, paralysis, ADHD and other learning disorders, and an inability to feel compassionate or connected to others.

TUBERCULINUM BOVINUM (tuberculosis nosode) This nosode and miasm have symptoms such as a tendency to catch colds easily, chronic enlargement of tonsils and glands, sensation of suffocation even when there is plenty of fresh air, dry hard hacking cough, mucus rattling in the throat with little or no expectoration. Emotionally, there is a deep feeling of being unfulfilled and a pressing need to move on or at least travel to some place different and new.

SULPHUR (Brimstone) The sulphur personality is absent-minded and indifferent to personal appearance—"a ragged philosopher" type. Sulphur is specific to complaints that seemed to be doing better and then relapse or just drag on and on. It is indicated when a carefully chosen remedy does not act as expected. A few keynote symptoms are dry and unhealthy skin and hair—every injury of the skin infects, pulse that is more rapid in the morning than in the evening, feels very weak and faint about 11 a. m. and must have something to eat immediate. The person sleeps in catnaps with the slightest noise awakening them.

THUJA OCCIDENTALIS (arbor vitae) A few keynote symptoms include polyps and warts, dullness of mind, depression, feels isolated but is averse to company, asthma in children, and chronic sinus infections. Thuja is considered a polycrest remedy for anything related to vaccine reactions or poisoning by drugs.

OLEANDER (rose laurel) Key symptoms of Oleander include weak memory, slow perception, sadness with lack of confidence, double vision, eruptions on scalp and behind ears, palpitations with weak, empty feeling in chest, involuntary urination, stiffness of joints, weakness of lower limbs, toothache when chewing, and very sensitive skin.

CICUTA VIROSA (water hemlock) This remedy is especially noted for convulsions after falls and concussions. The muscles become rigid and spastic, there are sudden violent shocks through the head, neck muscles become contorted, there is twitching of facial muscles, headache alternating with pain in the abdomen, and one-sided stupefying headache from a rush of blood to the head. Emotional symptoms include anxiety about the future, contemptuous, mistrustful, averse to company and especially shuns men. There is memory loss after an accident or injury with confusion of the present with the past. This remedy is listed as useful for cerebro-spinal meningitis.

MIGRAINE #1 (9X)

Useful for headaches with vision disturbances such as occur with migraines.

GLONOINUM (nitroglycerine) Used in both homeopathy and allopathic medicine for serious heart related issues, nitroglycerine has many circulatory symptoms, many of which play out in the head. There is sudden vascular congestion, violent pulsations, blood rushes to head and heart, congestive headaches, bursting sensations in the head, threatened strokes, high blood pressure, and complete collapse.

BELLADONNA (foxglove) Belladonna situations and symptoms manifest with sudden throbbing violence. Symptoms include congestive headaches with a red face, a throbbing hammering headache, severe neuralgic pain, throbbing in carotid and temporal arteries, pupils dilated with frequent and profuse urination.

GELSEMIUM SEMPERVIRENS (yellow jasmine) I consider Gelsemium to be a remedy with a strong affinity for the convalescent stage of illness and for "never the same since" an illness or an accident. A few symptoms of this remedy are nervous headaches from emotional excitement, pain in the temples that extends into the ear and nose and even to the chin, muscular weakness, dizziness, drowsiness and trembling, and excessive fatigue and weakness of all of the limbs with numbness.

NUX VOMICA (poison nut) The Nux vomica personality is very highly strung, fast-paced and competent. They are often very irritable—cannot handle noise or light, especially during a headache, and are angry and impatient when spoken to. They may be angry suddenly without provocation. Symptoms include migraines with vision disturbances, headaches brought on by sunlight, frontal headache with an urge to press the forehead against something, toxic headache from drugs or alcohol, headache from constipation, scalp sensitive to the slightest touch, and trigeminal neuralgia with numbness of the face.

IRIS VERSICOLOR (blue flag) The symptoms of Iris versicolor include migraines of gastric or liver origin. There is chronic pain in the forehead, frontal headache over the left eye with nausea, headache the alternates sides of the head, and ringing in the ears.

SANGUINARIA CANADENSIS (bloodroot) With Snguinaria, there are periodic sick headaches—pain begins in occiput and spreads upwards or spreads downwards centering over right eye. There is pain in the occiput like a flash of lightning, veins and temples are distended, and there is cough of gastric origin. This is a remedy where the symptoms are mostly on the right side of the body.

MIGRAINE #2 (9X)

BRYONIA ALBA (wild hops) The symptoms of Bryonia that apply to headaches include splitting headache that is worse from motion, bursting headache which feels like the brain is being forced out, the head feels as if hit by a hammer from within, pain over left eye, and frontal headache because of sinus congestion. Both mental exertion and motion aggravate the pain. The person just wants to be left alone.

CARBO VEGETABILIS (vegetable charcoal) Carbo veg is a remedy for a state of complete collapse with the body becoming blue and icy cold. Head symptoms include the head being hot with the limbs being very cold, dull compressive headaches, the head feels as if there is a heavy weight there, headaches from overindulgence in something, and cold sweat on the forehead indicating the onset of weakness and collapse.

GELSEMIUM SEMPERVIRENS (yellow jasmine) I consider Gelsemium to be a remedy with a strong affinity for the convalescent stage of illness and for "never the same since" an illness or an accident. A few symptoms of this remedy are nervous headaches from emotional excitement, pain in the temples that extends into the ear and nose and even to the chin, blurred vision with pain above the eye, muscular weakness, dizziness, drowsiness and trembling, and excessive fatigue and weakness of all of the limbs with numbness

NATRUM SULPHURICUM (sodium sulphate) A major action of this remedy is for head injuries and the serious headaches that follow them. When a person has sustained a head injury it is often dangerous to allow them to take pain medications, at least in sufficient quantity to handle the horrific pain. Nat sulph relieves much of the pain while helping stop any bleeding in the head and healing the nerves.

Nat sulpl also sets to work dealing with the mental effects of the injury to the brain. Some of this symptoms include depression, insomnia, confusion, irritability, suicidal impulses and, as the medica words it, "periodical attacks of mania." This is something we have experienced in our family and this remedy was amazing and a great blessing to us.

It should be noted that a person who is being benefitted by Nat sulp rarely commit suicide. They express a longing to commit suicide but also say that they are sure the family (or the business or the world in general) could not carry on without them. This is a very great comfort if you are the mother of the person with the head injury and you see how depressed and despairing of recovery they have become.

Headache symptoms include depression after head injuries, blindness after head injury, eyes sensitive to light, boring in right temple preceded by burning in stomach, and excessive salivation with headache.

PHOSPHORICUM ACIDUM (phosphoric acid) The symptoms of Phosphoricum acidum are often brought on by grief or shock. There is mental debility and emotional issues such as apathy and indifference followed by physical weakness. Headache symptoms include a feeling of a crushing weight on top of the head, pain as if temples were being crushed, and a dull headache from eyestrain.

MUSCULAR ACHES AND PAINS #1 (6X)

ARNICA MONTANA (leopard's bane) Arnica is the leading polycrest remedy for all things that have to do with trauma and all its effects—recent or long past. Of particular note is Arnica's effect on bruises, muscles that feel sore and bruised during illness or following overexertion, for pain in the teeth and gums following dental work (take before going to the dentist to avoid pain and soreness), hematoma from head injury, black eye from injury, and as a remedy for stroke victims.

Since the heart is also a muscle, Arnica can be of great value for strain of the heart muscle from violent running, any type of heart muscle weakness, and palpitations of the heart after an emotional shock or a physical injury. There is an unusual symptom of the pulse being quicker than the beat of the heart.

BRYONIA ALBA (wild hops) Many of the symptoms of Bryonia alba that are concerned with muscles have to do with back injuries. These symptoms include severe and painful muscles from back injuries, slipped discs with sharp pains, sharp pains and stiffness in lumbar region, vertebrae out of place causing much pain and immobility,and painful stiffness of neck. All symptoms are worse from motion and better from lying on the painful side. (How strange is that!)

CIMICIFUGA RACEMOSA (black cohosh) Some muscular symptoms include pain across pelvis from hip to hip, displaced labor pains that are focused in hips, thighs or back, muscular cramping pains that are of nerve origin, stiffness and contraction in neck and back. Emotionally, Bryonia is keynoted by gloom and dejection, as if there were a black cloud over everything.

MAGNESIA PHOSPHORICA (magnesium phosphate) Magnesium is a necessary mineral for bones and muscles. Symptoms include cramping of muscles with radiating pain, and neuralgic pains that are relieved by warmth. There is oversensitivity to pain and great anxiety from the pain.

RHUS TOXICODENDRON (poison oak) Rhus tox is a remedy for all afflictions of the nerves and the spinal cord. This include stiffness of muscles and joints in cold damp seasons, stiffness which motion "limbers up," pain from straining or lifting, and stiffness felt particularly in the sacrum. Afflictions of nerves and spinal cord. Paralysis is listed under Rhus tox in the medicas.

RUTA GRAVEOLENS (garden rue) Ruta is excellent for injured joints and bruised bones. It is listed for injuries to tendons and for tendonitis. Tendons have a more limited blood supply than do muscles and are, as a result, much more difficult to heal. Other symptoms include backache from injury or strain, vertebrae slipping out of place easily, eyestrain with headaches, and bruised feeling of the entire body.

MUSCULAR ACHES AND PAINS #2 (6X)\

VALERIANA OFFICINALIS (Valerian) Valeriana is a relaxant and moderate stimulant depending on the amount used. It is a mild stimulant to the circulatory and nervous systems. Valerian acts as a nervine and anti-spasmodic to muscles and introduces quiet and calm to the brain. Symptoms include sciatic pain that is worse for standing and for sitting on hard surfaces. Pain in heels, cramping pains in calves that are worse when the legs are crossed. There is constant jerking of muscles and cramps in the hands and the feet.

PASSIFLORA INCARNATA (Passion flower) Although it has not been proven as a homeopathic, passion flower is a safe and well known herbal remedy. It is useful for nervousness and problems with the brain and central nervous system. Passiflora is sedative, mildly narcotic, anti-spasmodic, and is listed for insomnia and convulsions in children. The convulsions and spasms of Passiflora are centered mainly in the muscles of the trunk. Passiflora should be given *before* the convulsions come on, if possible.

MAGNESIA CARBONICA (Magnesium carbonica) This remedy is calming to the nerves that control the muscle groups. There is violent bruised pain in the back during the night and heavy, tired, painful legs and feet during the day.

MUSCLE WEAKNESS (6X)

ALUMINUM OXYDATA (aluminum oxide) Aluminum poisoning lodged in the cerebrospinal axis causes disturbances in coordination as well as weakness and partial paralysis of muscles. This remedy is a specific for these types of problems. There is either extreme dryness of mucus membranes or excess salivation with partial paralysis of involuntary muscles. Senility and dementia are also listed as symptoms oaf Aluminum and, therefore, as side effects of aluminum poisoning.

CAUSTICUM (caustic potash) One of the first and very important keynotes listed for Causticum is weakness with loss of muscular strength. There is localized paralysis of muscles and even paralysis of some organs that are muscular in nature.

GELSEMIUM SEMPERVIRENS (yellow jasmine) Gelsemium is a remedy specific to paralysis of any kind in muscles. Symptoms include muscular weakness and trembling in the limbs, lack of muscular coordination, heaviness in the body as though the muscles cannot keep the body upright, and weakness and soreness of muscles. There is also a lot of symptoms having to do with nerve issues and damage as it affects muscles.

NUX VOMICA (Poison nut) This remedy is for irritable people with hypersensitive nervous systems which make them and overly impressionable emotionally. The nerve problems also produce cramps and spasms of muscles, contractions and tenseness in muscles, muscular weakness from over stimulation with sudden loss of muscle strength in arms and legs early in the morning, bruised pains in t he muscles, sudden sharp pains in the back when turning, and dull pain when sitting.

SILICA TERRA (pure flint) Some symptoms related to muscle issues include legs feeling paralyzed, trembling while walking, loss of power in legs, calves tense and contracted, and curvature of the spine.

ZINCUM METALLICUM (Zinc metal) Some symptoms related to muscle issues include the spine being very sensitive—cannot bear having it touched, general weakness, trembling and twitching of various muscles, nape of the neck feels weary and tired, pain the cervical muscles at night, stumbling, a spastic gait, and totters while walking.

NERVE #1 (9X)

CHAMOMILLA VULGARIS (German chamomile) Chamomilla is particularly suited to irritable, sensitive, discontented, whining children and their adult counterparts. I would have to list Chamomile has a very mild, but extremely important, polycrest for any hypersensitivity of the nervous system. A keynote is that the person lives in the past, dwelling on past irritations and slights by other people.

CUPRUM SULPHURICUM (copper sulfate) While Cuprum metallicum is a well-studied remedy, little is known about Cuprum sulphuricum. There are indications of nervousness, restlessness, irritability. and headache with shooting, nerve-type pain. The pain is better after resting.

KALI TELLURICUM (potassium tellurate) There is very little known about this remedy and I have no idea why it was included here unless the sleepiness of the remedy was believed to be caused by nerves.

NATRUM SULPHURICUM (sodium sulphate) This is a remedy for head injuries and the congestion of the blood in the brain as well as the damage done to delicate nerves. Headache with drowsiness, such as is seen in concussion, is a keynote of this remedy.

RANUNCULUS SCELERATUS (marsh buttercup) Nerve pain most often manifests with throbbing or shooting pains. This remedy is for those times when the muscles are twitching or burning. A keynote that should be present if this remedy is to be useful is a great intolerance of and aversion to mental effort. There are also some back pain symptoms that could be nerve related.

SCUTELLARIA LATERIFOLIA (skullcap) Scutellaria is a noted nervine and nerve sedative. Symptoms include nervous fear of some calamity that is about to come, inability to stay focused on anything, restlessness, twitching muscles, chronic fatigue, nervous headache at the base of the brain where the cranial nerves exit the head, irritability of the heart's electrical system, and unrefreshing sleep with much tossing and turning. The nervous exhaustion of this remedy is often brought on by overwork and lack of rest. The two—overwork and lack of rest—become a vicious cycle with one feeding the other.

NERVE #2 (7X)

CHAMOMILLA VULGARIS (German chomomile) Chamomilla is particularly suited to irritable, sensitive, discontented, whining children and their adult counterparts. I would have to list Chamomile as a very mild, but extremely important, polycrest for any hypersensitivity of the nervous system. A keynote is that the person lives in the past, dwelling on past irritations and slights by other people.

CUPRUM SULPHURICUM (copper sulfate) While Cuprum metallicum is a well-studied remedy, little is known about Cuprum sulphuricum. There are indications of nervousness, restlessness, irritability. and headache with shooting, nerve-type pain with pains better after resting. Perhaps there is a proving of which I am unaware available somewhere.

HELIANTHUS ANNUUS (sunflower) Headache. Drowsiness. Helianthus is considered a spleen remedy but is used externally, much like Arnica montana and Calendula, for arthritic pains and internally for headache and drowsiness.

STERCULIA ACUMINATA (kola nut) "Kola nut regulates the circulation and the heart rhythm and gives power to endure prolonged physical exertion without taking food and without feeling fatigued." (Murphy's Materia Medica).

NATRUM SULPHURICUM (sodium sulphate) This is a remedy for head injuries and the congestion of the blood in the brain as well as the damage done to delicate nerves. Headache with drowsiness, such as is seen in concussion, is a keynote of this remedy. The nervous conditions of this remedy are made worse by mental exertion. There is a fear of crowds that did not exist before the injury and great sleepiness during the day.

NERVE#3 (8X)

HYOSCYAMUS NIGER (henbane) Hyoscyamus is a deep-acting remedy for brain and nervous system disorders of some desperation. The symptom picture includes such things as mania of a particularly obscene and quarrelsome nature, lack of modesty with the improper display of the body, extreme jealousy and suspicion, nervous agitation, twitching of tendons, tremulous weakness or muscles, and hallucinations and delusions.

MORBILLINUM (measles nosode) The remedy symptom picture includes nervous fretfulness in children, and irritable moodiness in adults with constant fault-finding.

VENUS MERCANARIA (American scallop) Venus mercanaria is above all a remedy for things going on in the head. Symptoms include mental confusion, boredom, and incoordination of the mind and the body (hands) when trying to write.

NEURALGIA (8X)

GALEGA OFFICINALIS (goat's rue) Galega is a remedy which has been used extensively for diabetes and increasing the milk supply in nursing women. It is also listed for anemia, debility, and backache. I can find no mention of it for nerves or neuralgic type pains.

PISCIDIA ERYTHRINA (Jamaica dog-wood) Piscidia acts as a nerve sedative and pain killer and is listed for insomnia, neuralgia, pains, and nervous spasms.

CROTON TIGLIUM (croton oil seeds) Croton is listed for neuralgias of several types including neuralgia of the tongue, peculiar feelings as if parts were being drawn such as a drawing pain through the left chest and into the back. Symptoms are better after sleep or after gentle rubbing. Croton is listed as a remedy for Rhus poisoning from exposure to poison oak and poison ivy and has similar symptoms to Rhus tox.

PROZAC (fluoxetine thydrochloride) The symptom picture of this remedy includes changes in sleep habits, increased fatigue, difficulty concentrating, slowed thinking, feelings of guilt or worthlessness, suicidal thoughts, lack of muscle coordination, nervousness, enlargement of the thyroid gland, weight gain or loss, fluid retention, dehydration, kidney disorders, diabetes, pelvic pain, premenstrual syndrome with anxiety and depression, anger, persistent mood swings, joint and muscle pain, obsessive-compulsive disorder, bulimia, chronic fatigue, headaches and migraines, too low or too high blood pressure, irregular heartbeat, heart attack, heart failure, gout, arthritis, bone pain, muscle spasms, leg cramps, impotence, bleeding gums, gingivitis, slurred speech, convulsions, decreased reflexes, insomnia, marked inability to fall asleep or stay asleep, inflammation of the stomach, stomach ulcers, nausea, vomiting of blood, difficulty in swallowing, muscle spasms and weakness, tissue inflammation just below skin, and colitis.

I have listed a great many—not all—of the symptom picture of Prozac (homeopathic) because I wanted to use it as a forum to remind us that all drugs have side effects! And Prozac has more than most!!

Homeopathy works on the "law of similars," If a substance produces certain symptoms in a well person, it will alleviate those same symptoms in a person showing those symptoms when prepared and potentized following the protocols of homeopathy. In other words, the reason the homeopathic Prozac works against these symptoms is because it creates these problems in well people!! (Just in case you don't have enough problems with the problems that you have, take a drug with the above listed side effects in an attempt to make your life better!

PAIN REMEDY #1 (10X)

LOBELIA INFLATA (Indian tobacco) Lobelis is a vasomotor stimulant and has action on the nervous systems producing a relaxed condition. Pain is focused in the sacrum and in the neck, indicating that the nerves of the spine are involved. The pain in the sacrum is so severe that it cannot tolerate any touch and sitting is nearly impossible. There is dull, heavy head pain and shooting pains throughout the body.

RANUNCULUS SCELERATUS (marsh buttercup) Ranunculus is a remedy which affects first the nerves and then the muscles, eyes, serous membranes, chest, skin, fingers and toes, and the left side of the body. The pains are gnawing and boring with an overall sore feeling.

THUJA OCCIDENTALIS (arbor vitae) Some of the pains of Thuja include pulsing back pain with a bruised sensation in back and pain in heels and the Achilles tendon.

VINCA MINOR (lesser periwinkle) The symptoms of Vinca minor include painful tension and stiffness of the cervical muscles with an illusive sensation as if a weight were lying on the muscles which creates tearing pain in vertex of the head.

PAIN REMEDY #2

ASAFOETIDA (Gum of the Stinkasand) This remedy is good for the pains of such things as bone diseases and bone decay, headaches, and spasmodic tightness of muscles. The pains change and are better by touch and much worse at night.

KALMIA LATIFOLIA (mountain laurel) With Kalmia, large parts of a limb or several limbs and the joints that connect them become swollen and painful such as with arthritis. There is pain along the ulnar nerve going into the third or fourth fingers, sharp pains in the heart that take the breath away, and neuralgias. The pains shoot downward creating numbness, and the pains shift about rapidly.

CAUSTICUM (caustic potash) The pain associated with Causticum includes contracted tendons, muscle pain, paralysis of individual parts, burning with rawness and soreness, weakness and loss of muscular strength that creates unsteady walking and easy falling, and pain in the spine.

FERRUM METALLICUM (iron metal) With Ferrum there is pain in the shoulders, the neck is sore and stiff, there is pain in the scapula, heel pain, and headache that is hammering, pulsating, and congestive. The arthritis that is extremely painful. Ferrum also has action on the blood and on the thyroid so the symptoms include great fatigue.

RHUS TOXICODENDRON (poison oak) Rhus is for the pains of dislocated joints, ankle injuries, arthritis, back injuries, bone pain, gout, and stiffness in the sacrum. The pains are tearing, shooting, stitching and worse for exposure to cold and wet.

LITHIUM BENZOICUM (lithium benzoate) A keynote of Lithium is deep-seated pains in the small of the back as the result of gallstones and kidney stones. Lithium is not just a pain reliever. It acts on the free hippuric acid of the urine.

SPIRAEA ULMARIA (meadowsweet) Dullness and heaviness in the head and heaviness in all limbs. There are convulsions and possible epilepsy. The convulsions are worse on the left side.

PANCREATIC DISTRESS (10X)

TOXOPLASMOSIS (gondii nosode) This nosode remedy is made from a coccidian parasite that is found in cat feces. The most important thing to know about this parasite is that it has been linked, in pregnant women, to spontaneous abortion due to neonatal death and to difficulties with labor and delivery.

This parasite is particularly fond of the pancreas. Some sources claim that as much as 75% of hypoglycemia can be linked to it to the presence of this parasite in the pancreas. My father suffered from hypoglycemia and what appeared to be heart problems until the discovery and eradication of this parasite removed all of these symptoms.

LATHYRUS SATIVA (wild vetch) Sympoms of Lathyrus include emaciated limbs, infantile paralysis, spinal sclerosis, trembling of the arms, and pain in back so severe as to prevent movement. There is excessive rigidity of legs with spastic gait.

PARASITES

In one of Hanna Kroeger's repertories, Gretchen Lalik Wiegers said, "Parasites are more welcome when there is stagnation, which can even come in the form of negative thoughts."

An improperly functioning thyroid increases susceptibility to parasites. Proper minerals in the diet and the proper intake of them is the best preventative—and certainly aids the cure.

I have found that herbal remedies strong enough to deal with parasites are often too strong for the good bacteria in the intestinal tract, especially for use with children. Homeopathic remedies and the homeopathic versions of herbal parasite cleanses are more appropriate and create less damage to the digestive and intestinal systems because they strengthen the system against the invaders rather than kill the invaders outright.

PARASITES #1 (7X)

This is an herbal remedy used for the expulsion of parasites that has been potentized into a homeopathic remedy. Many of the ingredients, however, are homeopathics in their own right.

LAPPA ARCTIUM ***(burdock)*** Symptoms include flatulent dyspepsia, pain in heart with strange movement under sternum, frequent yellow stools in forenoon with some nausea, ringworm. Pain in the heart is a scary symptom since parasites have the ability to move into other body tissues.

CASSIA ACUTIFOLIA (senna) Symptoms include colic, constipation, infantile colic, with a sensation of coldness in abdomen.

GAULTHERIA PROCUMBENS ***(Wintergreen)*** Very severe pain in the abdomen that is much worse by the pressure of even a finger, prolonged vomiting, uncontrollable appetite with an irritable stomach are some of the symptoms of Gaultheria procumbens.

JUGLANS NIGRA (black walnut) Juglans is especially noteworthy because it affects the spleen and the liver in repair as well as in the expulsion of worms. Symptoms include bloating, flatulence, nausea, violent nausea, and emaciation. The symptoms can become quite serious in children.

TANACETUM VULGARE (tansy) Tansy as an herbs is well-renowned for the expulsion of worms. Symptoms include dysentery, pain in the bowels that is relieved by stool, a desire for stool immediately after eating (actually, unless tied to worms, this is a good and natural thing), faint and sick at the stomach, constant belchings, nausea and vomiting, mental fatigue, abnormal lassitude, inability to think coherently, and sadness that comes with a desire to be let entirely alone.

FOENICULUM SATIVUM (fennel) Moderates the griping pains of parasite expulsion, nausea, diarrhea, and improper excitement of the vascular and the respiratory organs.

ARTENSIA ABSINTHIUM/ABSINTHIUM ARTEMISIA (wormwood) This homeopathic remedy has been used to treat worms, and the rest of the symptom picture of this remedy certainly matches that of a parasite infestation. Absinthium artemisia, in the herbal world, is considered stronger for the purpose of expelling parasites than Artensium annua (sweet wormwood).

PARASITES #2 (7X)

This combination of homeopathics targets threadworm, the little white pinworms seen at the anus at night—often in children.

ENTEROBIUS VERMICULARIS NOSODE (pinworms) Symptoms include frequent and strong itching of the anal area, restless sleep due to the itching and discomfort of the anal area, and pain with rash and skin irritation around the anus. Pinworms can be identified by checking the child's anus during the night when the pinworms exit the body.

FILIX MAS (male fern) The symptom picture of Filix mas includes many abdominal and stomach disorders. Some of them are a match for a parasite infestation. Symptoms include great pain in the abdomen with gnawing and boring pains, and torpid inflammation of the lymph glands.

BRAYERA ANTHELMINTHICA (KOUSSO) Kousso symptoms include thirst, nausea, vomiting, vertigo, exhaustion, and fatigue. Kousso expels worms, but causes no improvement in the emaciation and weakness that the worms have created. All parasite cleanses need to be followed with healing remedies and good nutrition.

PARASITES #3 (8X)

This remedy is specific for whipworm infestation.

Symptoms in small children are gastrointestinal in nature. There is abdominal diarrhea, possible growth retardation, mucus in the sinuses, asthma, and nervousness.

VIOLA ODORATA (sweet-scented violet) This homeopathic remedy is well known for the expulsion of worms, particularly in children. Symptoms include distension of abdomen, bed-wetting in nervous children, violent itching at the anus, and the urine is milky with a strong smell.

NATRUM MURIATICUM (sodium chloride) Children with worm infestations are often late in learning to talk and walk. Other symptoms include abdomen that is swollen with colic, rumbling, constipation and diarrhea on alternating days, and unquenchable thirst.

SYZYGIUM AROMATICUM (clove oil) There are no homeopathic provings of clove oil yet but t he oil is widely used in the expulsion of worms and parasites and relieves gas pains and cramping.

ARTEMISIA ANNUAM (sweet wormwood) Artemisia annua has no homeopathic provings but is closely related to Artemsia vulgaris which is well-renowned for the expulsion of parasites.

CHELIDONIUM MAJUS (greater celandine) Symptoms of this remedy include rumbling and diarrhea, distention of the abdomen, tenderness in the epigastrium region, alternating diarrheas and constipation, crawling and itching in the rectum, and a sensation as if the anus were contracted alternating with itching during stool.

PREGNANCY (6X)

This remedy is intended for the relief of mild, early-stage toxemia.

EUPHRASIA OFFICINALIS (eyebright) Symptoms include catarrhal headache, painless swelling in hands and feet, stitches in the hips when walking, frequent waking during early morning hours, and dim or blurred vision.

IRIS VERSICOLOR (blue flag) This remedy is indicated for morning sickness, abdominal tenderness, chronic indigestion of milk products, throbbing headache—usually on right side and often beginning with vision disturbances, and vomiting with burning pain.

NATRUM SULPHURICUM (sodium sulfate) Symptoms include frequent urination, early diabetes, glucose, bile, and sediment in urine, gout, uric acid crystals in tissues of extremities, pain in the hip joints on rising or sitting down, edema of the feet, and liver and gallbladder disorders during pregnancy.

THUJA OCCIDENTALIS (arbor vitae) Thuja, as it relates to pregnancy, usually has to do with emotional symptoms. The woman feels isolated and alone yet is averse to company. Physically, there is pain in the hip joints which give way when walking. Often when there has been toxemia early in pregnancy, there is post-partum depression after the birth of the child. This remedy, taken when the toxemia first appears, may prevent post-partum depression later on. See Section Two: Remedies for Pregnancy and Childbirth. This remedy is very strong and caution is always advised when pregnant when taking any remedy. Muscle testing to confirm remedy choice is advised.

RESCUE REMEDY (Five-Flower Formula (4X)

Rescue remedy can be regarded as a single remedy although it is a composite of 5 flower essences.

Rescue Remedy is most effective when used on the occasion of any profound trauma or emergency in helping the person cope with extreme pain and shock. Rescue remedy brings immediate calm and helps with the physical and emotional aspects of shock.

This formula is also useful for energy work when the client becomes too involved in the trauma they are trying to work on. I have also found this remedy to be a wonderful resource for children that are upset or frightened.

CHERRY PLUM (flower essence) Cherry Plum increases feelings of being guided and protected. It nourishes spiritual surrender and trust, allowing for stability even in times of crisis. This remedy alleviates fears of losing control in stressful situations and calms the mind during times of extremes of tension and fear.

CLEMATIS (flower essence) Clematis is for states of shock where there is a need to bring the person into focus on the present moment because it encourages practical and helpful responses to stress and injury.

IMPATIENS (flower essence) Impatiens helps to inspire patience and acceptance of circumstances and the flow of things around them. (I love that the name *impatiens* reminds me of the lack of patience I so often display when I am under stress!) Impatiens is in this remedy to provide the calm assurance that things are being taken care of in a timely, or at least acceptable, fashion and that things will turn out OK.

ROCK ROSE (flower essence) Rock Rose is a remedy for the inspiring of courage, inner peace, and tranquility when facing great challenges or even injuries. This remedy helps to bring calmness in the face of deep fear, terror, panic, and the fear of death or serious pain. Rock rose is of value whenever there is extreme fear, pain, grief, or loneliness.

STAR OF BETHLEHEM (flower essence) Star of Bethlehem increases a person's ability to accept help from the spiritual realm. Star of Bethlehem is a deeply restorative remedy—can bring a sense of calm peacefulness and the assurance that there is help from loved ones beyond the veil. This remedy is useful for any shock or trauma—makes little difference whether the event was recent or was in the distant past.

All five of these remedies may be used on their own, but they are particularly effective when combined into a single bottle and administered together in this manner.

RESPIRATORY DISTRESS #1 (12X)

This remedy is useful for extreme lung problems with symptoms as extensive as those of Cystic Fibrosis.

FILIX MAS Symptoms of this remedy include clogging of the lymph glands and thickening of and clogging of mucosa throughout the body, including the lungs. Normally, mucus is watery. Mucus keeps the linings of certain organs moist and prevents them from drying out or getting infected. Sticky mucus builds up and can block airways, tubes and ducts throughout your body. Blocked ducts in the pancreas keep digestive enzymes from reaching the small intestine and this, in turn, keeps the intestines from absorbing fats and proteins properly.

NATRUM SALICYLICUM (sodium salicylicum) Symptoms concerning the lungs include great difficulty breathing, breathing very noisy with hallow gasps for air, panting respiration, and dryness in mouth and throat with great thirst.

Consider trying the Butterfly Express, llc, essential oil called [Le]Stefanie along with this remedy.

RESPIRATORY DISTRESS #2 (8X)

This remedy is potentized from herbal remedies.

LIGUSTICUM PORTERI (osha) Herbally, osha is considered one of the best treatments for viral infections. It is also used for eliminating toxins through sweating, as a stomach remedy where there has been much vomiting, for lowering blood pressure, inducing uterine contractions, and for the slowing os post-partum bleeding.

PULMONARIA OFFICINALIS (lungwort) This plant has been cultivated for centuries as a medicinal herb. Its symptoms include many pulmonary complaints, it stops bleeding, improves tissue firmness., alleviates cough, helps with hoarseness. aids mild lung problems, and sooths throat irritation.

RESPIRATORY #3 DISTRESS (6X)

This remedy is meant to alleviate smoker's cough and similar afflictions.

IODUM PURUM (iodine) This remedy affects all glandular structures. Symptoms include many acute disorders of the respiratory system, acute catarrh of all mucus membranes, dry irritated cough which is worse at night, suffocating cough—and hardly get breath, and pneumonia. Other symptoms include weight loss in spite of good appetite. The weight loss often continues to the point of emaciation.

MYRTUS COMMUNIS (myrtle) This remedy has a powerful action on the upper part of the *left* lung and is indicated for dry hollow cough from upper anterior portion of lungs, dryness in the throat, stitching pain running from left breast through to the scapula, cough with great tightness in the lungs, and coughing of blood. The symptoms of Myrtus are worse from changes in atmospheric pressure.

RANUNCULUS SCELERATUS (buttercup) Symptoms include anxious oppressed breathing with a great desire to get a deep breath, gnawing pain in the left palm (this is the heart region in footzone and reflexology), and sore burning behind the sternum. The symptoms are worse for deep breathing and are triggered by anger. The symptoms are mostly right-sided.

THIOSINAMINUM Thiosinaminum as a dramatic action on the lymphatic glands. The only lung symptoms are accelerated respiration and lack of elasticity in tissues and organs, including the lungs. Thiosinaminum dissolves scar tissue and keloids and is said to work with tumors and enlarged glands.

RESPIRATORY #4 DISTRESS (7X)

This remedy is specific for respiratory ailment with emotional drivers.

PINE The Pine Bach Flower Essence was listed by Back in the group of *For Those Who suffer Despondency and Despair.* Pine is useful for states connected to guilt, regret and self-reproach and an inability to objectively acknowledge one's faults. This remedy includes nervous breathing syndrome and insomnia. Gastric and duodenal ulcers and an irritable colon are also common.

TEPLITZ AQUA (Teplitx Mineral Springs) The symptoms of Teplitz aqua include tearfulness, low spirits, irritability, and speech difficulties. This remedy is particularly indicated for gout. The symptoms are worse at night and better by drinking cold water.

VESPA CRABRO (wasp) The symptoms of Vespa crabro include hurried respiration, hoarseness, loss of voice, stinging and burning pains, pale face with drops of sweat on the forehead, arms thrown out from the body in an attempt to gasp for more air, sleepless and restless all night, and nerve and muscular excitement and irritability. Cold water first relieves and then irritates.

RESPIRATORY DISTRESS #5 (12X)

This remedy is for respiratory distress that comes with kidney ailments and early diabetes.

FERRUM IODATUM (iron iodide) The symptom picture of the remedy includes chronic pneumonia., shortness of breath—must take deep breaths in order to get oxygen, and enlarged glands.

EQUISETUM HYEMALE (horsetail) The purpose of Equisetum hyemale in this remedy is to support the kidneys through the rigors of a respiratory illness.

FUMARIA OFFICINALIS (fumitory) This remedy also has action on the kidneys. Symptoms include backache, bloating, flatulence, headache, confusion and great difficulty concentrating.

NASTURTIUM AQUATICUM (watercress) As an herbal remedy, watercress is related to strictures in the urinary/bladder system.

NATRUM SULPHURICUM (sodium sulfate) Symptoms include asthma that is worse in damp weather, pain in the lower left chest, cough with roughness in the throat, eyes sensitive to sunlight, and depression.

CALCAREA PHOSPHORICA (calcium phosphate) Symptoms include rattling of mucus in the lungs, enlargement of tonsils, breathing is more frequent than it should be and is short and difficult, a child loses breath on being lifted up, suffocating attacks in children following nursing—the breathing is made worse by crying. There is a predisposition to glandular and bone diseases. Ailments of this remedy are brought on by grief, either recent or unprocessed.

SCARS/ADHESIONS (10X)

HISTAMINUM MURIATICUM (histamine) There are symptoms in nearly every system and organ and for venous structures in the symptom picture of Histaminum muriaticum. A keynote is numbness of areas of skin or muscles. This wide variety of action may give this remedy the capability of repairing scaring that occurs in the outer layers of the skin, the muscle layers beneath, the veins and arteries, and even heal internal organs as well.

MALATHION Malathion is an insecticide of relative high human toxicity. It weakens the immune system and creates havoc with the bowels and the bladder. ***Malathion converts to malaoxon, which is 60 times more poisonous than malathion itself, during the chlorination process imposed on drinking water***. Besides immune compromise, these chemicals cause adhesions (scar tissue in the intestines) and muscle twitching elsewhere. This remedy is an excellent choice for scarring anywhere in the body.

RESERPINUM (***alkaloid of Rauwolfia serpentina)*** The picture of Reserpinum includes dry, hard scabs and hard, abnormal growths following the swelling of tissues with edema. The mental picture is alarming as it lists anxiety with suicidal tendencies.

THERIDON CURASSAVICUM (orange spider) The picture of this remedy lists thickening of muscle or skin tissue but it also lists tuberculosis, making this remedy useful for scar tissue in the lungs. Emotionals include a highly sensitive nervous system. There is a strange sensitivity to noise in which the vibrations of the music are felt penetrating into the teeth.

THIOSINAMINUM (mustard seed) Quoting Murphy's Materia Medica, "Thiosinaminum has been effective in curing adhesions, scars, lupus and enlarge lymphatic glands. It is a dissolvent, externally and internally, for ***dissolving scar tissue and keloids."*** This remedy is also listed for wounds that are slow to heal and for wounds that form a lot of scar tissue. Also useful to granulations, scars, and keloids after burns and for scarred eardrums or eardrums that thicken causing hearing loss.

SINUS (9X)

EUPHRASIA OFFICINALIS (eyebright) Symptoms include allergies and hay fever, feeling as if there is sand in the eyes, catarrhal conjunctivitis, catarrhal headache with profuse discharge from the nose, eyes water all the time, and burning and swelling of the lids.

HYDRASTIS CANADENSIS (golden seal) Symptoms that apply to the sinus cavities include thick, ropy discharge from the nose, frontal headache from catarrh, eustachian catarrh, and tinnitus from catarrh of the inner ear.

KALI BICHROMICUM (potassium bichromate) The symptoms of this remedy include coryza, perforation of the nasal septum, headaches over the eyebrows, migraines in small spots from the catarrh, pressure and pain at root or bridge of the nose, sinusitis, post-nasal drip of thick catarrh, large mucus plugs, loss of smell, and the nasal septum becomes ulcerated.

PULSATILLA NIGRICANS (windflower) Pulsatilla people are mild, emotional, and tearful with consolation improving all symptoms. The symptoms that apply to sinus issues are catarrhal conjunctivitis, profuse bland yellow discharges, ear infections that are worse at night, nose stopped up when indoors but running profusely outside, and large green fetid scales in the nose.

SKIN ERUPTIONS (8X)

GINKGO BILOBA (maidenhair tree) Although Ginkgo biloba is indicated for the circulatory system and the brain. Tthere are symptoms such as burning, itching eye sockets, transient pox-like eruptions, and eczema. Exhaustion is also part of the picture. Symptoms are worse from walking.

MENTHA PIPERITA (peppermint) Peppermint has a very clear emotional pattern. The physical symptoms that pertain to skin issues found in this remedy include muscles around the neck are very painful to touch, every scratch becomes a sore, and there is much itching especially by the ears.

TEREBINTHINIAE OLEUM (oil of turpentine) With this remedy the sensitivity of the skin in increased, there is a feeling of heat under the skin, vesicular eruptions, aching soreness of the muscles, and red spots created from bleeding capillaries that spreads over the body.

MERCURIUS SOLUBILIS (mercury vivus) This is a very restless remedy. The person must move from place to place. The skin feels constantly moist with itching that is made worse from the warmth of the bed, moist vesicles surrounded by dry scales the bleed easily. This remedy has a relation to chicken pox and the varicella virus.

SLEEP (9X)

CHAMOMILLA VULGARIS (German chamomile) The symptoms of Chamomilla include being oversensitive to caffeine—high, then total crash, tired but cannot rest, sleeplessness due to pain of any sort, and anxious frightened dreams with half-open eyes.

EPHEDRA VULGARIS (ma huang) Ephedra, in herbal form, has long been used as a tonic and mild stimulant for those recovering from a debilitating illness. There is apathy and deep fatigue with a great longing for sleep that does not come.

HEPAR SULPHURIS CALCAREUM (calcium sulphide) Hepar is noted for great debility. The eyes and eyelids become inflamed. The person experiences a lot of vertigo and falls asleep at inappropriate times and places.

STERCULIA ACUMINATA (kola nut) There is very little known about this remedy either as an herb except that it gives the power to endure prolonged physical exertion without taking food and without feeling fatigued. The homeopathic remedy is for exhaustion after prolonged exertion and for blood sugar issues that become worse when meals are missed.

NATRUM NITRICUM (sodium nitrate) Natrum muriacticum has a list of symptoms related to sleep. I can find none on record for this remedy. It is good for great irritability and dull headache.

TEETHING (MIXED POTENCIES, 6X AND 12X)

Hyland's teething tablets are absolutely amazing! They make the teething time of a baby's development so much easier. This remedy is in liquid form, as are all of the homeopathic remedies that I use. There are those that believe that the tablets are more effective because they dissolve in the mouth, coating the gums as they do so. This makes no sense according to homeopathic principles and I did not find it to be true with my own children. Remaking them in tablet form (or buying them that way from Hyland's) is a simple procedure if you want to use them that way.

CALCAREA PHOSPHORICUM (calcium phosphate) (6X) Calcarea phos supports the proper development and formation of the teeth and builds a degree of immunity to tooth decay. It is also included in this formula because it is known to relieve the irritability too often common with children during the teething months and is said to relieve pain, particularly at night.

CHAMOMILLA VULGARIS (German chamomile) (6X) Chamomilla is one of the leading polycrest remedies for irritable, fussy, and whining children. Keynotes of this remedy include the child being dissatisfied, and demanding and wanting to be carried or held all of the time. A child who would benefit from Chamomilla is extremely sensitive to every type of pain.

COFFEA CRUDA ((unroasted coffee) 6X) Coffea is included for oversensitivity, intolerance of pain, and sleeplessness. Coffea is an excellent preventative of fever and would help allay convulsions if the child were so inclined.

BELLADONNA (deadly nightshade) (12X) Belladonna is included to relieve the redness, inflammation swelling, and discomfort commonly associated with teething.

TENSION #1 (6X)

This remedy is for safe and natural relief of stress, nervousness, anxiety, pressure headaches in back of neck, and post-partum depression.

CHAMOMILLA VULGARIS (German chamomile) Chamomilla is particularly suited to irritable, sensitive, discontented, whining children and their adult counterparts. I would have to list Chamomile as a very mild, but extremely important, polycrest for any hypersensitivity of the nervous system. The person is dissatisfied with everything and can turn suddenly spiteful and irritable. A keynote of this remedy is that the person lives in the past, dwelling on past irritations and slights by other people.

KALI PHOSPHORICUM (potassium phosphate) Like all remedies containing phosphorus, this is a remedy for mental and physical exhaustion caused by overwork, overexcitement, or worry. There is a great sensitivity to light and noise and sleeplessness because the mind is over-active with worry.

HUMULUS LUPULUS (hops) The Humulus person is highly excited and excitable. Other symptoms include mental confusion, violent pulsating of temporal and carotid arteries, frequent startling from deep sleep, dull headache with dizziness, and a weak and slow pulse.

RED CHESTNUT (flower essence) This Bach flower was listed under the group *For Those Who Have Fear* by Bach. There is extreme physical nervousness, with tightening of the stomach from fear. The fear of this remedy is fear for the welfare of others, particularly family and friends. There is a very great difference that is experienced by the energy system when we move from loving compassion to the counterfeit emotion of worry. Unless our worry moves us to appropriate action, it harms us while doing no good for the person about whom we are worrying.

WILLOW (flower essence) The negative emotions of Willow flower essence are despondency and despair, resentment, bitterness, chronic repression of aggressive or irritable impulses, suppressed anger resulting in indigestion, headaches, irregular heart action, and chronic cough.

TENSION #2 8X

Aids with stress and tension which can lead to chronic pain, neck and back tension and MS.

AMBRA GRISEA (ambergis) Applicable symptoms include extreme hypertension, anxiety, weakened by age or overwork, cramps in hands with the arms numb, stiffness in loins from sitting very long, and a sensation of coldness and numbness in spots. The symptoms are worse from the presence of others and worse from embarrassment or any type of worry.

CINCHONA/CHINA OFFICINALIS (Peruvian bark) Cinchona is a remedy for debility and exhaustion from loss of vital fluid due to diarrhea and hemorrhages. A few of the many symptoms of this polycrest remedy are insomnia from fantasies, oversensitivity to noise, intense throbbing of the head and the carotids, sleeplessness from an overactive mind, irritability, heavy pressure on the sacrum, and cold hands and feet.

CUPRUM ACETICUM (copper acetate) A great many of the symptoms of Cuprum are in the head. A few of these are violent throbbing and sharp pains in the forehead, head reels when in a large room, brain seems to be gone, vertigo, constant protrusion and retraction of the tongue, and inclined to gape and cry.

PHOSPHORUS (the element) The debilitating diseases of Phosphorus are keynoted by the insidious onset, gradually increasing debility with a sudden slide in to severe prostrations. This pattern often follows on the heels of a serious emotional shock of some sort.

TRAUMATIC EXPERIENCES (7X)

CHERRY PLUM (flower essence) This essence is specific for severe pain, where one feels almost unable to bear the strain. Cherry Plum is used in drug rehabilitation. Prolonged mental effort leads to failing nerves and exhaustion and there is great anguish and distress seen when a person would benefit from this remedy.

RED CHESTNUT (flower essence) This Bach flower was listed under the group *For Those Who Have Fear* by Bach. There is extreme physical nervousness, with tightening of the stomach from fear. The fear of this remedy is fear for the welfare of others, particularly family and friends. When someone we know has been seriously injured there can be a serious response within our own bodies.

FERRUM PHOSPHORICUM (iron phospate) The person for whom this remedy will be appropriate will have been nervous and sensitive before the trauma occurred. The skin will be pale but flushed at the same time with sweaty hands. Look for vertigo and fainting, particularly at the sight of blood. They person may complain of great dizziness with everything spinning around them. Muscle weakness will always be present. Physically, this is a remedy for anemia and for fresh wounds, contusions, and sprains.

KALI IODATUM (potassium iodide) One of the emotional symptoms of this remedy is that troublesome experiences and impressions stay with the person for a long time, becoming the basis of many emotional symptoms. Some of these symptoms are startling at sudden noises, light-headedness, fluttering of the heart, palpitations, weak pulse, and vertigo. The person needing this remedy is often troubled, and despondent.

NARCOTINUM (opium alkaloid) This remedy is interesting in that it has been extensively proven, but very few distinctive and notable symptoms were noted. Those that were seen include vertigo from the least movement of the head, confusion, no mental grasp of anything, brain fatigue, dullness of the senses, loss of consciousness, trembling, and cold sweat with all of these symptoms leading the person toward a state of total collapse.

ZINCUM PHOSPHORICUM (Zinc phosphate) Zinc phos symptoms include nervousness, vertigo, hysteria, restlessness, repetitive movements, forgetfulness, fearfulness, anxiety, and nervousness when any event is being anticipated. Vertigo. There are claims that this remedy relieves the mental depression and paralysis following strokes and other forms of cerebral congestion.

This remedy is changeable with opposites such as being happy, open, and enthusiastic one moment then becoming gloomy and discontented without warning or obvious reason. There may be laughing that turns suddenly to hysterical screaming.

VAGINITIS (9X)

KALI SULPHURICUM (potassium sulfate) This is a remedy for anemia, loss of memory, and anxiety from the anticipation of some event or experience. A keynote of this remedy is restless, repetitive movements. Applicable symptoms include backache during menses, leucorrhea, eruptions and itching on vulva, with yellow mucus and discharges. The anxiety is better for being in the open air.

POPULUS CANDICANS (Balm of Gilead) Balm of Gilead is mentioned in the Bible in the context of relief from despair and anguish. An important symptom of this remedy is erratic menstrual cycle—scant and delayed, then early and abundant. Symptoms applicable to this combination include burning in vaginal area with strong and highly colored urine.

YUCCA FILAMENTOSA (bear grass) Yucca is predominantly a liver remedy. Symptoms include despondent, irritable, unable to remember what was read, seems unable to understand when spoken to, various types of headaches and throbbing of the temporal arteries.

VENOUS CONGESTION (12X)

POPULUS CANDICANS (Balm of Gilead) Balm of Gilead is mentioned in the Bible in the context of relief from despair and anguish and is used as a symbol for the Savior. Symptoms include venous congestion, such as varicose veins, that are better for application of hot cloths. The sound of the heart is irregular and muffled.

THERIDION CURASSAVICUM (orange spider) Spider remedies always have an action on the blood and on the nerves. Symptoms for Theridion are burning feeling in legs and arms, peculiar pain around the heart, and cardiac symptoms are the result of anxiety and stress. Symptoms are better for lying down and worse for walking, particularly up stairs.

VINCA MINOR (lesser periwinkle) Vinca shows a wide range of symptoms in any blood disorder or blood clotting/hemorrhaging problem as well as a tendency to passive uterine hemorrhages. Vein weakness is displayed as capillary problems leading to nosebleeds

Warts (Wart Formula) (10X)

Aids in the elimination of warts and growths on the skin. Warts are often a symptom of problems in the Psora miasm, which is common to all of mankind and rears its ugly head from time to time in all of us.

LACTICUM ACIDUM (lactic acid) Acidity of the body with aching pains, nausea, itching and burning of the skin, red spots or blotches on thighs and lower limbs, constant cough that is worse in the spring and the fall are symptoms of Lacticum acidum. All symptoms are made worse by cold.

SCROPHULARIA NODOSA (knotted figwort) Symptoms include eczema, lymphoma, enlarged glands, skin burns when rubbed, itching that is worse on the back of the hands, the inside of wrists and between the fingers. There are painful hemorrhoids and great drowsiness in morning.

THUJA OCCIDENTALIS (arbor vitae) Interesting to this remedy's symptoms are brown spots on the hands and arms, birthmarks, impetigo with itching, anal warts, the formation of cysts, moles, polyps, and venereal warts. There is rapid exhaustion and emaciation.

CAUSTICUM (caustic potash) Symptoms include seedy warts, itching, soreness in folds of skin and between thighs.

DULCAMARA (woody nightshade) Dulcamara is a glandular and lymphatic remedy. Symptoms include swollen glands, herpes, warts, sore throat, severe itching of the skin and red spots that are worse in wet and cold weather or brought on by it, eczema, rash on infants, skin callous, nettle rash over the whole body, and little boils.

CALCAREA CARBONICA This is a very important polycrest remedy that constitutes one of the three pillars of Hahnemann's homeopathic practice. Symptoms of Calcarea carb include abscesses, polyps, worms, psoriasis, swollen glands, small wounds that do not heal well, recurring blood boils, and ***warts on the face and the hands.*** This is an anti-psoric remedy which means that there is a plethora of skin symptoms.

NAJA TRIPUDIANS (cobra venom) This is a rare snake remedy that does not have hemorrhage listed in its symptom picture. Symptoms of Naja include skin that is swollen and mottled with small white itching blisters on the inflamed base of the neck and on the nose and on the body. These symptoms occur most often in the afternoon. There are scars that itch and an irritating, dry cough.

NATRUM SULPHURICUM (sodium sulphate) With this remedy the skin is jaundiced, there is eczema that is moist and oozing profusely, watery, yellow blisters, and itching pimples. All symptoms are worse from damp weather and worse from the head injuries that are the common cause of symptoms with this remedy.

WEAKNESS #1 (12X)

This remedy supports against symptoms similar to those of radiation sickness.

CITRUS LIMONUM (lemon) Symptoms include sore throats, excessive menstruation, powerful effect on blood and circulation, inflammation, daily headaches, stiff, bruised feeling in joints, aintness with a weak pulse, hemorrhage, and painful enlargement of the spleen.

FAGOPYRUM ESCULENTUM (buckwheat) Symptoms of this remedy include stiffness, bruised feeling in muscles and neck, headache with tired neck, throbbing sensation in arteries, pain in the shoulder, pain along the fingertips, and pain in liver region.

FUCUS VESICULOSUS (sea kelp) This is a tissue remedy of great power. Symptoms include constipation followed by watery diarrhea, swelling of the neck around thyroid, indigestion, flatulence, obesity related to low thyroid function, headache as if the head were being compressed by an iron ring, urine contains blood, nosebleed, and anemia.

Kelp, from which this remedy is made, contains iodine and the actions of these two remedies are comparable.

HYDRANGEA ARBORESCENS (seven-barks) Much of the purpose of this homeopathic remedy being placed in this combination would be to support the kidneys. Symptoms include bladder catarrh and stones in the bladder and kidneys with bloody urine, abdominal symptoms with sharp pains that are most often on the left side, enlarged prostate, great thirst, and burning during urination.

CALCAREA FLORATA (flouride of lime) Murphy's Materia Medica lists burns from X-ray and radiation. Other symptoms include sharp pains in hepatic region, bony growths and spurs, deficient enamel of teeth, weakness, nausea and distress—especially when fatigued and gouty enlargements of fingers.

NATRUM MURIATICUM (common salt) This remedy has specific action on the emotions, heart, kidney, and the spleen. There are pages of symptoms listed in the materia medicas. Among them are blinding headaches, faint feeling, fluttering heart, and heartburn with palpitations.

PHOSPHORUS (the element) Phsphorus is indicated for people who are—or have become as the result of illness—excitable, impressionable, and very weak. The debility of phosphorus often comes on slowly with gradually increasing debility that ends in severe or rapid disease. Profound shock is often the cause. Some of the symptoms of phosphorus are inflammation of mucus membranes and nerves with effects on bone, blood and circulation. The muscles become flabby and weak.

STRONTIUM NITRICUM (strontium nitrate) There are no provings that I can find, just some case histories. The symptoms noted include anemia, fatigue, kidney distress, headache, shock after surgical procedures, high blood pressure with flushed face, pulsating arteries, and threatened stroke. The person may become very forgetful and irritable with a tendency to fly into a rage.

URANIUM NITRICUM (uranium nitrate) This remedy, because of its position on the periodic table, is one for use in situations and illnesses that have become very serious. Symptoms include emaciation, debility, nausea, vomiting, kidney distress with bed-wetting at night, sugar in the urine, headache over the left eye, general acidity, gastric ulcer, pain in pyloric region, nausea and vomiting.

WEAKNESS #2 (7X)

This remedy is useful for sunburn, flu-like symptoms after a weather change, and heat exhaustion.

FERRUM PHOSPHORICUM (iron phosphate) Ferrum is considered useful for anemia and debility and weakness. According to Robin Murphy's materia medica Ferrum phos stimulates the blood to increase hemoglobin. This remedy is useful for the first stages of all inflammatory disorders, fresh wounds, contusions, sprains, and bruised soreness on the chest, shoulders, and muscles. A keynote symptom is vertigo with rush of blood to the head.

IPOMOEA PURPUREA (morning glory) Some symptoms that apply to this remedy are heaviness in the back and the neck, thoracic spasms, headache first in the right and then in the left temple, pulse accelerated with extra systole, kidney disorders and stones with pain in the back, agitation, mental confusion, and neuro-muscular and arthritic pains.

KALI SULPHURICUM (potassium sulfate) Symptoms include a sensation of heaviness and weariness, vertigo, chilliness, palpitations of the heart, anxiety with the symptoms being worse for heat and better in the open air.

WEAKNESS #3 (4X)

This remedy is for support of immune system with symptoms similar to radiation sickness. It is also for coping with fear and panic.

This remedy is meant to be similar to the Deva flower essence that was created to clear fears of the future of life on this planet and fears about the effects of electromagnetic, toxic, and environmental pollution. I find it effective when there are fears about one's own future. Fear weakens the immune and the nervous systems and this remedy strengthens those systems.

AGRIMONY (flower essence) Listed by Bach in the group *Oversensitive to Influences and Ideas*. There is denial of one's own opinions and emotions, restlessness in mind and body, and craving for stimulants. Agrimony will greatly ease the pain of a patient who is smiling despite pain and anxiety.

CRAB APPLE (flower essence) The negative aspects of Crab Apple are self-centered, with obsessiveness or shame about appearance their appearance. A tendency to obsess about weight—anorexia and bulimia being common. The emotional pattern manifests in the physical body as accumulated wastes in the blood stream, chronic poisonings due to environmental hazards, vomiting, nausea, and emaciation.

ROCK ROSE (flower essence) Rock Rose is an ingredient in Rescue Remedy (Five Flower Formula). Although is is indicated for calming the victim after a traumatic injury or experience, it is just as useful for times of weakness and prolonged illness.

Some symptoms associated with Rock Rose include fright and heightened anxiety, prolonged fearful worry, chronic loss of sleep, anger, hatred, irrational resentment, impatience, aggressiveness, feelings of helplessness, desire for peace and rest, lack of physical/mental/emotional endurance, digestive problems, sensitivity to noise and touch, frequent nightmares, and renewed fear of any contact with the person or the situation that originally engendered fear and trauma.

MIMULUS (flower essence) The negative emotions of Mimulus include constant fear, dread of things, persons, or events, anticipatory fears, chronic phobias, nervousness, lowered stamina and decreased vitality, frequent loose bowels, griping intestinal pains during acute states of anxiety, emotional diarrhea, and duodenal ulcers. This remedy is useful during physical rehabilitation after accidents, surgery, sickness, and is excellent for the debilities of old age.

The balanced state of Mimulus is courage and confidence to face life's challenges.

WHITE OLEANDER (flower essence) The negative emotions of White Oleander are fear of being left alone and uncared for during an illness, fear of feeling inferior to others gingivitis, tooth decay due to improper nutrient balance caused by a clogged and congested colon, poisons from the colon lodging in joints, fatigue and weakness, and injury to ligaments.

EUCALYPTUS (flower essence) Symptoms of Eucalyptus include gastrointestinal distress with sleeplessness and restlessness. There is relapsing of ailments that go away then come back again and again. Other symptoms include dull, congestive headache, nervous headache, suppurative inflammation of the kidneys, acute diarrhea, and digestion that is slow, difficult and painful. eucalyptus is said to be a preventive for influenza.

WEAKNESS #4 (4X)

This remedy is meant to bring a measure of comfort and relief from the pain of cancer and cancer treatments.

SARCOMA (nosode) There is nothing in the literature about this remedy. I can only assume that it is meant to act along the same lines as other cancer nosodes act. Remedies for the cancer miasm usually fit the profile of highly intelligent, very driven individuals who must always do everything that they do to the very best that it can be done. They also have a great tendency to take on the responsibilities of others as if it is somehow their job to do everything for everybody.

EUPHORBIUM OFFICINARIUM (gum euphorbium) According to Robin Murphy's Materia Medica this remedy would be useful for the pains of cancer, spasmodic flatulent colic, burning pains in the abdomen, bruised pain in occiput and forehead, red swelling of the cheeks, boils and carbuncles. There is sleepiness during the day and chilliness and shivering over the whole body first thing in the morning.

CARCINOSIN (cancer nosode) Being a nosode, it is usually used intercurrently (along with) another remedy which closely matches the symptoms. Symptoms of Carcinosin are contradictory and alternating states of mind, polyps, keloids, brittle bones, hemorrhoids, chronic or acute insomnia, chronic fatigue, excessive weariness and fatigue, multiple allergies. This remedy is for persons who have lived under great fear for long periods of time. There is usually a great craving for chocolate.

WEAKNESS #5 (4X)

This remedy is especially useful for chronic fatigue and exhaustion with no other known cause than geopathic stress and hyper-sensitivity to electric and electronic devices.

FERRUM METALLICUM (iron metal) Ferrum met is leading polycrest for anything having to do with the uptake of iron and the debilitating anemia that results from poor absorption of iron. This type of weakness is accompanied by extreme weakness and sensitivity to noise. Even though the person is extremely weak and tired, there is always a large degree of restlessness with the person being driven from their bed to walk about restlessly. There is a tendency to bleeding and hemorrhage and any blood seen will be watery and very thin looking. Ferrum is a remedy for blood diseases of any description.

Ferrum is a very emotional remedy. It is as though the person is just too tired—and too discouraged from the overwhelming tiredness—to keep their emotions in check.

SILICA TERRA The materia medicas describe the pattern of Sillica terra as a tendency to easy exhaustion and eventual prostration of mind and body. These extreme states are linked to defective nutrition due to imperfect assimilation of nutrients, often beginning in childhood. Silica terra is keynoted by loss of self-confidence, performance anxiety, and the continual anticipation of failure at the beginning of any enterprise. There is a distinct inability to focus and concentrate and there will be mental difficulties from overexertion of their minds.

CUPRUM METALLICUM (copper metal) This remedy is particularly effective when there are problems with the nerves of the cerebro-spinal axis. There will be spasms in the related muscles with violent muscles cramping being common. The cramps are often felt in the toes, fingers, and calves, where the muscles feel knotted. Cramping sensations may also occur in the chest, being felt behind the sternum.

A deficiency of copper is also associated with the rupturing of blood vessels in the backs of the hands and elsewhere, including rupture of veins and arteries in the head—the definition of stroke. The ruptures in the head may trigger convulsions.

YEAST (6X)

This remedy is for the symptoms associated with candida (yeast) infections

ALOE SOCOTRINA (common aloe) Aloe socotrina is an anti-psoric remedy, giving it a great action on issues of the skin since one of psorsas main characteristics is the pushing out of a symptom from deep within the body to the outside of the body—often on to the skin. A keynote symptoms is itching of the skin which appears each year just as winter approaches. There are often hemorrhoids which look like a bunch of grapes and are made better from cold. This remedy affects all of the veins in the abdomen and the pelvic area, the liver, colon, and rectum. Emotional symptoms include being insecure and dissatisfied with self.

ALUMINUM OXYDATA (aluminum oxide) Aluminum poisoning lodged in the cerebrospinal axis causes disturbances in coordination as well as weakness and partial paralysis of muscles. This remedy is a specific for these types of problems. There is either extreme dryness of mucus membranes or excess salivation with partial paralysis of involuntary muscles. Senility and dementia are also listed as symptoms of Aluminum and, therefore, as side effects of aluminum poisoning. Other symptoms include memory weakness or loss, forgets things or loses their way (as in Alzheimer's disease), confusion as to personal identity, and great exhaustion brought on by menstruation—barely recovers before the next cycle begins.

ANTIMONIUM CRUDUM (native sulphide of antimony) Symptoms include irritability and fretfulness, abdomen is very distended, there is itching and pain of neck and back, yellow crusted eruptions on face and chin, brittle nails, eczema with gastric problems, tenderness of ovarian region with nausea and vomiting, and watery vaginal discharges which sting down the thighs. This is truly a remedy for yeast infections all by itself and should be considered in a stronger potency if the mental and emotional patterns (looked up in a materia medica) match closely.

ARGENTUM NITRICUM (silver nitrate) A keynotd of Argentum nitricum is a really great desire for sweets. The person is full of fear, phobias, and anxieties. There is flatulence causing extreme abdominal distension, hypoglycemia, diarrhea from emotions, menses with headache, menses that is irregular or lasting only one day, extreme mucus and erosion of the cervix with bleeding. There is heavy bleeding mid-cycle, usually about 2 weeks after menses.

CHELIDONIUM MAJUS (greater celandine) Chelidonium is a major liver remedy with symptoms more pronounced on the right side. Some symptoms that might apply here are acrid leucorrhea that stain underwear with burning of the vaginal area. The woman is cross and irritable and often suffers from hypoglycemia either just before menses or all of the time. There is a headache that is better after eating and nausea and vomiting with sick headaches.

GAMBOGIA MORELLA (gummi gutti) The main symptom of a yeast infection which is mentioned with Gambogia is violent itching in various parts of the body. There is also profuse, watery diarrhea, gnawing pains in the coccyx, with burning pains and soreness all through the body.

GRAPHITES NATURALIS (black lead) Graphites is a mineral carbon and is related to Carbo animas and Carbo vegetabilis. Graphites, in non-homeopathic form, also contains a small percentage of iron and so is also related to Ferrum in its homeopathic symptom picture.

Some symptoms include a tendency to cracks or fissures at corner of the eyes, the nose, and behind the ears, thickening and scarring of the skin, ***alternating digestive and skin problems***, sensitivity to cold, better after weeping, cannot bear tight clothes around the waist, painless, swollen glands on the side of the neck, itching pimples that are moist after scratching, and unhealthy skin—every cut infects.

LYCOPODIUM CLAVATUM (club moss) Lycopodium is one of 3 basic remedies around which the remedy groups in materia medicas are placed. Symptoms include fear of public speaking, love of power, bloated abdomen with food allergies, diabetes, involuntary urination, and great weakness of digestion with much bloating.

SILICA TERRA (pure flint) A very important keynote of Silica as it relates to yeast infections is that the skin is unhealthy with suppurative processes that are stubborn in clearing. Yeast infections for which many things have been tried with little success often respond to Silica as one of the primary actions of Silica is to push foreign objects and toxic conditions out of the body. There is poor assimilation of nutrients, felons and abscesses, and parts lain on go to sleep or become painful. This remedy is also listed for the ill effects of vaccinations.

Section TWO

Remedies for Pregnancy, Childbirth and Infant Care

Chapter Two

MATERIA MEDICA OF COMMONLY USED REMEDIES FOR PREGNANCY, CHILDBIRTH AND INFANT CARE

In homeopathy we find a gentle, safe way to treat the interconnected physical and emotional concerns of pregnant women and their newborns. Homeopathic remedies are part of a whole person—holistic—approach to care because they impact not just the physical symptoms, but underlying emotions, absorption of nutrients, placental and uterine tone, fetal growth, and a host of other aspects of childbearing and infant care.

Low potencies (30C, possibly 200C and the tissue salt remedies), unless quite experienced with homeopathic remedies, are advised for use in most instances and with most women and children. A 200C is usually strong enough for even emergency situations. Tissue salt remedies are usually given 3 or 4 times a day for up to 4 weeks, depending on the severity of the symptoms and the progress of the healing. Remedies in 30C and 200C potency are given as needed, as recommended by a homeopathic physician or experienced person, or as recommended in accepted and common literature.

ACHILLEA MILLEFOLIUM *(yarrow)* Please see: Millefolium achillea

ACONITUM NAPELLUS *(monkshood)*

This is predominantly a remedy for acute conditions of many varieties such as a miscarriage or a threatened premature birth that may have come on suddenly with little warning. There will be sudden hemorrhage of bright red blood with faintness and panic, shock, and urine retention in mother or baby. Other symptoms include loss of milk in the nursing mother after a fright or exposure to cold and inflammation of the breast that comes on suddenly and is usually accompanied by fever. In babies and children especially, there will be fever that is sudden and goes high quickly.

There will be a lot of fear and worry with the mother continually asking, "Am I going to be OK?" During labor, there will be vaginal dryness and slower than optimal dilation. Circulation and nerve issues may manifest as numbness and tingling of hands and feet.

Keynotes of Aconite are always centered around the situation being brought on by, or accompanied by, the symptoms coming on very suddenly and rapidly. There remedy is particularly useful if the mother is frightened by the thought of labor or has been fearful throughout the pregnancy. Aconite is also excellent following an emergency such as a shoulder dystocia, where panic, palpitations, and rapid pulse are present and remain even after the crisis has passes. ***The suddenness and violence with which symptoms come on is the most important keynote of this remedy and the sooner the remedy is given, the better will be the results!***

AETHUSA CYNAPIUM *(fool's parsley)*

This remedy is particularly useful when an infant has been or is ill and cannot, for a time, tolerate their mother's milk. The keynote and most reliable indicator for Aethusa is projectile vomiting or diarrhea within a few moments of nursing This cycle brings about dehydration and exhaustion with the baby falling asleep for a short while afterwards and then waking hungry as ever only to repeat the cycle until they become very dehydrated and too weak to nurse at all.

ANACARDIUM ORIENTALE *(marking nut)*

Anacardium is ***not*** a polycrest for pregnancy but is extremely useful for those conditions in which it is indicated, usually by observing the mental and emotional symptoms. These symptoms include lack of confidence in themselves and extreme mood swings. There is often a history of verbal, physical, and/or sexual abuse with humiliation and punishment as part of the picture.

Some conditions for which Anacadium may be helpful include: morning sickness accompanied by dry heaving, headache from strong smells or mental exertion with the headache improving upon eating, constipation, and itching of the skin.

Anacadium acts on the nerves, muscles, and joints. All symptoms are better for eating. Symptoms are described as a feeling of being plugged up or having a plug blocking some passageway.

ANTIMONIUM TARTARICUM *(tartar emetic)*

During labor this remedy may be useful for rigidity of the cervix with pelvic inflammation.

A newborn who might benefit from this remedy will be pale, gasping, breathless, usually as the result of meconium aspiration during the birth. These symptoms may also indicate immature or improperly developed lungs and if often indicated for bronchitis and other respiratory ailments in babies and children.

An important keynote is rattling of mucus with little expectoration. The person will become increasingly weak and drowsy, with lack of reaction to stimuli. A nursing infant will let go of the nipple as if the are needing to take a breath.

APIS MELLIFICA *(honey bee)*

Since Apis is an insect remedy it will have the general symptoms of burning, stinging, swelling and any pain that is present will have a bruised quality to it. There will be a distinct lack of thirst and all conditions will be aggravated by heat and better for cold applications. Other indicators may include irritability, tearfulness, weepiness—cannot stop crying—and vertigo that is worse when sitting and extreme when lying down.

Some conditions for which Apis might be indicated—if the general symptoms match—include cystitis, urine retention, toxemia with swelling, edema of extremities, puffiness of the face, high blood pressure. Apis should be considered if there is any blood flow early in labor. (Bleeding early in labor is never a good sign.)

ARNICA MONTANA *(leopard's bane)*

Arnica is a leading first-aid remedy for any kind of trauma and bruising of muscles and soft tissues. Arnica should be used during labor in conjunction with other chosen remedies for hemorrhage or for fetal distress during or following a difficult birth. The remedy is given to the mother during the labor and to both mother and baby following the birth. Mother and baby will be benefitted greatly.

When arnica is indicated at such times, the person's (or baby's) head will be hot but the body will be cold. When we, as midwives, began using arnica oil on our hands when checking dilation during labor, we discovered that any swelling or bruising of those soft tissues just melted away and stopped impeding the descent of the baby's head which shortened the length of the pushing stage of labor dramatically.

During labor, Arnica is indicated whenever there is soreness in the back as well as for both feeble and irregular labor pains or violent pains that accomplish very little.

Arnica is ***always*** indicated, not just during labor, for shock accompanied by a dazed appearance. There will be some degree of denial—the woman will be insisting that she is really OK. (Give the remedy to her anyway.) Arnica may also be used to prevent shock when it is pending and for bleeding, varicosities, hematomas, aching legs that are worse from pressure, after pains, urine retention.

ARSENICUM ALBUM *(white oxide of arsenic)*

Arsenicum album is a true polycrest, with pages of symptoms listed in materia medicas.

Keynotes of Arsenicum include being chilly, fearful, restless, anxious, unable to sleep with all symptoms worsening after midnight. This remedy is indicated—strongly—if the mother is obsessively cleaning house or trying to feed the midwives during a labor that is intermittent, stopping and starting with no clear pattern. This seems like a strange symptom but I have seen it and I have also seen a dose of 200C Arsenicum turn it right around. The mother slowed down, slept for a couple of hours, and then went into serious labor and delivered well.

Arsenicum album is used for newborn resuscitation if the baby has poor color and respiratory responses.

AURUM METALLICUM *(gold metal)*

The keynotes of Aurum in any situation are violent hysterics, anguish of mind, and great grief, with a negative view of every situation. The person will weep continuously and, whether so inclined or not, often prays. Other keynotes include congestion in the head and heart with heart palpitations. The face will be pale and swollen and the exhaustion may lead to fainting.

During labor there will be lack of confidence in herself and in the progress of the labor. Labor pains will often be irregular and there will be a marked inability to tolerate pain. There may even be remarks made that she wishes she could die or even talk of killing herself because of pain. The vagina will be rigid and unresponsive, leading to exhaustion and lack of progress. The woman will probably be chilly, wanting to be wrapped up, but will be asking for frequent sips of cold water.

During pregnancy, Aurum is indicated only for those situations that are quite dire in nature, such as severe morning sickness, really nasty heartburn, severe vomiting and diarrhea—possibly leading to miscarriage or early labor.

BELLADONNA *(deadly nightshade)*

Belladonna is a remedy of heat and intensity with symptoms coming on suddenly and in extremes. Belladonna situations are made worse from light, motion, noise, and touch. During pregnancy there may be varicose veins that are hot and swollen. Pains, during labor, or at any time, are pulsing and throbbing and are often neuralgic in nature.

During labor, the contractions come and go suddenly and are accompanied by intense bearing-down sensations. Gushing hemorrhages with bright red bleeding—quite frightening—are seen when this remedy is needed. If retained placenta occurs—and it likely will if other symptoms have been present and no remedy has been given to break the pattern—there will be a profuse flow of hot blood when the placenta finally detaches. There may be convulsions during or after delivery and blood pulses rather than flowing freely.

There will be a copious flow of milk as the breasts 'let down' and mastitis is common when this picture was present during labor. Belladonna, along with Bryonia, are polycrests for mastitis. (Phytolacca follows both Belladonna and Bryonia well in mastitis.) Twitching and jerking of muscles, due to nerve issue, may be present during pregnancy, labor, delivery and the post-partum period.

BELLIS PERENNIS *(English Daisy)*

Many of the keynote symptoms and actions of Bellis are similar to Arnica but Bellis is specific to abdominal and pelvic regions, making it of great benefit during pregnancy and childbirth.

Symptoms include pain down outer thighs making walking difficult, weak and tender abdominal muscles, prolapsed rectum, easy bruising, and hematomas. There is often a bearing-down sensation and the woman feels as if she must hold up her belly. (Sepia has similar bearing down sensations but the emotional symptoms are quite different.)

This remedy is also good for stagnant blood situations such as varicose veins, sprains, bruises, and swelling due to accidents.

BORAX VENETA *(sodium biborate)*

This remedy is often effective when an infant seems to have a fear of falling or becomes panicky at any downward motion—baby clings tightly and cries when being placed in the crib or with any forward/downward motion. There may also be a distinct sensitivity to noise, with startling and startling awake at the slightest sound.

Borax is also a remedy for thrush in babies—baby cries when nursing or refuses to nurse with the infection passing back and forth from baby to mother. In mom the infection manifests as blisters on the nipples. With or without infection there may be shooting pains in the breasts—worse directly after nursing.

BRYONIA ALBA *(wild hops)*

Bryonia is one of the leading remedies for inflammation of the membranes which line the lungs, heart, abdominal, and pelvic regions. It is among the leading polycrest remedies for mastitis, pleurisy, peritonitis, and post-partum infections of any kind.

All symptoms are worse for motion—mother usually supports breasts when moving at all. There will be irritability and a desire to be left alone. The symptoms of Bryonia come on slowly. Follow this remedy with Phytolacca, especially with breast infections. With breast infections there will be fever, stony hardness, and sharp pains. Hot, aching, red, swollen veins, if the emotional patterns fit, respond well to this remedy.

CALCAREA CARBONICA *(calcium carbonate)*

Calcarea carbonica is an especially important polycrest remedy and, along with Sulphur and Lycopodium, stands at the head of anti-psoric miasmic remedies. The psora miasm shows up from time to time in all of us but is especially likely to appear during pregnancy as childbearing is such a "mortal sphere" energy.

Keynote of cravings for indigestibles such as dirt, chalk, coal, pencils, are often seen, especially in children. This is a polycrest remedy—useful and effective in many conditions of pregnancy and for responsible, dutiful mothers who have worked or worried themselves to exhaustion. Malnutrition or lack of absorption of nutrients are also key factors in the exhaustion and there is an odd keynote of the head sweating abnormally.

Some other symptoms and issues occurring in the mother include: shortness of breath that is worse climbing stairs, constipation that is not uncomfortable, varicosities of the vulva, blood in the urine, and insomnia, often with nightmares.

Symptoms and issues in the baby include diaper rash, umbilical hernia, colic, thrush, developmental delays, difficult or late teething, milk allergy with chronic congestion, and cradle cap.

CALCAREA FLUORATA *(fluoride of lime)*

This cell salt governs the elasticity of tissues and the walls of blood vessels, making it of vital importance during pregnancy. Calcarea fluorata improves poor circulation and strengthens vein and artery walls.

Situations in which this remedy may prove useful include varicose veins, hemorrhoids, stretch marks, and uterine fibroids. This remedy may prevent the formation of adhesions following a C-section.

CALCAREA PHOSPHORICA *(phosphate of lime)*

Calcarea phos improves digestion and increases the absorption of necessary nutrients, especially calcium and is indicated for any weakness of bones or lack of circulation. For leg cramps alternate this remedy with Mag Phos. Other major symptoms include Pain in the symphysis pubis, insufficient milk supply, teething problems, and delayed development.

In babies and children, there may be failure to thrive—wants to nurse a lot but does not seem to be up-taking sufficient nutrition or the baby vomits easily after nursing. Alternately, the child refuses the breast to the point that sufficient nutrition is not being accomplished. This remedy is useful for children that are peevish and fretful or are prone to temper tantrums.

CANTHARIS VESICATORIA *(spanish fly)*

There is anxious restlessness that eventually leads to anger or outrage all through the various symptoms of this remedy—picture a fly buzzing and buzzing about, becoming ever more agitated by the minute. Cantharis is a leading remedy for cystitis, all kidney and bladder problems including dribbling urine. Like all insect remedies, there will be burning pain and intense urging. Cantharis is sometimes useful for retained placenta if the keynote restlessness has been present throughout the labor.

CARBO VEGETABILIS *(vegetable charcoal)*

Carbo veg is a remedy for undernourished blood and weakened blood vessels and for states of complete collapse. It should be used during labor if the fetal heart rate slows below normal rates. Carbo veg should be on hand for use immediately following the birth if the keynotes of paleness, cyanosis, collapse state, lethargy, and icy coldness are present in baby. If a very stressed and compromised baby is making any attempt whatsoever to breathe, this remedy can be truly remarkable in stimulating the child to accept life.

Carbo veg can be a wonderful remedy for many complaints of pregnancy such as indigestion and especially anything to do with veins—varicose veins, hemorrhoids, etc. With any ailment which will respond well to Carbo veg, there will be shortness of breath and exhaustion with lack of energy and stamina. Carbo veg is an excellent choice, if other keynotes match, for edema and hemorrhage.

CASTOR EQUI *(rudimentary thumbnail of horses)*

Castor equi acts on the nipples, the nails, and the bones and is useful for cracked or ulcerated nipples, itching of the nipples, weakness of the spine, brittle nails, psoriasis, and pain in the coccyx.

CAULOPHYLLUM THALICTROIDES *(blue cohosh)*

Caulopyhyllum is likely the leading polycrest for late pregnancy and preparing for labor. Caulophyllum is indicated for an exhausted, out-of-tone uterus, either during labor or post-partum and, occasionally, during the later months of pregnancy. This remedy is useful for uterine weakness and the prevention of early miscarriage due to uterine atony. Conditions such as excessive toning contractions in weeks prior to labor, rigid cervix during labor, hemorrhage with no contractions, uterine inertia, lack of progress during labor, and retained placenta in an exhausted mother usually respond well to Caulophyllum.

Caulophyllum is renowned as a labor regulator, especially when alternated with . Caulophyllum is often—should be always—given during the last two weeks of pregnancy as it will likely shorten labor and prevent many unwelcome situations from arising.

Symptoms include painful swollen joints of fingers or toes. The woman is usually nervous, irritable, apprehensive, and easily annoyed.

CAUSTICUM *(Caustic potash)*

Causticum should be considered for uterine inertia during labor. Uterine inertia is keynoted by irregular and insufficient contractions with no bearing down direction to the energy of the contraction. Causticum is also indicated for urinary incontinence or retention of urine due to lax bladder muscles or for the holding urine for too long during labor. Outside of childbirth, this is a remedy for any muscle paralysis, including Bell's palsy and similar conditions.

Women needing this remedy feel great sympathy for the suffering of others. Another keynote of Causticum is the improvement of all symptoms when cold drinks are given.

CHAMOMILLA VULGARIS *(German chamomile)*

Chamomilla vulgaris is one of the leading remedies for infants and children. Chamomilla is useful for infant jaundice with irritability, colic with arching of the back accompanied by kicking and screaming, teething problems with fever, and many other common complaints. An unusual keynote is fever with one cheek red and hot, the other cheek pale and cold. Children, especially when ill, wake often during the night and symptoms are worse in late evening.

A laboring woman will be hyper-sensitivite to pain—labor seems intolerable while still in early stages and often becomes unproductive. The woman will be restless, impatient, wanting attention but never satisfied, whiny, and having a lot of low back pain. This remedy is often helpful with headaches brought on by stimulant withdrawal and for many other types of headaches also.

CHELIDONIUM MAJUS *(greater celandine)*

This is a major organ and venous remedy, specific especially to the gall bladder and liver. Imbalance in these areas leads to irritability and outbursts of temper. There is often a desire to weep without any reason and a great need for sleep but sleep is un-refreshing to them. Other important keynotes for women during pregnancy or during labor are headache with nausea and vomiting and pain under the right scapula.

Chelidonium is indicated for persistent jaundice in a newborn and for babies who do not nurse well, exhibit poor muscle tone, and are abnormally sleepy.

CHINA OFFICINALIS *(peruvian bark)*

The chronic picture of this remedy in childbirth is extreme and prolonged fatigue following a difficult labor or birth or following a delivery which involved loss of blood or fluids resulting in shock. Symptoms, during the labor, include a dislike of being touched and sensitivity to noise. Shock, should it occur, will be from loss of body fluids and have the basic symptoms of cold sweat, weakness, paleness, ringing in the ears, thready pulse, and very low blood pressure.

CIMICIFUGA RACEMOSA *(black cohosh)*

Cimicifuga is a polycrest, alternating with Caulophyllum, during labor for lack of progress with erratic contractions and pains appearing in varied locations and for retrogression in dilation of cervix during labor. Emotional symptoms include foreboding, especially if there were previous difficult labors, anxiety, even hysteria.

CINNAMONUM CEYLANICUM *(cinnamon tree)*

Some of the keynotes of this remedy include weak or false labor pains, spasms or fainting, severe, bright red hemorrhage after only a few pains in first-time mothers, placenta previa, lax tissue, poor circulation, and—importantly—hemorrhage a few days after delivery that is passive and unaccompanied by pain.

COCCULUS INDICUS *(Indian cockle)*

Some keynote symptoms of Cocculus, present during pregnancy or at any time, include nausea aggravated by motion and motion sickness, nausea accompanied by vertigo, and sensitivity to smells or the thought of food. In labor, the cervix is rigid. Other keynote symptoms include insomnia, un-refreshing sleep that is interrupted by dreams with all symptoms greatly aggravated by even the slightest bit of sleep deprivation (a vicious cycle). There are often headaches that are made worse for the motion of riding in a car.

COFFEA CRUDA *(unroasted coffee)*

Keynote symptoms include being nervous, fearful, hypersensitive to noise or vibration, having thoughts that race about with an overactive mind, and being awakened by the slightest noise.

Labor pains will seem agonizing and often be felt, intensely, in the back and along the sciatic nerve. There is a decreased milk supply due to excitement and nervousness.

COLCHICUM AUTUMNALE *(meadow saffron)*

The most frequent use of Colchicum in pregnancy is for nausea with great sensitivity to odors. The mother will also complain about achiness in her joints when moving and will usually be found lying quite still as far away from the smell of food as possible. Along with nausea, there may be abdominal distension, gas, vomiting, diarrhea. Colchicum may be a useful remedy for toxemia with protein in the urine, edema, joint pains, and headaches with all symptoms appearing to have an underlying problem with the kidneys.

With this remedy there is a particular aversion to meat, eggs, and fish. Even the thought of food, or having to prepare food, is nauseating and distressing. Symptoms are often accompanied by internal coldness, great exhaustion, feelings of depression, irritability, discontent, and peevishness.

COLOCYNTHIS *(bitter cucumber)*

One of the principle uses of this remedy is for an infant with colic that can only find relief if lying facedown on the parent's knees and having the firm pressure of a hand placed on his back. There are several instances where the colic seemed to be tied to the mother having ingested milk products. The giving of the remedy to the baby as needed with each instance resulted in the colic episodes disappearing in a few weeks regardless of whether or not the mother drank milk or ingested foods containing milk products.

CONIUM MACULATUM *(poison hemlock)*

During labor and delivery there will be vertigo, exhaustion, sensitivity to light, with spasmodic contractions that accomplish little good. Retained placenta, after pains moving from left to right when baby nurses.

Keynotes of this remedy, in general or during pregnancy and labor, are great dizziness that is worse for lying down and moving the head or eyes even slightly, urine flows in stops and starts, heartburn, face may become bluish or reddish-yellow, ringing in the ears, and indifference.

CROCUS SATIVUS *(saffron)*

Movements of fetus are violent and painful to the mother and there is a sensation of rolling or bounding of the baby in the uterus. Crocus sativus is a remedy for miscarriages, effective when the presenting blood is black and stringy with the tails of the clots adhering to symptoms. Crocus sativus is also effective for retained placenta with ice-cold extremities and hemorrhages coming in dark, large, stringy clots. Palpitations with anxiety.

General symptoms include hysteria, alternation of sudden anger with talking and laughing, dry eyes that burn, weakness in knees and legs, and obstinate constipation. Physical symptoms rapidly change sides and mental symptoms alternate from one extreme to the other, and there is great forgetfulness.

ERIGERON CANADENSIS *(fleabane)*

Symptoms of this remedy include weak uterus, bright red hemorrhage early and/or late in labor due to uterine atony, and characteristic very profuse flow of bright red blood that comes in a great gush and then stops temporarily but begins again—alarmingly—with the slightest movement. There is pallor and weakness due to loss of blood and often great irritation of the rectum and bladder.

Painful urination which sometimes comes with blood in the urine, congestion in the head with red face and nosebleed, fever, and violent vomiting are other conditions that, when seen, would respond well to this remedy.

FERRUM PHOSPHORICUM *(phosphate of iron)*

This remedy increases the capacity of the blood to carry oxygen by improving the absorption of iron. Ferrum is an excellent remedy for re-building hemoglobin after hemorrhage or during pregnancy. More general symptoms include anemai, fever, headache, vomiting of undigested food, and sour belchings.

GELSEMIUM SEMPERVIRENS *(yellow jasmine)*

Gelsemium is a wonderful remedy for dysfunctional labor with failure to dilate because of a thick and rigid cervix. Dysfunctional labors usually end with great fatigue which includes weakness with trembling, especially of the legs. (Oh, how I remember that!) The pain of Gelsemium contractions moves up and down the back. Gelsemium is one of the best remedies that I know of for retained urine after delivery.

Outstanding and definitive emotionals that indicate the need for this remedy include performance anxiety in either the mother or the midwives. (Yes, the midwives can take a dose too if the tenseness of the situation is creating anxiety in them.) The urge to push the baby out is absent and the baby moves upward, instead of downward, with contractions. The mother, or the midwives, may find themselves chattering nervously about inconsequential thing!

GLONOINUM *(nitroglycerine)*

Symptoms that may occur during pregnancy include headache, congestion of blood to head and chest, and eclampsia with urine that is copious and albuminous. Headache is often a problem during labor with the headache appearing or becoming intense after profuse hemorrhage. If these symptoms have been seen, a rush of blood to the head with convulsions or unconsciousness may follow delivery of the baby. Glonium, given earlier in the labor, will prevent the appearance of these more serious symptoms later on.

Some general, non labor, symptoms include hot flashes during menopause (a polycrest for this), throbbing in temples that is made worse for walking, veins of the temples become distended, there may be violent irregularities in the circulation with the face becoming deep red, flushed, and hot. Flashes of lightning-like sparks before the eyes and laborious actions of the heart are indications of serious issues.

GOSSYPIUM HERBACEUM *(cotton plant)*

Pregnancy and labor symptoms include morning sickness with copious saliva that is worse for the slightest motion or for attempting to sit up or get out of bed. This remedy may be useful for a sluggish second stage of labor and retained placenta, especially after a miscarriage or premature delivery.

General symptoms—can be present when pregnant or when not—include frequent desire to urinate, intermittent pain in the ovaries, uterine fibroids with gastric pain, and frequent urination with burning pain. The pains of this remedy jump rapidly from place to place.

GRAPHITES NATURALIS *(black lead)*

Symptoms Graphites are sore, cracked, blistered nipples, sores and eruptions under the breasts and in the arm pits, leucorrhea, tenderness in the abdominal region. These symptoms are more common in overweight women. All symptoms are better for a bout of weeping. There may be obstinacy and moodiness, and hot drinks and sweets will disagree.

Graphites may help with the re-absorption of scar tissue (see also Silica and Thiosinaminum).

HAMAMELIS VIRGINIANA *(witch hazel)*

Hamamelis is a remedy to be considered for physical issues such as venous congestion, varicose veins, varicosities of the vulva, bleeding hemorrhoids, laxness in ligaments and tissues, prolapsed rectum, and nosebleeds. Symptoms of a more emotional nature include being forgetful of words when talking, a tendency to be irritable, depressed, or gloomy. The sadness of Hamamelis is usually based on feeling unappreciated by to others.

HEPAR SULPHURIS CALCAREUM *(calcium sulphide)*

Some symptoms of this remedy include vaginitis with curdish, cheesy, sour smelling discharge, itching and irritation of vaginal tissues, cracked nipples, and mastitis. The person, mom or baby, will tend to be irritable and very sensitive to pain and to being touched. Hepar is useful for conjunctivitis (eye infection) in infants with discharge and redness of the upper eyelid. Pulsatilla is the keynoter remedy for this condition but if Pulsatilla fails or is not indicated because other symptoms do not match the Pulsatilla picture, Helpar sulpuris calcareum should be considred. Symptoms are better for warmth.

HYDRASTIS CANADENSIS *(golden seal)*

The most common use of this remedy is with cracked or retracted nipples or with severe constipation during pregnancy that creates hemorrhoids. Hydrastis, being golden seal in English, has many uses for things that have to do with infection and any condition with mucus present.

HYOSCYAMUS NIGER *(henbane)*

Early symptoms, perhaps indicating trouble coming on, include headache and twitching of facial muscles during labor, cold sweat with a pale, bluish face, eelings of suffocation, and nervous irritability.

More serious symptoms include unconsciousness or loss of sight and hearing during labor or miscarriage, bright red, continuous hemorrhage, jerking and twitching of limbs, delirium, and retained placenta. Great restlessness runs through every symptom and situation with Hyoscyamus niger.

HYPERICUM PERFORATUM *(St. John's wort)*

Hypericum is a polycrest for anything to do with the nerves. Indicated for convulsions from trauma to the head, making it useful for the baby that has experienced shoulder dystocia or some other type of difficult delivery and is a remedy for a broken tail bone or pain in tail bone after delivery. Also useful for pinched nerves in the back, neuralgias, breast disorders, and spinal injuries.

This is an important remedy for trauma to nerve-rich areas of the boy—pains shoot from the site of the injury toward the back of the head. This remedy has often brought relief from pain due to anesthesia that was injected along the spine. The person often uses wrong words when speaking with symptoms arising or worsening following a scare of some sort.

IGNATIA AMARA *(St. Ignatius bean)*

As always Ignatia complaints are characterized by having been brought on by disappointment or grief. There will be weeping, but usually only when alone because sympathy is both unwelcome and likely to make things worse. Symptoms are often contradictory and relieved in unexpected ways.

Symptoms pertaining to pregnancy and childbirth include threatened miscarriage as the result of grief, loss of appetite to the point where the health of both mom and baby are threatened, twitching and spasms of muscles during labor contractions, post-partum depression that is most likely when the birthing experience did not meet the woman's expectations, and decreased milk supply from emotional upset.

IPECACUANHA *(ipecac root)*

Symptoms include nausea from smell of food, great aversion to any type of food, morning sickness with excessive salivation, incapacitating nausea and vomiting, migraine with nausea and vomiting, threatened miscarriage due to extremes of nausea and vomiting with vomit consisting of blood, bile, food, and mucus. The vomiting continues throughout the pregnancy and may even become repeated vomiting during labor. If there is hemorrhage after the birth it will come with more nausea and vomiting. The hemorrhage will be profuse, gushing, and the blood will be bright red.

KALI CARBONICUM *(potassium carbonate)*

Kali carbonicum resembles the picture of Arsenicum album with aggravation in the wee hours of the morning. All symptoms are worse for changes in the weather.

Symptoms seen that are related to the childbearing years include severe backache during pregnancy, labor, or miscarriage, sciatica that is right-sided, backache severe enough to disturb sleep, back labor which radiates to gluteal muscles and upper legs that is relieved by pressure, and post-partum depression with irritability and back pain.

KALI PHOSPHORICUM *(phosphate of potash)*

Kali phos is a nerve remedy and can be useful for women who are very nervous, overly sensitive, in a weakened state, and easily exhausted. All remedies which contain phosphorus are useful for exhaustion due to nervous conditions.

Kali phos symptoms that are seen in women duirng childbearing include exhaustion in labor (frequent, low-potency doses are best here), nervous exhaustion during the early post-partum days, fatigue, headaches, and insomnia.

KREOSOTUM *(beech wood kreosote)*

Symptoms of Kreosotum include offensive, burning, foul-smelling discharges during pregnancy, violent itching of vulva and vagina that occasionally extends to the thighs, and a burning sensation with urination. There is little warning of the need to urinate which creates panic and emotional distress for the woman.

Emotional keynotes include willful and obstinate and insisting that all is well when, in reality, the person is quite sick. There is an unusual layer to this remedy for children. The child often dozes or naps with the eyes half open and, sometimes, while making a moaning sound. This remedy removes that symptom while making a difference with the underlying emotional pattern of willfulness

This remedy is listed in homeopathic Materia Medicas for use with uterine and cervical cancers.

LAC CANINUM *(dog's milk)*

Symptoms include vertigo, headache with blurred vision, nausea, and vomiting. The person craves milk and drinks a lot of it even though it aggravates the digestive system. Mastitis that begins in left breast and then occurs on the right side also. The mastitis may be difficult to treat as it continues to alternate sides instead of clearing up altogether. Symptoms are worse after sleep.

This remedy is used to dry up milk at conclusion of the nursing period but is also used to stimulate milk production when it has fallen off for no known reason. (Remember, these types of opposite reactions are normal in natural medicine.)

Emotional symptoms include despondent, nervous and easily startled, oversensitive, and can't bear to be touched by anything or anyone when not feeling well.

LAC VACCINUM DEFLORATUM *(skimmed cow's milk)*

Symptoms include migraine headaches with visual aura that are worse during pregnancy and during menses, one-sided throbbing frontal headache, nausea during pregnancy that is made worse for motion in cars, boats, or airplanes, constipation, loss of appetite with special aversion to milk, great thirst, and mouth very dry with offensive breath.

Several of the 'Lac' remedies show states of imbalance related to being alone/being with others. This remedy has a pronounced aversion to company—doesn't want to see or talk to anyone. Like Lac canninum, this remedy restores the flow of milk when it has become scanty. Symptoms are worse in the morning and from motion and the person always feels chilly.

LACTUCA VIROSA *(acrid lettuce)*

The dominion of this remedy is for breast feeding disorders (galactagogue) and is reported to have been used successfully to stimulate milk production in adoptive mothers who want to nurse their new baby. Lactuca is useful for some very specific menstrual issues, and for insomnia.

LAUROCERASUS OFFICINALIS *(cherry laurel)*

This is a remedy for very serious resuscitation situations in which a newborn or infant is having difficulty breathing, is gasping for breath, pulse is failing, and the child is turning blue. Laurocerasus is absolutelly amazing for these types of situations. Heart abnormalities may—are likely to—be present. This remedy is used to stabilize the infant, if it is possible to do so, and then transport for medical intervention. I would never want to be without this remedy at a birth, just in case!

LILIUM TIGRINUM *(tiger lily)*

Symptoms include pains extending down into inner thighs, constant pressure in rectum with the desire for a stool, uterine inertia, failure of uterus to fold and harden properly after delivery, uterine prolapse, heavy dragging sensation in hypogastric region, feeling of unusual fullness in chest, and constant pressure on the bladder. After the birth the after pains will hit peak intensity a few days after delivery instead of kicking in immediately as is usual.

Many of these symptoms are present for the woman at times in her life other than pregnancy and labor. The woman, both during labor and when ill, will be very sensitive to the touch of clothing or bed covers.

LOBELIA INFLATA *(Indian tobacco)*

General symptoms of Lobelia include pain through head in sudden shocks, fear of death, violent nausea, profuse sweat which disappears suddenly, and urine that is deep red in color with red sediment.

Lobelia is not a commonly used remedy but has an important place with vagus (pneumogastric) nerve related disorders. (The vagus nerve plays a role in every body system.) The morning sickness for which this remedy would be useful would include some degree of shortness of breath. In labor, the symptoms pertaining to this remedy include a rigid and thick cervix and an inflexible perineum, great shortness of breath with each contraction, violent pains in sacrum and back, shooting pains through whole body, weakness, despondency, and sobbing.

LYCOPODIUM CLAVATUM *(club moss)*

Common symptoms of Lycopodium include food allergies, a large appetite with abdominal pain, gas, and bloating after eating, heartburn, varicosities in the legs which are very painful, gallstones, and kidney problems. The symptoms are usually right-sided symptoms, or symptoms begin on the right and move to the left. Emotional symptoms include indecisiveness and lack of self-confidence.

Lycopodium is a polycrest remedy for infants. Some keynote symptoms are chronic colic and stuffiness of nasal passages, rapid nursing followed by hiccups, jaundice, ***abnormalities in the urogenital tract from birth, including undescended testicles and right-sided hernias***, and very poor absorption and assimilation of nutrients.

MAGNESIA MURIATICA *(Magnesium chloride)*

General emotional symptoms include a deep dislike of any type of confrontation or discord, and overwhelming anxiety. General symptoms include, among others, flatulence, congestive headache, sense of great fatigue in the legs even when sitting, and palpitations that are worse when sitting or lying on left side but better by moving about. Interestingly, other symptoms are often worse when lying on right side.

With Magnesia muriactic contractions of the uterus extend outward to the hips and thighs, severe pain in the back, labor that is interrupted by muscle spasms (rather than effective contractions), the laboring woman becomes hysterical from the pain, and labor ceases altogether or pains become very weak.

MAGNESIA PHOSPHORICA *(phosphate of magnesia)*

Mag phos is antispasmodic—and is a major remedy for any complaint that comes with spasms and is often used alternately with Calc phos for leg cramps in pregnancy or in labor. Mag phos benefits the nervous system, ensuring rhythmic contractions during labor. Thois remedy is also used for sciatica, twitching of muscles, and headaches accompanied by stabbing pains. ***Mag phos is especially useful for afterbirth pains, especially those experienced when nursing.***

MEDORRHINUM *(gonorrhea nosode)*

This remedy is nearly always indicated if there is any history of sexually transmitted diseases, or herpes of any type. Other issues treated by Med are chronic sinusitis, vaginitis, or cystitis—with vaginal discharges having a fishy odor, and infertility.

This remedy is the #1 nosode for the sycosis miasm identified by Hahnemann and considered basic to all homeopathic treatment. The emotional symptoms are many, distinctive, and quite deep. Some of them are difficulty concentrating, panic attacks with fear in the dark and fear that someone is behind her, and despair of recovery or returning to a normal state after childbirth,

In infants, the keynote symptom of Med is chronic diaper rash. A distinctive aspect of this remedy is that the infant sleeps in a knee-chest position with the knees drawn up under the body and the baby has thrown off any covers.

MILLEFOLIUM ACHILLEA *(yarrow)*

Sudden, bright red, profuse, constant hemorrhage after childbirth or miscarriage. The blood will be very fluid and without any indication that it is going to clot off ever! Yarrow is suited to any situation where bleeding is sudden, heavy, and bright red. Millefolium is particularly useful in the passing of fibroids but please seek professional help to cope with the bleeding that may (is likely to) occur.

Millefoilim is distinguished from Aconite by the absence of the mental/emotional symptom of restless anxiety.

NATRUM MURIATICUM *(sodium chloride)*

Infertility, excessive dryness and lack of fluids anywhere in the body—too little or too much amniotic fluid, mal-presentation of baby, heartburn, and constipation are a few things for which Nat mur might be suited if these issues present as the result of grief or loss. Nat mur is also a remedy for herpes that is aggravated by stress and fatigue. Coldness of the body that is especially pronounced in the legs and intense cravings for salt are also indicators.

Natrum muriaticum is a polycrest remedy for lack of amniotic fluid and for turning a mal-positioned baby if the emotional patterns fit!

All Natrum remedies have an underlying element/cause that has to do with grief and loss. There is often deep depression and fear of failure and rejection. The mother will be stoic and somewhat walled-off, wanting to be alone with her pain and will be annoyed and even aggravated by consolation from others.

NATRUM PHOSPHORICUM *(phosphate of soda)*

Nat phos is an acid neutralizer, and aids in the assimilation of fats and sugars, making it useful for any condition that is the result of an acidic state of the body or blood. Symptoms include acid indigestion, heartburn, vomiting of sour-smelling material, stiffness and swelling of joints. A strange keynote is a thick yellow coating on the tongue.

NATRUM SULPHURICUM *(sodium sulphate)*

Common symptoms include nausea, gas, bloating, and headache with constipation. As a tissue salt, this remedy affects liver function and regulates the water in the tissues. I suspect it does this in higher potencies also. Because of the effect of this remedy on the liver, it should be looked at seriously whenever there is jaundice in newborns. The trip into the world, leading with one's tiny head, can be traumatic.

Nat mur is a polycrest remedy for head injury and a history of head injury. A head injury can leave a person unusually susceptible to the emotional patterns of this remedy and is something a midwife should be aware of if it applies. Some of those emotional patterns are post-partum depression, feeling overburdened and overwhelmed—life (and this pregnancy) is seen as a struggle. All symptoms are worse for hot, humid weather and there is a craving for sweets.

NITRICUM ACIDUM *(nitric acid)*

Acid remedies always have an underlying element of fatigue and nitricums always have an element of opposing extremes—tension/relaxation, control/abdication of all responsibility, and congestion-holding in/explosion. Some symptoms include anal fissures, hemorrhage, hemorrhoids, the need for a recovery period when having over-indulged in sugar, and tendency to canker sores.

Keynotes can be a fear of death, irritability, pessimism, holding grudges and being unaffected by apologies, vindictive, craves chalk, dirt, and other indigestibles, and loves fat and salt.

NUX VOMICA *(poison nut)*

Nux is a remedy for hard-driving people who feel a lot of stress and need to work too hard. These people are ambitious and competitive, often impatient, fault-finding, and quarrelsome but also easily offended

Other pertinent symptoms include morning sickness, any type of nausea, vomiting, dry heaves, constipation, dull headache from some sort of toxicity, insomnia from chattering mind that grows worse after 3 AM, hypersensitivity to noise and odors, and irritability with spasms in the back.

Constipation and straining in infants who are restless and active is also an indication for this remedy.

OPIUM *(poppy)*

Opium is a resuscitation remedy which, hopefully, you will never see needed. The symptom picture includes obstructed slow respiration, deeply flushed red or purple mottled face, eyes heavy and half closed with pupils constricted and staring, sweaty skin, and twitching limbs. This remedy is also good for constipation or urine retention in a newborn. This is a deep acting remedy—the symptom picture must be a close fit and a low-potency remedy is recommended and, usually, only one dose is required.

PHOSPHORUS *(the element)*

Bleeding gums or nosebleeds during pregnancy, excessive vomiting and diarrhea during pregnancy, hypoglycemia during pregnancy, vomiting in labor if food is taken, profuse,bright red hemorrhage especially in tall, slim women, post surgical vomiting resulting from reaction to anesthesia are a few of the situations for which Phosphorus might prove useful.

Desires salt, ice cream, sweets, very cold drinks, cheese, and chocolate. Becomes very anxious when alone—wants sympathy and is better for comfort, consolation, and other people around her.

An obvious and unusual keynote is that water is often vomited as soon as it gets warm in the stomach.

PHYTOLACCA DECANDRA *(poke root)*

Phytolacca is a glandular remedy with powerful effects on fibrous tissues and the sheaths and fascias of muscles. Phytolacca is a polycrest remedy for recurrent mastitis (consider higher potency). Other issues treated well by Phytolacca are fissured nipples, glandular swellings, intense pain when nursing with pain radiating throughout the body, lumpy, nodular,hard breasts with blocked ducts, and is used for slowing excessive milk flow. Phytolacca follows well or should be used intercurrently with Belladonna or Bryonia.

Some of the emotional patterns of Phytolacca include feeling irritable, restless, and feeling sure that she will die of whatever condition she is currently suffering from.

PLATINUM METALLICUM *(platina metal)*

Symptoms that need Platinum include painful, ineffective labor pains that are mostly on left side, genital area very sensitive, any bleeding will contain hard black clots, retained placenta, localized numbness and coldness.

The emotional symptom picture includes being greatly troubled by past events, wounded pride, being disdainful of others. Platinum emotionals include a lost sense of proportion in emotional areas with an interesting corollary to depth perception problems in physical vision.

PLUMBUM METALLICUM *(lead metal)*

With plumbum there is a tendency to miscarriage because uterine growth and elasticity is insufficient—baby grows fine but uterus does not. This will result in a feeling of constriction (not enough room) in the abdomen with pain being felt from abdomen to backbone

Depression, terrible colic and gastric distress, face pale and yellowish in color (pregnant woman), cramps in the calves, feeling that she must constantly stretch in every direction (which she does), shortness of breath, and jaundice in the newborn are additional parts of the Plumbum symptom picture.

PULSATILLA NIGRICANS *(wind flower)*

Many women fit the Pulsatilla profile during pregnancy, making this one of the truly polycrest remedies. Remember this one, especially for fetal mal-presentations.

Symptoms common to Pulsatilla are nausea later in the day, nausea after eating fatty foods, persistent headaches during pregnancy that usually manifest with nausea, and vaginitis with changeable discharge.

Pulsatilla is used with miscarriage with intense downward pressure—either to stop the spotting or to help carry the miscarriage to completion. Can also help with lack of progress in labor. Post-partum Pulsatilla is useful for hemorrhage which starts and stops repeatedly (usually beginning again when midwife puts her attention elsewhere), weepiness, overabundant milk supply and overactive letdown response, and for cracked nipples with pain down the back or pain moving from place to place. In the child of a mother who is deep into the Pulsatilla picture, breast milk or enlarged breasts in a newborn—male or female (I have seen this) somtimes occurs. The baby may also be prone to conjunctivitis.

If the woman fits the general emotional picture of Pulsatilla—either most of the time or just during this pregnancy—Pulsatillla can be a great help. I have even seen it turn a persistently transverse, post-dates baby and initiate labor in just a few minutes after the remedy was given.

A great number of mild, but annoying and potentially serious conditions, which change or move around the body, being weepy and emotional, and wanting constant reassurance. Symptom are always aggravated by heat, especially by a stuffy room and are better for distraction or going somewhere

PYROGENIUM *(rotten meat pus)*

One of the most important remedies for uterine infection and sepsis. There will be a low fever with rapid pulse or a high fever with a slow pulse. The blood will be dark and offensive-smelling. Pyrogenium infections always include a throbbing headache with body aches—the bed suddenly feels too hard.

This remedy is especially useful for sepsis due to retained placental pieces or for a miscarriage in which tissue is retained and is decomposing. All symptoms of Pyrogenium are better from heat, hot baths, and motion such as rocking.

RHUS TOXICODENDRON *(poison nut)*

The symptoms associated with Rhus tox are often brought on or made worse by exertion, especially if the exercise is done in cold or damp weather with the expected modality of symptoms being better for hot baths, warmth in any form, massage, and movement. There is great apprehension at night, restlessness, inability to stay in one position, and dwelling on unhappy parts of the past.

Other symptoms include insomnia that is worse around midnight, aching in back and joints, sciatica, restless legs at night, stiffness on sitting which gets better as one moves around again, fingers that are swollen and stiff in the morning, threatened miscarriage after exertion, and chilliness after long labor.

This remedy is the only one that I know of—and is very effective—for the temporary paralysis of the lower legs after childbirth that is occasionally seen, This paralysis is more common when the labor and delivery have been conducted with the woman lying flat on her back, causing the weight of the baby to push on the nerve bundle that lies in the small of the back.

RICINUS COMMUNIS *(castor oil bean)*

Ricinus is useful for increasing the milk supply and producing milk in women who have not been able to nurse a baby previously. A keynote symptom is the swelling of the glands auxiliary to the breasts accompanied by pain running down the arms.

Ricinus also has a use in a small percentage of women for persistent nausea, vomiting, and diarrhea accompanied by chilliness. There will be rice water stools (pale, nearly clear, and very liquid) and nearly clear vomit.

RUTA GRAVEOLENS *(garden rue)*

Ruta is not a polycrest remedy but is absolutely essential in the event of a miscarriage (or a history of miscarriage) at seven months. Other symptoms include bleeding that signals an impending miscarriage, prolapsed uterus after delivery, and stiffness in muscles and tendons following an injury.

Keynote emotional symptoms include feelings of intense weakness and despair with sadness and dissatisfaction with life in general and with herself especially. These symptoms are always worse when the woman is tired. Everything is better from rest, especially reclining or lying down, and symptoms become worse from exertion.

SABINA OFFICINALIS *(savine)*

Sabina is useful for completion of a miscarriage with bright red bleeding containing clots (helps clot the blood and assists the folding and clamping of the uterus), retained placenta, and uterine atony

Sabina is also used for a chronic tendency to miscarry in the third month (also use tinctures of false unicorn and lobelia for this). Endometriosis is the source of many uterine problems for the woman.

SAMBUCUS NIGRA *(elder)*

The major use of this remedy is nasal obstruction in a newborn that is so severe it is preventing proper nursing. Other symptoms include cold feet with warm body and perspiration over the whole body except the head. Symptoms are better for motion and when the person is upright.

SANICULA AQUA *(mineral springs)*

This is a constitutional remedy with a wide range of action. It is said to be effective in the treatment of venereal warts and for vaginitis with discharges that smell like old cheese or spoiled fish.

SARSAPARILLA OFFICINALIS/SMILAX OFFICINALIS *(wild licorice)*

Symptoms of Sarsaparilla include cystitis with pain at the close of urination, frequent urge to urinate with burning on urination, and retracted, inverted, or withered nipples.

The emotional patterns of Sarsaparilla include being despondent and gloomy without cause, being overly sensitive and easily offended, and feeling left out of things or even pushed out and unneeded

SECALE CORNUTUM *(ergot of rye)*

Prolonged bearing-down urges without results during labor (except that if the woman is allowed to push too soon there will be swelling of tissues), hemorrhage with flow of dark, thin blood often from a low-lying placenta, continuous oozing of small amounts of thin blood between periods, miscarriage, and nosebleed are a few of the symptoms of Secale's remedy picture.

Contracts the blood vessels and the uterus, particularly the lower segment, and is especially useful for worn and tired multipara (multiple previous pregnancies) women. Internal burning heat with icy coldness externally but the person is better for being uncovered is a keynote symptom.

SEPIA SUCCUS *(cuttlefish ink)*

Sepia is one of the top 3 polycrests for women and is useful for most women at sometime in their lives when the basic, and distinctive, mental and emotional patterns fit. Issues include hormonal imbalances, infertility or miscarriages due to hormonal imbalances, poor muscle tone, uterine prolapse and prolapse of other organs such as the bladder, incompetent cervix, placenta previa, urinary incontinence, and bearing-down sensations in the pelvis as if everything will fall out. Emotionally the woman feels overwhelmed by and resents the demands of family and home. She just wants to be left alone for a few days or weeks.

Some especially important keynotes of Sepia are that the woman has never been well since puberty, pregnancy, weaning, menopause, or taking birth control pills (any major hormone change) with symptoms being better for vigorous exercise—really.

SILICA TERRA *(pure silica)*

Silica stimulates the absorption of scar tissue (see Graphites and Thiosinaminum) and stimulates the body to reject and eliminate foreign objects such as slivers and bit of glass.

Silica is effective for the sore, cracked, ulcerated, difficult to heal nipples of nursing mothers and for breast abscesses with the baby rejecting nursing on that side. Emotional symptoms are easily exhausted, poor assimilation of nutrients, cold and lacking in vital heat even when exercising, and loss of self-confidence.

Symptoms in newborn baby for which Silica is indicated include plugged tear ducts, failure to thrive, especially in premature babies, vomiting of breast milk with weight loss, and infected umbilical area with pus. Most babies who will respond to Silica are chilly and weak

STAPHYSAGRIA *(stavesacre)*

The ailments and emotional symptoms of Staphysagria are tied to abuse (real or perceived) and the anger that the woman feels about it. This anger is sometimes even experienced by the baby as colic each time it nurses. An indication of the woman's anger is that she does not want to be touched, even the necessary amount, during her labor. The woman often takes the role of silent martyr in her family.

Other symptoms include obstructed labor especially in women with a history of abuse and can bevery useful for the trauma of cut or torn tissues during labor, delivery, or C-section. Staphysagria has been know to relieve pain at the incision site even months later. This remedy is useful for post-partum depression manifesting with suppressed anger, for pain as milk begins to flow, colitis, and for backache that is worse in the morning while still lying in bed

SULPHUR *(brimstone)*

Keynotes of Sulphur include complaints that clear out but then relapse,being absent-minded and easily bored, and usually feeling too warm. The ailments of Sulphur are always aggravated by heat. This remedy should be used when a carefully selected, closely matched remedy fails to act as promptly as it should.

Other symptoms requiring treatment with Sulphur include itching and burning skin eruptions of all kinds which are aggravated by heat or taking a bath, diarrhea, frequently interrupted sleep patterns, and toxemia of late pregnancy with edema and hypertension.

SYMPHORICARPOS RACEMOSUS *(snowberry)*

During pregnancy Symphoricarpos may be useful when there is an extreme aversion to all food, persistent nausea and vomiting of pregnancy with the nausea worse from even the slightest motion, a bitter taste in the mouth, and persistent constipation. Symptoms will be better for lying down, especially when lying flat on the back.

THIOSINAMINUM *(mustard seed oil)*

Thiosinaminum dissolves scar tissue (see also Silica and Graphites) and abdominal adhesions caused by endometriosis, and often helps with pelvic inflammatory disease (PID) and keloids.

Thiosinaminum is indicated for chronic ruptured eardrums in children, the formation of calcium deposits on bones of the ears, scarred eardrums or eardrums that thicken causing hearing difficulties.

THUJA OCCIDENTALIS *(arbor vitae)*

Thuja is an efficient hemostatic (stops bleeding) and is indicated if the fetus moves about more violently than seems normal, there is threatened miscarriage in the third month which began with spotting for 4-5 days, and with the bleeding gradually increasing until profuse bleeding and miscarriage occurs.

Never well since a vaccination, history of rapid onset exhaustion often followed by complete prostration, difficulty concentrating, slow speech, self-contempt, and deep depression are a few other common symptoms associated with this remedy.

TRILLIUM PENDULUM *(lamb's quarter)*

Trillium is a remedy for women who habitually hemorrhage after delivery. There will be gushes of blood at the slightest motion with pain in the back and very cold legs.

A keynote of this remedy is dizziness and feeling very faint from the loss of blood. Trillium may also be useful for threatened miscarriage.

TUBERCULINUM BOVINUM *(tuberculosis nosode)*

This is a miasmic remedy often indicated for birth defects, especially those occurring along the midline, the spine, or the palate (examples: hair-lip, extra or missing teeth, or tongue-tied situations). An indication for this remedy is that the baby is born with fine hair along the spine and abnormally long eyelashes.

URTICA URENS *(stinging nettle)*

Urtica urens acts on the breasts, glands, liver, spleen, and genitourinary organs. Urtica is sometimes used to stop the flow of milk when wanting to cease nursing although Urtica can stimulate the milk supply as long as baby is being put to the breast. Urtica is a useful for skin eruptions with sensitivity, itching, and burning. Urtica urens antidotes ill effects of eating shellfish and relieves severe allergic reactions—particularly food allergies, and relieves acute and chronic gout, kidney stones, and fever blisters.

USTILAGO MAYDIS *(corn smut)*

Labor: Cervix is soft and pliable but contractions are insufficient to cause dilation due to uterine inertia and lack of proper uterine tone. Hemorrhage, if it occurs, will likely be dark and continuous but not profuse, or it may be bright red gushes—contradictory symptoms that may be confusing in trying to decide on a remedy. The after pains will be lengthy with much bearing-down sensations.

This remedy is sometimes used in early stages of a miscarriage as a preventative. If that is not possible, it may aid in bringing completion that includes all tissues being passed. Ustilago is also used for bleeding fibroids. Two keynote symptoms are that the eyes feel hot when closed and the face pales suddenly.

This remedy has many symptoms in menstruation and should probably be used much more often than it is. Some of the symptoms include heavy bleeding, light periods with vicarious bleeding from the lungs or the rectum, bleeding between periods with characteristic pain in the left breast, suppressed menses with no obvious cause, and bearing down sensations during the bleeding part of the menstrual cycle.

VERATRUM VIRIDE *(American hellebore)*

Labor: Arterial pulse is full, hard, and quick, blood is congested in head and chest, and a constant burning distress in cardiac region with excessively strong beating of the heart. There is a feeling of impending stroke or convulsion, cold clammy sweat, face is cold and bluish with paleness around the lips and nose, labored breathing, faintness, and even temporary blindness.

The description above indicates a potential crisis situation. Immediate medical attention is advised.

VERATRUM ALBUM *(white hellebore)*

Veratrum symptoms include excessive weakness, weak pulse, violent palpitations, thirst for ice-cold water, cramps in calves, miscarriages accompanied by exhausting diarrhea, and shortness of breath. This remedy is marked by cold sweat on the forehead and great exhaustion. The face may be red when lying down but becomes pale and bluish on rising

VIBURNUM OPULUS *(cramp bark)*

Spasmodic cramping pains with colic, violent cramping of calves and legs, false labor pains during any part of the pregnancy, pains shooting from uterus into the legs and thighs, unable to sit still because of the intensity of the pains, and a tired bruised feeling in the back are some of the symptoms of this remedy.

This remedy is often very useful for women who have had more than one early miscarriage.

VIBURNUM PRUNIFOLIUM *(black haw)*

Viburnum is primarily a remedy for threatened miscarriage, especially for women who have miscarried before or had an early baby who did not survive. Also useful in a labor and delivery situation that has suddenly become dangerous when there is a rupture of membranes (bag of waters) accompanied by a gush of bright red blood. Other alarming symptoms will include partial loss of speech or a low, indistinct voice, partial loss of consciousness, vertigo, and the throat and mouth are very dry

This is a remedy to be used at any time during a pregnancy at the onset of very painful, labor-like pains with terrible cramping of the legs. A second dose should be given if the pains and cramping continue, becoming so severe as to threaten the rupture of the membranes and to bring on a miscarriage. If rupture occurs there will be a keynote and frightening gush of bright red blood.

(Immediate medical attention is required unless labor is far advanced and delivery can be accomplished immediately. If this is a miscarriage situation and bleeding remains heavy, medical attention may also be required.)

Chapter Three

PRENATAL PROBLEMS
INCLUDING
PREGNANCY, CHILDBIRTH, WOMEN'S HEALTH AND INFANTS

Amniotic Fluid Levels

NATRUM MURIATICUM Nat mur is useful when fluid levels are either too great or have become insufficient. The driving emotional patterns of Nat mur are always something to do with grief or loss.

Anemia

FERRUM PHOSPHORICUM This remedy builds hemoglobin and increases the ability of red blood cells to carry oxygen and nutrients to the tissues and to the placenta.

Back Pain

KALI CARBONICUM Kali carb is useful after a difficult birth or following a miscarriage, as much for emotional recovery as for physical return to health.

NUX VOMICA Symptoms include sudden sharp pains when turning, dull pain while sitting, and a bruised feeling in lumbar region. This is a remedy for driven, work-a-holic people who are a bit on the tense side all of the time.

SEPIA SUCCUS This is a very important polycrest remedy for women. There will be sudden stabs of pain causing nausea and a feeling of weakness in the small of the back.

Bearing-Down Sensation in Pelvis

BELLIS PERENNIS The woman feels as if she must support and hold up her belly in order to walk or move about.

SEPIA SUCCUS The feeling is as if everything is about to fall out the bottom. There will need to be the very specific emotional patterns of Sepia for it to be effective in any case.

Bleeding Gums / Nosebleeds

PHOSPHORUS This remedy has a very distinctive emotional pattern of restless anxiety and putting others 'needs before her own which must match for this remedy to be effective

Blood Pressure (high) (see Toxemia)

Braxton Hicks (toning contractions)

CALCAREA PHOSPHORIA A remedy to slow or stop contractions that are the result of calcium deficiency.

CAULOPHYLLUM THALICTROIDES This is an amazing remedy for toning contractions that are very weak and irregular. If these irregular contractions come with bearing-down pains they may be cause for alarm—take this remedy immediately and lie down to rest until the bearing down sensations subside.

MAGNESIA PHOSPHORICA The contractions of Mag phos are more like a muscle cramp spreading sideways than a productive contraction.

Chloasma (mask of pregnancy)

SEPIA SUCCUS This is a polycrest remedy for many situations of pregnancy and women's health because it brings balance to the hormones and tone to sagging tissues.

Constipation

ANACARDIUM ORIENTALE With Anacardium, even a soft stool passes with great difficulty.

CALCAREA CARBONICA Severe constipation that is not uncomfortable is a keynote of Calcarea carb.

LAC VACCINUM DEFLORATUM Very persistent constipation that is accompanied by violent headaches.

NATRUM MURIATICUM Two symptoms of Nat mur here are constipation on alternate days and alternating with diarrhea and the anus becomes torn and bleeds.

NUX VOMICA With Nux there is constant uneasiness in rectum, passing only small quantities of stool with each attempt, itching, and blind hemorrhoids.

SEPIA SUCCUS Sensation of hard ball in rectum, shooting pains, prolapsed rectum or anus, and hemorrhoids.

SYMPHORICARPUS Symphoricarpus is for constipation with disgust at the thought of any food at all.

Fetal Movements (painful)

ARNICA MONTANA There is a sensation of being bruised internally from the baby's motions and the mother often experiences heart palpitations when the baby is in motion.

CROCUS SATIVUS The movements of fetus are violent and painful and there is a sensation of the baby rolling and bounding about in the uterus—more than a sensation, the baby is actually moving a lot.

SEPIA SUCCUS Sepia is keynoted by bearing-down sensations, feelings of being overwhelmed by family responsibilities, and over sensitivity to any pain set Sepia apart.

Food Poisoning

ARSENICUM ALBUM This remedy is for stomach and intestinal sickness from ingesting bad meat, water, vegetables, melons, or fruits, and for nausea from any cause at all where the nausea comes with a sweet taste in the mouth. Sometimes there is vomiting, sometimes not.

CARBO VEGETABILIS With Carbo veg the abdomen is greatly distended, the person is very weak, there is a blue cast to the skin, and they feel very faint.

Gallbladder Pain

CHELIDONIUM MAJUS The symptoms of Chelidonium are the typical symptoms of gallbladder distress with severe pain, vomiting, and headache.

VERATRUM ALBUM Veratrum symptoms include a cold feeling in the stomach, gastric irritability with pain in region of gallbladder, and chronic vomiting of food with great weakness after vomiting.

Headaches

BELLADONNA Belladonna headaches are made worse for stimulants such as caffeine. Headache is often the result of fatigue, and will be better when the mind is occupied. Strangely, the headache is usually worse in the morning when first waking, gets better during the day, then worse again in the late evening.

CHAMOMILLA VULGARIS Chamomilla is most often suitable for delicate, fatigued women. The headache is accompanied by and caused by persistent constipation and the headache that is made worse from caffeine.

LAC VACCINUM DEFLORATUM These are intense migraines with blindness and with coldness all through the body. The headache is most often in the left eye and left temple.

NUX VOMICA Frontal headache from toxicity, drugs, alcohol, or caffeine in intense, hard-working women with an almost driven need to succeed is the picture of the Nux headache.

Heartburn

ARSENICUM ALBUM The heartburn is usually from vinegar, acidic food, ice cream, or ice water. There will be belching of acid which hurts the throat.

CALCAREA CARBONICA The heartburn will come with frequent loud, sour belching and is most common in women who worry over-much about their duties and responsibilities. There is usually a history of difficulty with calcium absorption.

LYCOPODIUM CLAVATUM The heartburn comes with sufficient pressure as to make breathing difficult. The belches rise only to the pharynx and get stuck there.

NATRUM MURIATICUM There is always an element of grief or loss to the symptoms of Nat mur. The heartburn is accompanied by heart palpitations.

NATRUM PHOSPHORICUM Nat phos heartburn is the typical acid indigestion with sour belching after eating and a feeling of great fatigue.

Hemorrhoids

AESCULUS HIPPOCASTANUM Aesculus hemorrhoids may be internal, blind hemorrhoids with bleeding, or the hemorrhoids may be external and made worse by standing and walking.

SEPIA SUCCUS These hemorrhoids produce a sensation of a weight or ball in the anus. They bleed when walking and are very sore.

SULPHUR The hemorrhoids typical of Sulphur ooze fluid all the time, come in great bunches that are sore, tender, raw, burning, and often bleed quite heavily.

Herpes

MEDORRHINUM Medorrhinum is an important nosode but other symptoms need to match the remedy picture closely (as always in homeopathy). There usually has been a poor reaction or a poor result from other remedies that were tried first because they seemed to be a better match. Medorrhinum, being a nosode, is best used inter-currently with another remedy whose picture, mental or emotional, matches very closely the physical and emotional symptoms that the person is experiencing at the moment and in the past.

MERCURIUS SOLUBLIS Open sores, especially in the mouth and throat, enlarged lymph glands, vaginitis with itching, extreme sensitivity to both hot and cold are part of the symptom picture of Mercurius. A keynote is that the person changes their mind constantly and restlessly—changing position and location

NATRUM MURIATICUM The keynote is acute and chronic grief but with a grim determination to survive. The eruptions are worse from stress or emotional upsets.

PHOSPHORUS The basic symptoms of thirst, over-sensitivity to external impressions, noise, odors, and people must be present, along with dryness of mucous membranes. There will always be some degree of fatigue

THUJA OCCIDENTALIS Thuja is marked by excessive growth of warts and eruptions and is a polycrest remedy for anything that has come about as the result of a reaction to vaccination and/or drugs.

Hyperemesis (severe vomiting)

IPECACUANHA The picture of Ipecac includes severe weakness, light-headedness with overactive imagination, and many exaggerated fears and concerns. The woman is usually sickest on waking but feels better after eating a little bit of something.

PHOSPHORUS With phosphorus there is constant nausea with mental confusion, great sensitivity to odors, and cravings for cold things but vomits them as soon as they warm in the stomach.

Insomnia

ARSENICUM ALBUM The sleeplessness is from anxiety and nervous exhaustion.

CALCAREA CARBONICA With Calcarea carb the drowsiness occurs in the early part of the evening and the woman wakes frequently during the night.

CHAMOMILLA VULGARIS The symptoms of Chamomilla include being tired and drowsy but cannot sleep, being sleepless from stimulants like caffeine or chocolate, having anxious frightened dreams, sleeps best with a pillow between the thighs, and sometimes weeps during sleep without realizing it.

COCCULUS INDICUS Sleepless from mental or physical exertion, anxious frightful dreams, sleep frequently interrupted by startling awake, slightest loss of sleep irritates and makes other symptoms worsen, and constant drowsiness after slight loss of sleep are all part of the Cocculus picture.

COFFEA CRUDA A person needing Coffea sleeps well until 3 am but then only dozes afterwards. The sleeplessness is from the incessant flow of thoughts and ideas.

IGNATIA AMARA Ignatia symptoms arise from grief, worry, anxious thoughts, relationship or business cares. The person has the same nightmares over and over again, night after night.

KALI CARBONICUM Waking about 2 am and having difficulty sleeping again with the result that there is extreme sleepiness during the day is the classic picture of Kali carb insomnia.

NUX VOMICA Nux people are always better for taking a nap! They are sleepless from the rush of ideas or from mental strain. They often awaken about 3 am and lay awake the rest of the night.

RHUS TOXICODENDRON Restless sleep with much tossing about trying to get comfortable, dreams of great effort and exertion, dreams of working hard at daily tasks, waking feeling stiff and sore and sometimes with heart palpitations. Stretching relieves the stiffness and palpitations.

SULPHUR The sleep patterns of Sulfur includes such things as sleeps in catnaps, drowsy during the day but wakeful at night, and having many vivid dreams. The woman is particularly wakeful from 3 to 5 am.

Itching of the Skin (Pruritis)

APIS MELLIFICA Apis is an insect remedy so automatically comes with burning no matter what other things may be going on. Some symptom are hives and skin rashes with burning and stinging. Apis symptoms are always worse at night.

RHUS TOXICODENDRON Rhus tox is effective for many types of skin rashes and eruptions while being of benefit for any nerves involved—a true polycrest.

SULPHUR With Sulphur there is unhealthy skin with every little injury becoming infected. The burning sensation created by the rash becomes worse from scratching and from any type of warmth.

URICA URENS This remedy is for itching with raised, red blotches. The itching is often accompanied by joint pain.

Joints Stiff or Painful

CALCAREA PHOSPHORICA The pain of Calcarea phos is located in the symphysis pubis.

CIMICIFUGA RACEMOSA This is a polycrest remedy for displaced labor pains going to the hips and thighs. It is also useful for stiffness and contraction of the muscles in the neck and back.

IGNATIA AMARA With Ignatia, the joints feel dislocated, the back is stiff with sciatic pains that worsen during labor, violent sacral pains

NATRUM PHOSPHORICUM Swelling of joints, especially fingers or toes, legs give way when the mother attempts to walk about. Be sure to match with the basic emotional patterns of this remedy.

NATRUM SULPHURICUM The pain for which Nat sulp is indicated is in the hip joints and is worst when rising or sitting down.

RHUS TOXICODENDRON Rhus to is indicated when there is stiffness in nearly all joints with the stiffness being better for warmth, motion, and massage. There is audible cracking of the joints when stretching. Sciatic pain often responds well to this remedy.

RUTA GRAVEOLENS Ruta grav is specific for knees that are weak and give out when walking up stairs. There is aching but with great restlessness that prevents the stillness needed for healing.

Leg Cramps

The following two remedies are often used alternately with each other

CALCAREA PHOSPHORICA Calcarea phos is indicated when there is stiffness and pain with coldness and numbness. The legs become very weary when going upstairs.

MAGNESIA PHOSPHORICA With Mag phos there are shooting pains in nape of the neck and in the lower part of the back. There is stiffness of all of the joints.

Malpresentation of the Baby

PULSATILLA NIGRICANS Pulsatilla will turn a breech or transverse baby about 40% of the time. This is probably because about 40% of these situations are out-of-balance hormones and emotions in ways that match a Pulsatilla emotional picture.

CARBO VEGETABILIS Carbo veg often corrects an abnormal presentation if the rest of the picture matches. Important emotional symptoms include a strange mix of indifference to things usually loved but anxiety on waking in the morning.

NATRUM MURIATICUM Nat mur balances the fluid levels (either too much or too little amniotic fluid) which may be contributing to either failure of the baby to remain in correct position or inability to turn to a proper position.

Check the symptom picture of the polycrest pregnancy remedies against the woman's other symptoms and proceed with the best match.

Morning Sickness

ANACARDIUM ORIENTALE The Anacardium picture includes nausea in the morning that is better for getting a little food into the stomach. The woman feels better after eventually vomiting and the giving of Anacardium may produce the result in order for the woman to feel better.

ARSENICUM ALBUM The nausea of Arsenicum in pregnant women comes with burning pain in the stomach and a complete aversion to the sight or smell or thought of food

CARBO VEGETABILIS Nausea with chest pain, distension of abdomen, and shortness of breath are characteristic of the morning sickness made better by Carbo veg.

COCCULUS INDICUS Nausea aggravated by motion sickness, nausea with vertigo, sensitivity to smells or the thought of food are some of the many types of nausea found in the Cocculus symptom picture.

COLCHICUM AUTUMNALE Colchicum morning sickness includes nausea from odors, icy coldness of the stomach, sometimes even swallowing their own saliva causes vomiting and the nausea get worse from the slightest motion.

IGNATIA AMARA With Ignatia, the morning sickness is always connected to suppressed grief or disappointment.

KALI MURIATICUM Fatty or rich foods cause nausea, morning sickness with vomiting of white phlegm, and nausea and vomiting with shivering are indications for Kali mur.

LAC VACCINUM DEFLORATUM Nausea and vomiting with a sensation of deathly illness and incessant vomiting with no relation to eating are keynotes of Lac Vaccinum.

LYCOPODIUM CLAVATUM The Lycopocium picture includes vomiting first of undigested food—sour and acidic—then of bitter tasting water. The nausea and vomiting are made worse by motion of cars.

NATRUM SULPHURICUM Green bilious vomiting with bitter taste in the mouth, acid indigestion, frequent hiccups after eating breads and pastries are keynotes of Nat sulph.

NUX VOMICA The Nux picture includes nausea and vomiting every morning with great sensitivity to pressure in region of the stomach, region of the stomach very sensitive to the pressure of clothing, and cramps in stomach after eating especially in the morning.

PULSATILLA NIGRICANS Vomiting after fruits, fats, pastry, ice cream, or iced drinks, vomiting with pale face and chilliness, and vomiting of food eaten long before due to insufficiency of the digestion are keynotes of the Pulsatilla picture.

SEPIA SUCCUS Nausea, vomiting, and bloated abdomen after eating. The vomiting of Sepia typically occurs in the late afternoon or evening, rather than in the morning—was certainly this way for me and I do wish I had known about Sepia in those days.

SYMPHORICARPOS RACEMOSA Nausea worse from even the slightest motion, bitter taste in the mouth, persistent morning sickness, and averse to all food with the smell and thought of food very repugnant and causes immediate nausea and vomiting are part of the Symphoricarpos picture.

Phlebitis (swelling caused by a blood clot)

ACONITUM NAPELLUS Aconite is a useful emergency and first-response remedy—consider Byonia alba as a follow-up.

BELLADONNA The onset of anything Belladonna will be sudden and the area will always be red and hot to the touch.

BRYONIA ALBA With Bryoinia, the heart and circulation are profoundly affected. Bryonia is not as rapid in its effects as Aconitum but is deeper. Bryonia is often used as a follow-up remedy to Aconitum.

CARBO VEGETABILIS This resmedy is useful as a "kick-start" when there is lack of reaction to chosen remedies. It's picture with phlebitis is very general.

HAMAMELIS VIRGINIANA This is witch hazel and the principal action of this remedy is on venous congestion, blood clots, varicose veins, hemorrhoids, and hemorrhages Hamamelis is often the best choice for this condition.

PULSATILLA NIGRICANS The Pulsatilla picture includes pain in the extremities that is worse from letting the affected part hang down and there may be numbness or pulsations throughout the whole body.

CALCAREA CARBONICA As always with Calcarea carb there has been cravings for indigestibles such as dirt, chalk, coal, pencils, usually caused by a nutritional deficiency or the inability to absorb nutrients. The plebitis is usually from insufficient nutrition and from the stress on the kidneys from the ingestion of these things.

NITRICUM ACIDUM Like Calcarea carb, there are cravings for indigestible, non-food items. Along with the phlebitis there are keynote symptoms of anxiety about health, pessimism, the holding of grudges, vindicative, being headstrong and irritable. These symptoms must be present for the remedy to be effective.

Prolapse—Rectal

RUTA GRAVEOLENS Before actual prolapse there may be a pulling sensation felt in the back which is aggravated by sitting and relieved by hot baths. The sooner the Ruta is given, the better will be the results.

Prolapse—Uterine

SEPIA SUCCUS This polycrest remedy is the first thing to reach for whenever there is heaviness or bearing-down sensations in the pelvic organs. Sepia has no equal in the treatment of uterine prolapse.

Prolapse—Umbilical Cord

No known homeopathic solution

The birth attendant must, with sterile hands and arms, coil the umbilicus and place as much of it as possible inside the vaginal vault. This is best done with the mother in a knee/chest position. The cord must be kept moist by the application of wet towels until the baby can be delivered. Transport should be immediate. This is a life-threatening situation for the baby.

Restless Legs

RHUS TOXICODENDRON Numbness and prickling sensation that affects sleep will often be helped by Rhus tox.

Scar Tissue / Stretch Marks

CALCAREA FLUORATA Calcarea fluorata helps dissolve scar tissue, has been effective even when the tissue is raised and stony hard, and may prevent scar tissue forming at tear and incision sites.

GRAPHITES NATURALIS This remedy is particularly effective on old scars that are raised, oozing, or ulcerated.

SILICA TERRA Silica promotes the expulsion of dead or scarred tissue—literally brings it to the surface and causes it to sluff off. It may take a little bit of patience to obtain the results wanted.

THIOSINAMINUM Thiosinaminum is for wounds that have formed a lot of scar tissue and granulations and is useful for lack of elasticity in injured skin. If tears or surgical scars occur, Thiosinaminum might be tried as a preventative to scar formation.

Sciatica

CIMICIFUGA RACEMOSA This remedy is a polycrest for the childbearing years and is the most effective remedy known for labor pains that displace to the hips, thighs, back, and legs, and are violent and shooting.

COFFEA CRUDA The person needing Coffea is intolerant of pain and despairing of it ever getting any better. The sciatica is worse for motion and worsens in the afternoon and evening and is accompanied by restlessness and sleeplessness at night.

KALI BICHROMICUM Kali bi is for left-sided sciatica that is better for motion or from stretching the legs but is made much worse by standing or lying in bed

KALI CARBONICUM Withe Kali carb it feels like the lower back is broken. The person must lie down or lean on something to relieve the pain.

RHUS TOXICODENDRON The sciatica of Rhus tox is worse for cold, damp weather and gets worse at night. The pain is much relieved by warmth and by exercise.

Shortness of Breath (dyspnea)

CALCAREA CARBONICA The shortness of breath is caused by the constriction of the lungs from the distension of the abdomen created by gastric gas and bloating.

CARBO VEGETABILIS In the materia medicas, Carbo vegetabilis, often thought of as a digestive remedy, has more symptoms under lung than under any other body system including the digestion.

Sugar in the Urine

PHOSPHORUS Phosphorus profoundly affects the nutrition and function of all tissues and cells and is an organ and endocrine system remedy.

PULSATILLA NIGRICANS Pulsatilla is a polycrest hormone and endocrine remedy.

Toxemia

APIS MELLIFICA Stinging pains, localized swelling with redness and heat, thirstlessness, intolerance of heat, and slow or nonexistent urination are some of the symptoms of Apis. Natrum muriaticum is complementary to Apis and should be considered for use at the same time.

COLCHICUM AUTUMNALE A few symptoms of Colchicum include kidney failure with high uric acid content in the blood, swelling and coldness of legs and feet, depressed, irritable, and peevish

NUX VOMICA A few symptoms are paralysis of bladder leading to uric acid poisoning, headache from toxicity, varicose veins. Look for the very definite mental picture of Nux as symptoms need to match, of course.

SULPHUR Symptoms of Sulphur include hypertension, edema, proteinuria, great thirst, and excessive heat production throughout the body. Mental/emotional symptoms of a sensitive, excitable, and impressionable personality must be present.

Urinary Tract Infections

APIS MELLIFICA Apis is keynoted by urine that is scanty or suppressed or urine may be profuse—much more than fluid intake accounts for. In either case, urine has deep color and causes burning.

CANTHARIS VESICATORIA With Cantharis the urine is burning with cutting pains and intolerable urging. It passes drop by drop, dribbling and bloody.

CAUSTICUM Paralysis of bladder and retention of urine after labor, and involuntary passage of urine when coughing, sneezing, and walking are the primary keynotes of Causticum.

LYCOPODIUM CLAVATUM Pain in the back before urinating, retention of urine, and hot urine with heavy red sediment are some of the urinary tract symptoms of Lycopodium.

MEDORRHINUM After stooping, there is violent pain in region of kidneys on rising. Urine flows very slowly and may be either colorless or intensely yellow with Medorrhinum.

SARSAPARILLA OFFICINALIS Pain from right kidney spreading downward and gravel in the kidneys are seen when Sarsaparilla is needed.

Vaginitis

HEPAR SULPHURIS CALCAREUM This picure is vaginitis with curdish, cheesy, sour smelling discharge, and itching and irritation of vaginal tissues.

HYDRASTIS CANADENSIS The vaginitis of Hydrastis comes with thick, ropy discharge and intense itching which is relieved, strangely, by intercourse.

KALI BICHROMICUM Itching and burning with thick, stringy, tough, yellow-green mucous keynote the vaginitis of Kali bichromicum.

KREOSOTUM With Kreosotum, there is offensive, burning, foul-smelling discharges with violent itching of vulva and vagina. The itching sometimes extends to the inner thighs. There is a keynote of needing to urinate whenever she hears water running or puts her hands in water.

MEDORRHINUM Intense itching, discharges have the characteristic fishy odor associated with Medorrhinum with the symptoms made better by bathing in lukewarm water.

NATRUM MURIATICUM Natrum mur is useful for genital herpes that is made worse by stress and for general burning and dryness of vaginal tissues.

NATRUM SULPHURICUM With Nat sulph there are herpes-type eruptions, with yellow-green mucous. The vaginal symptoms are accompanied by hoarseness in the throat.

PULSATILLA NIGRICANS Vaginal discharge with swollen vulva, pain in the lower back, and great exhaustion are the Pulsatilla vaginitis picture. Other unique Pulsatilla mental and emotional symptoms should be present.

SANICULA AQUA Venereal warts and vaginitis with discharges that smell like old cheese or spoiled fish are the keynotes here.

SEPIA SUCCUS There is much swelling of vaginal tissues with intense itching of the vulva in the Sepia picture. The emotional keynoteof annoyance with family responsibilities should be present.

Varicosities

CALCAREA CARBONICA Calcarea carb types tend to fibroids, cysts, polyps in the kidneys, prolapse of the anus with burning, and stinging, and hemorrhoids which are painful when walking but better sitting.

CARBO VEGETABILIS With Carbo veg, the varicosities are usually burning, bluish-white hemorrhoids which cause great pain during and after a stool.

HAMAMELIS VIRGINIANA Vague discomfort with mild symptoms of congestion, heaviness, swelling, or soreness in veins of the lower body including the rectum are keynotes of Hamamelis. This is the best remedy, in low potency, if other distinctive symptoms are lacking—follow with appropriate remedy as the symptoms are clarified by the taking of this remedy.

LACHESIS MUTA A Keynoted of lachesis is that the constriction of clothing irritates the veins. There is sensitivity to touch in genital areas, symptoms are often left-sided and are aggravated by sleep and made better for being up and walking about.

PULSATILLA NIGRICANS Pulsatilla is known for the wide variety of varicose veins and hemorrhoids. Look for the distinctive mental and emotional symptoms.

SEPIA SUCCUS Varicose veins with related Sepia symptoms of bearing-down sensation in pelvis and rectum, ambivalence and annoyance at family responsibilities, and always better for exercise are the types of varicosities that will be helped by Sepia.

Chapter Four
MISCARRIAGES

Miscarriages—Threatened and the Prevention of Miscarriages

ACONITUM NAPELLUS Aconite is for threatened miscarriage following a scare or a miscarriage manifesting with fright, anxiety, and great restlessness. The pains will be shooting, sharp, and centered deep in the uterus. There will probably be great fear of her own impending death as well as very low tolerance for and despair at the pain.

ARNICA MONTANA Arnica is for threatened miscarriage following a fall or accident. Contractions may be weak and lead one to believe that all will be fine. Arnica will help with the soreness or bruising of the fall—there is no reason not to use this remedy following a trauma when pregnant, just in case.

ARSENICUM ALBUM Arsenicum is used as a complementary remedy, in low potency, if there is extreme anxiety, exhaustion, restlessness, and fear of death. Look for the characteristic digestive disturbances.

CAULOPHYLLUM THALICTROIDES Caulophyllum should be considered when contractions are sharp, spasmodic, very low in pelvis with excessive weakness, fatigue, and trembling. This remedy is also for use in the completion stage to expel placental tissue and can be used as a preventative if there is a history of miscarriage due to lack of uterine tone.

CHINA OFFICINALIS CINCHONA Excessive loss of blood, with chilliness, thirst, faintness, and shock, and low or absent blood pressure preceded by a rapid and thready pulse are keynotes of China. It is also indicated for extreme and prolonged fatigue following a miscarriage.

CIMICIFUGA RACEMOSA Cimicifuga symptoms include lack of uterine tone with jerky, uncoordinated uterine spasms. The pain radiates across the abdomen from hip to hip. There is an emotional black cloud coloring everything with feelings of gloom and dejection.

IGNATIA AMARA Ignatia always includes a history of grief or disappointment. The symptoms will present with a contradictory pattern. This may be a follow-up remedy, helping the mother to cope with the loss and disappointment of the miscarriage. An appropriate remedy to the original cause and picture, not including the grief and loss, should have already been given.

IPECACUANHA Ipecac contractions will be centered at the navel and travelling inward. The bleeding will be profuse and bright red—coming in either gushes or a steady flow and be accompanied by headache.

PULSATILLA NIGRICANS Pulsatilla is indicated by the rapid changing of the symptoms and by the usual distinctive mental/emotional picture.

RHUS TOXICODENDRON Rhus tox should be considered for miscarriage from a strain, from lifting, or overexertion. The pains often begin as back pain late at night or in the early morning hours and soon feel as if one is being torn asunder. The woman will find she cannot rest comfortably in any position.

RUTA GRAVEOLENS Ruta miscarriages begin with slight bleeding at irregular intervals as a forerunner of a miscarriage. A miscarriage that Ruta will be indicated for often occurs around the seventh month.

SABINA OFFICINALIS Consider Sabina for excessive and painful uterine bleeding of any kind.

Miscarriage contractions of Sabina extend from the sacrum to the pubis, at regular intervals, with the gushing of clots and tissue. Sabina may be useful for prevention if a miscarriage of this description has occurred sometime previously and it is given at the first sign of trouble.

SEPIA SUCCUS Use Sepia for threatened or incomplete miscarriage where there is the characteristic sensation of heaviness or bearing-down. There will usually be nausea and irritability.

SECALE CORNUTUM The miscarriages of Secale usually occur about the third month.

VIBURNUM PRUNIFOLIUM Very painful, labor-like pains with terrible cramping of the legs are typical of Viburnum at odd times during the pregnancy. There is cause for concern if the pains become severe enough to threaten the rupture of the membranes (bag of waters) and to bring on a miscarriage. If rupture occurs there will be a gush of bright red blood. Immediate medical attention is advised because the bright red blood indicates a problem with the blood already seen being the only indication of a compromised cord or placental site. There is never a good reason for blood at this stage although some causes are worse and more dangerous to the baby than others.

Miscarriages—Chronic Tendency to Miscarry

CAULOPHYLLUM THALICTROIDES Caulophyllum is indicated for women who have habitually miscarried from lack of uterine tone. The woman may have had several children or may be a younger woman who is simply out-of-shape.

RUTA GRAVEOLENS The habitual miscarriages of Ruta typically occur at seven months, possibly from a combination of hormonal imbalance and lack of uterine tone.

SABINA OFFICINALIS Often a history of bleeding between periods and/or a copious amount of vaginal discharges precede this type of miscarriage.

SEPIA SUCCUS Sepia is the leading polycrest remedy for women and is useful when the other symptoms of the Sepia picture have been present. These symptoms include never really well since puberty or childbirth, heaviness and bearing-down sensations as if everything is going to fall out through the vagina, ambivalence toward family or annoyance at the demands of family life upon her time. .

Miscarriage—To Assist Completion

See previous section for ***Aconitum napellus, Arnica montana, Caulophyllum thalictroides, Pulsatilla nigricans, Sabina officinalis and Sepia succus*** picture descriptions. These remedies, while often preventing a miscarriage by correcting the underlying problem, also effectively assist the body in the completion of the miscarriage should that outcome be unavoidable. Clean bleeding away of placental tissue, cord, and conceptus are necessary if septicemia is to be avoided.

BELLADONNA With Belladonna there will be profuse flow of hot blood usually accompanied by twitching and jerking of muscles.

CANTHARIS VESICATORIA This is a remedy for retained urine and a urinary tract infection following a miscarriage. There will be dribbling of urine with burning pain.

CONIUM MACULATUM The Conium picture includes vertigo, exhaustion, muscular weakness, and ringing in the ears.

GOSSYPIUM HERBACEUM Gossypium should be considered when there is retained placenta or pieces of placenta following a miscarriage. There is usually back pain and a dragging pain in the pelvis.

KALI CARBONICUM This remedy is for use when there is impending miscarriage with pains moving from back into buttocks and thighs. After miscarriage there will be great weakness and pain in the back.

Chapter Five

PREPARATION FOR LABOR AND DELIVERY

Polycrest Female Remedies

Natrum muriaticum, Pulsatilla nigricans, and ***Sepia succus*** are the leading polycrest remedies for women during pregnancy. Care-givers and pregnant women should make themselves very familiar with the symptom pictures of these three remedies, especially as they relate to pregnancy.

Many women will display the symptoms of Pulsatilla during pregnancy. This pattern will usually be seen in the mental and emotional realms first and happens even when this insecure, changeable pattern is not at all who they are when not pregnant. The hormones of pregnancy which create the laxness of tissues that allows for uterine and abdominal growth often move out of balance and create the physical (and emotional) symptoms of the Sepia picture.

The Pulsatilla hemorrhage or Sepia's uterine prolapse may be prevented if remedies are given during the pregnancy when the mental and emotional symptoms first present themselves. Using homeopathic remedies in this way may prevent a multitude of woes and will have done no harm, especially when prescribed on early, mild, presenting symptoms. Since it is impossible to walk two roads at once (one where the remedies were given and one where they were not), it is impossible to compile dramatic evidence of positive results for the practice of the art of prevention.

Suggested Remedies for the Final Weeks Before Delivery

CAULOPHYLLUM THALICTROIDES Caulophyllum aids the body in producing oxytocin, encourages regular contractions with effective downward expulsive force, and may relieve excessive pre-labor toning or false labor contractions.

CIMICIFUGA RACEMOSA Cimicifuga is excellent for fear of labor and delivery. It complements the action of Caulophyllum, especially for women with a past history of dysfunctional labor and a fear of the upcoming one.

ARNICA MONTANA Arnica, in low potency, prevents excess blood loss, shock, and excessive trauma to soft tissues and should certainly be considered if there is fear of the coming labor based on past traumatic experiences.

Chapter Six

LABOR
ONSET THROUGH SECOND STAGE
(Full Dilation of Cervix)

Anger/Irritability

CHAMOMILLA VULGARIS The symptoms of chamomilla include irritable, whining, discontented, demanding, and extremely sensitive to pain. The woman may be cross, rude, quarrelsome, obstinate, and express dissatisfaction with everything and everyone around her and everything being done for her.

NUX VOMICA A woman who would benefit from Nux is very irritable, offended by every harmless word, cannot bear noises, odors, light, being touched, or having music played to soothe her. The laboring mother will be headstrong, very self-willed, angry and impatient, especially when interrupted or spoken to.

STAPHYSAGRIA This remedy is often tied to humiliation, abuse, deep grief, or shame. There are times of violent, passionate outburst, but there is always anger just under the surface, even when she appears quite calm. She may alternate between gloomy and morose, and fits of anger—including throwing things—during the labor and will be morbidly sensitive and self-pitying.

Labor

Anxiety

ACONITUM NAPELLUS The Aconitum symptoms picture includes nightmares, phobias, and panic attacks. Fear of the future, often with a particular fear of death, will make labor an unpleasant experience unless the fear can be brought into perspective. This remedy may help with those emotions. There is also often a special fear of doctors and fears that she cannot possibly endure the pain. There will almost always be restlessness and the need to be doing something besides just waiting out the labor.

ARSENICUM ALBUM The laboring woman will be extremely nervous and anxious and will be continually changing body positions. She will be expressing, constantly, a fear that something is going to go wrong or that she is going to die.

CIMICIFUGA RACEMOSA Gloom and dejection with a black cloud of negativity over everything characterizes Cimicifuga. The laboring woman cries if questioned about the reasons for her sadness. The emotional "flip-side" of this remedy is nervousness, fidgeting, excitability manifesting by incessant talking while jumping from one subject to another. ***Hysteria*** is a very real possibility!

GELSEMIUM SEMPERVIRENS This is a remedy for "stage fright" or a jittery feeling from excited anticipation of the birth. Gelsemium is noted for muscular weakness and insomnia from excitement or anticipation. A person needing Gelsemium often chatters from nervousness.

The emotional "opposite" of this symptom picture is mental dullness and feeling drowsy and dazed. There may be apathy towards their physical condition except for concern that they are not strong enough to see the labor through. There is fear of and great reluctance about being seen by a doctor.

IGNATIA AMARA This remedy is always about grief, emotional shock, and disappointment. The woman will be over-sensitive, nervous, highly emotional, moody, and sometimes quarrelsome. Joking and laughter changing suddenly to tears and hysterical outbursts are common.

PULSATILLA NIGRICANS The laboring woman who needs Pulsatilla craves affection and sympathy and needs constant reassurance. Whiney—the world actually looks better to her after a bout of whining so sympathetic listening is always appropriate. Consolation, or a hug, improves all ailments. There is usually some history—real or just perception—of abandonment betrayal, or grief.

Note: During my own childbearing years I closely resembled a Pulsatilla personality except in labor. I preferred to go deep inside myself, laboring on my feet and being left to wander about the house by myself with the back of an over-stuffed rocking chair to lean over during contractions. I would maintain this attitude and preference until I could feel the baby's head between my legs. This is not un-typical for the Pulsatilla personality; it is the opposing pattern. Pulsatilla women complain about the little things and buckle right in bravely when there are hard things to be done.

Back Pain

BELLADONNA With Belladonna the lumbar region feels broken, sometimes with pain in the hips and the thighs. The lumbar vertebrae may even be curved improperly, adding to the pain. There is difficulty walking with pain in sacrum, swelling in glands of the neck with stiff neck and shoulder muscles. The shoulder stiffness is more often on the right side than on the left side.

CAUSTICUM The symptoms of Causticum include back pain and stiffness between the shoulders that is made worse by swallowing, pain in the hips with cramps in the lumbar region and buttocks, and stiffness of the neck or back when rising from a chair.

CHAMOMILLA VULGARIS The pain of Chamomilla, exactly opposite of Pulsatilla, will move to the opposite of that being lain on. If the woman lies on her left side, the right hip will begin to ache. There may be stiffness of the neck muscles and sever pain in the hips.

COFFEA CRUDA The keynote of Coffea pain is that it seems so intolerable and like it will never end. There is weakness and pain in the small of the back.

KALI CARBONICUM When Kali carb is needed there will be severe backache during labor with the back feeling stiff and almost paralyzed. The mother will want to lie down but, because of the weight of the baby and the labor pains, se will not be able to find a restful position.

Bleeding

More than a little bleeding (the bloody show of early labor) is a very serious thing during labor. There are only three possible causes—placenta previa, placental abruption and a split or cut in the umbilical cord. All of these situations are life-threatening to both mother and baby. Unless delivery is imminent, immediate medical assistance should be sought. Any remedies given will be an attempt to slow the bleeding until medical assistance is reached. The keynotes of these remedies are discussed in Chapter 7 under Bleeding/ Hemorrhage.

Bladder Paralysis

ARNICA MONTANA and CAUSTICUM The damage to the bladder is from pressure of fetus during the labor. Attempting to keep the bladder empty in order to avoid problems later on doesn't work very well since a keynote of these two remedies is an inability to pass urine during labor.

CAULOPHYLLUM THALICTROIDES Laboring women should be encouraged to keep the bladder empty as urine in the bladder can lead to paralysis of the bladder! In the case of a Caulophyllum personality, keeping the bladder empty can prevent post-partum problems.

Cervix—unyielding

ANTIMONIUM TARTARICUM Many times when the cervix is dilating very slowly, Antimonium is what is needed. The mother will be feeling nauseous and experiencing shortness of breath. There will often be a history of pelvic inflammation.

BELLADONNA Hot and moist are keynotes of the Belladonna picture and that is how the cervix will feel—completely different than is usual. The cervix will also be abnormally tender to touch and will make delivery very painful if not remedied before the infant's head is pushing against it. The cervix thins but remains rigid, with painful spasms.

CAULOPHYLLUM THALICTROIDES With this polycrest remedy the cervix is extremely rigid with pains going in every direction but not producing an effective downward momentum. The cervix feels, to the laboring woman, as though it is being pricked by needles.

CIMICIFUGA RACEMOSA The uterus and cervix seem to withdraw upward during contractions, which are almost continuous and unusually painful. The cervix spasms and is slow to soften and thin.

GELSEMIUM SEMPERVIRENS The cervix, in this case, feels round like a button or the tip of a nose (this how a *non-pregnant* woman's cervix is supposed to feel). The cervix remains hard, thick, rigid, and as though it cannot possibly soften and dilate. Labor pains seem to go through the uterus and up the back. Things will progress unusually slowly and the woman will eventually feel great weakness.

IGNATIA AMARA Rigid cervix, with faintness and trembling and there will almost always be a lot of sighing that sounds like, and probably is, driven by some sort of grief since Ignatia is a grief driven remedy.

JABORANDI Normal moisture and secretions from the vagina are missing, making the passages hot and dry. There will be profuse sweat with dryness of the tissues of the mouth. The cervix is unyielding to touch.

LOBELIA INFLATA With Lobelia thre is a thick, unyielding cervix. Nausea comes with each contraction and there may be breathlessness which seems to hamper the downward expulsion force of labor.

LYCOPODIUM CLAVATUM The force of the contractions goes upward or from left to right and the woman will lose confidence in her ability to "get labor right." The cervix remains rigid and hard.

NUX VOMICA Labor pains seem to constrict the pelvic muscles, impeding the dilation of the cervix and the downward movement of the baby. There may be sharp pains in the calves of the legs during contractions with painful tightening of muscles in the back and the thighs.

SECALE CORNUTUM When Secale is called for, there will have been several weeks of false labor before real labor begins. The uterus feels soft and flabby but there has been no softening or dilation of the cervix.

VERATRUM VIRIDE With Veratrum viride the cervix is rigid. The arterial pulse is full, hard, and quick. Blood is congested in the head and chest, there is a feeling of impending stroke or convulsion, and a cold clammy sweat may develop. (These are indications of a potential crisis situation. Immediate medical attention is advised if the situation does not show marked improvement immediately following the giving of the remedy.)

Convulsions

APIS MELLIFICA At the onset of the convulsion, the brain feels very tired with a dull, heavy sensation in the occiput as if from a blow. Triggers of the convulsion may be allergies, grief at bad news, or a fright.

BELLADONNA Throbbing, hammering headache with feeling of fullness, especially across the forehead, with the pain being worse for light, noise, and even for lying down. The congestion of blood to the head that is a keynote of Belladonna creates a feeling as if the head would burst.

HYPERICUM PERFORATUM Hypericum is often a remedy for the nerves and nervous system. Convulsions are most likely to be the result of a previous head injury or injury to spinal nerves. The injury may even have been to the tailbone during a previous labor or be the result of a whiplash injury. The convulsions are accompanied by throbbing pains, centering in the vertex of the head.

Cramping, Spasms

IGNATIA AMARA Ignatia is a remedy where cramping and spasms are seen in nearly every part of the body. For Ignatia to be effective as a remedy here, the emotional picture of Ignatia must be present—grief, emotional shock, disappointment, internal conflicts, irritable and quarrelsome. The person will be idealistic, sentimental, and romantic.

MAGNESIA PHOSPHORICA Mag phos is useful for cramping muscles, including the uterus from which pain will be with radiating with the spasms. The pains shift from place to place and are better for rest. The cramping often becomes worse at night. Magnesium is necessary for the uptake of calcium, and lack of calcium is often implicated in muscle spasms. Homeopathic remedies often have the effect of encouraging the body to utilize calcium more efficiently and to uptake more of what is available.

NUX VOMICA The person needing Nux always has an irritable nervous system. This may be a part of their basic nature or only a symptom of the present stress of labor. The cramps and spasms will be in the limbs, particularly in the calves and soles, and be similar to the "charley horses" experienced throughout the pregnancy—quite painful.

Delayed Onset of Labor

CAULOPHYLLUM THALICTROIDES Once again, the indicators for this remedy are weakness and atony of the reproductive and pelvic organs, often due to multiple births and miscarriages. There will be apprehension and nervousness and other aspects of this remedy's symptom picture.

CIMICIFUGA RACEMOSA Cimicifuga is often called for when there is a history of negative experience in childbirth or when there has been a previous miscarriage. Toning contractions will have been of an unusually erratic nature. There may be sciatic pain.

IGNATIA AMARA Ignatia should be considered when emotional factors such as grief seem to be playing a part in the delay of the labor. Part of the Ignatia picture is that physical symptoms seem to be opposites and almost "impossible" from an anatomical standpoint.

PULSATILLA NIGRICANS The delay may be due to hormonal imbalance. The baby's position should be carefully checked as this remedy is often needed for abnormal presentations and labor may be delaying because the baby is not in a workable position (transverse lie, for example). There will be the usual Pulsatilla emotional symptoms, including a need to whine and be emotionally supported.

Exhaustion

ARSENICUM ALBUM The Arsenicum picture can be one of collapse and total exhaustion. It is even considered to be a resuscitation remedy for extreme circumstances. A keynote is that the absolute prostration seems to be out of proportion to the problems being experienced.

CARBO VEGETABILIS This is very much a resuscitation remedy when a situation is critical. Symptoms include very low vitality from loss of fluids or dehydration with icy-coldness and a blue tinge to the skin and the person will be weak and very exhausted. Carbo veg is especially useful when there is any degree of sepsis. A keynote indicator is lack of expected and normal reaction after a trauma followed suddenly by the serious weakness described above.

CAULOPHYLLUM THALICTROIDES Symptoms include internal trembling with great physical weakness. Labor pains may be weak and of insufficient strength or they may stop altogether because of the exhaustion or because the woman will no longer endure the pain. ***This is a polycrest remedy and worth remembering***. Caulophyllum has been of value to me, and every other midwife, in many different situations many times.

GELSEMIUM SEMPERVIRENS The Gelsemiun picture includes dizziness, drowsiness, and trembling with mental as well as physical prostration. Slow pulse with a feeling of being tired all over and apathy towards developing situations. There may be twitches of single muscles and sluggish circulation with venous congestion.

KALI PHOSPHORICUM There will be the characteristic Phosphorus low vitality and nervous condition. The laboring woman will be sensitive, weak, and easily tired—at least at this moment. Phosphorus is especially suited to worn-out mothers, tired from too much to do and too little sleep before labor began. If not prevented, complete nervous prostration before the labor is finished is a distinct possibility.

Fetal Distress

ARNICA MONTANA Arnica is recommended for use following any traumatic or difficult birth.

CARBO VEGETABILIS Give this remedy to the mother, in quite high potency, at the first sign of elevated heart tones in the fetus. Typically, the heart tones of a fetus in trouble will speed up as the baby seeks more oxygen from poorly oxygenated blood. By the time they fall off (slow down) the situation is desperate and delivery MUST be accomplished quickly!

Fever

BELLADONNA This is the only remedy I could find mentioned in literature for fever during labor. I would repertorize all of the symptoms and proceed by also giving the best indicated remedy based on the woman's general picture and the symptoms that are unique to the present situation.

Heart Trouble or Failure

DIGITALIS PURPUREA There is sudden constant pain in the region of the heart. The pulse is weak and very slow, but becomes rapid with the slightest movement. This remedy should be given while seeking immediate medical assistance.

Lack of Progress

ANTIMONIUM TARTARICUM Pelvic inflammation may have been a problem throughout the pregnancy or is chronic to the woman even between pregnancies and is one of the keynote indicators for choice of this remedy over some others when the cervix is rigid and inflamed.

ARSENICUM ALBUM Sudden great weakness, fatigue, exhaustion, and prostration are keynotes of Arsenicum. Labor pains become weak with no downward force or they may stop altogether.

CAULOPHYLLUM THALICTROIDES Uterus may feel soft and spongy even at the height of a contraction and there is lack of uterine tone. Labor pains are weak and of insufficient strength. The woman is exhausted out of proportion to the energy having been expended or she may be having difficulty coping, mentally and emotionally, with the pain of labor.

This remedy seems to work best early on in the labor, especially if there is trembling and over-excitement. Excellent for use when the cervix is rigid and slow to dilate or is dilating in an uneven manner, more on one side than the other, or is forming a lip of some kind.

CIMICIFUGA RACEMOSA Contractions are irregular, erratic, violent, but with no effective downward power. The lavoring woman may be emotionally affected by a previous negative or frightening experience of childbirth and often appears gloomy with doubts and fears about her ability to continue. The contractions are usually accompanied by sciatic pain or headache. There may even be confusion and mental disassociation.

CAUSTICUM This remedy is characterized by weakness, loss of muscle strength, and contractions that have become weak. There may even be localized paralysis-type weakness in areas where the baby's head has been pressing.

CHAMOMILLA VULGARIS Chamomilla is always keynoted by hypersensitivity. In labor, the woman will be hypersensitive to pain—labor seems intolerable and so much worse than she expected. The woman may be irritable and vocally unsatisfied with the care she is receiving throughout the labor. She will often send the labor attendants away but then wants them right back again.

GELSEMIUM SEMPERVIRENS This is a wonderful remedy for dysfunctional labor with failure to dilate. The cervix is thick and rigid. Fatigue and weakness are always part of the Gelsemium picture. There will be trembling, especially of the legs. During the final stages, the urge to push the baby out is absent and the baby moves upward with contractions. Pain moves up and down the back. This woman should be encouraged to keep the bladder empty as bladder paralysis from retained urine is possible after delivery.

GOSSYPIUM HERBACEUM The labor may seem to have been going well but then becomes sluggish in the second stage. Focus of the pains seems to go from one place to another. The labor, left to proceed without homeopathic treatment, will be lengthy but relatively painless. The Gossypium will shorten the labor but will not increase the pain! There will be a frequent desire to urinate throughout the labor.

NUX VOMICA Nux is not a very common remedy in labor but may be called for if the tense and nervous emotional/mental picture fits.

PULSATILLA NIGRICANS The lack of progress may be due to mal positioning of the baby. Abnormal presentations are common among women matching the Pulsatilla mental/emotional picture. Labor may also cause heart palpitations. Another keynote of this remedy is labor pains which become weak with the mother becoming very sleepy—she may even sleep through the contractions. Pulsatilla women do not like to labor lying down as the pains feel much worse in that position!

SECALE CORNUTUM Labor is very relaxed with no downward, expulsive action. When bearing-down pain finally comes, the woman suddenly feels very cold. The strength of the uterus has often been weakened by weeks of Braxton Hicks (false labor) contractions.

STAPHYSAGRIA Extreme painful sensitivity of the genital area with this extraordinary painfulness remaining longer than is usual after the delivery is often seen when Staphysagria is needed.

Painful Labor Contractions (extremely)

CHAMOMILLA VULGARIS When Chamomilla is needed, the pains are spasmodic, rather than directed efficiently downward. The mother is very sensitive to the pain of the contractions and feels that she cannot possibly endure them. She may be frantic and impatient and will not tolerate anyone near her.

PLATINUM METALLICUM These contractions are spasmodic and very painful. The entire genital area is very tender and painful during contractions. A keynote symptoms is that contractions are usually more painful on the left side of the body than on the right.

PULSATILLA NIGRICANS Labor seems unusually painful, but the pain is relieved by walking about and/or supporting the underside of the abdomen.

VIBURNUM PRUNIFOLIUM Viburnum is keynoted by very painful labor pains with terrible cramping of the legs. The pains are so severe as to threaten the rupture of the membranes (bag of waters) too early in the labor. If rupture of the membranes occurs there will usually be a gush of bright red blood. This situation is cause for concern unless the bleeding stops immediately. May signal a partial early dislodging of the placenta or a tear in the cord and represent a serious risk to the mother or the child.

Perineum and Cervix (rigid)

LOBELIA INFLATA Thick, leathery, unyielding, almost undilatable cervix with a rigid and non-elastic perineum keynotes Lobelia. There is terrible pain in the sacrum and in the back during the labor. Often the mother will be apprehensive of her own death, sighing, or even sobbing about the pain and discomfort she is experiencing.

Placenta Previa

Placenta previa is a serious situation for both the mother and the baby and is not safely deliverable without medical intervention. Life-threatening hemorrhage will *always* occur and the baby will suffer oxygen deprivation in almost every case!

CINNAMONUM CEYLANCIUM The standard literature indicates that a frightening hemorrhage that begins after only a few pains will be seen more often than normal in first time moms. My experience does not bear this assessment out. Previous C-section, multiple previous miscarriages, or a large number of previous births that have left scars on the uterine wall often create a low implant of the placenta and lead to this kind of trouble.

SEPIA SUCCUS There is a feeling of great weight in the anus with an empty sensation in the pit of the stomach. As always with Sepia, there will be bearing-down sensations, with a feeling that everything may just fall out through the pelvic floor at any moment. Fetal movements may be very feeble and the baby's heart tones should be watched closely.

Precipitous Birth

ACONITUM NAPELLUS Fright or emotional trauma may have brought about early labor, with labor moving very quickly and violently. Aconite is a primary trauma, emergency, and first-aid remedy.

Sciatic Pain (See "Sciatica" in the PreNatal Section)

Trembling or shivers

CAULOPHYLLUM THALICTROIDES Internal trembling with weakness, exhaustion, nervousness, irritability, apprehension, and general debility are keynote indicators of Caulophyllum.

CIMICIFUGA RACEMOSA Symptoms include trembling or twitching in various places or of the part lain on, nervous shuddering, and gloominess.

GELSEMIUM SEMPERVIRENS Symptoms include dizziness, drowsiness, and trembling with tremors or twitching of single muscles.

Uterine Inertia or Fatigue

ARNICA MONTANA Arnica symptoms include weak or irregular contractions, with a sense of great weariness. Alternatively, there are violent pains which accomplish very little. The whole body feels sore and bruised in any position. There will be back pain from the intensity and misdirection of the contractions with intense soreness and tenderness of the inner edge of the cervix, even before labor begins, due to pressure of the baby's head. This tenderness is the result of a flabby uterus that has not kept baby properly up off cervix during the pregnancy.

CAUSTICUM Situations that respond to causticum are often the result of grief or intense efforts nursing or caring for another person. There will be distressing pain in the back and inability to urinate.

CHINA OFFICINALIS China symptoms include uterine fatigue and general exhaustion from a long labor or loss of fluids. There may be ringing in the ears, cold skin, cold sweat, and faint pulse.

GELSEMIUM SEMPERVIRENS With Gelsemium, the uterus feels heavy and sore, inefficient labor pains or labor that has stopped altogether from uterine atony and inertia, and overall muscular weakness.

PULSATILLA NIGRICANS Labor contractions stopping or becoming irregular and spasmodic due to uterine atony or fatigue.

SECALE CORNUTUM Symptoms of Secale include a flabby, relaxed uterus, weak, irregular contractions with little or no downward expulsive action, and a placenta that has gone septic.

Vomiting

ARSENICUM ALBUM A keynote symptom of Arsenicum is burning pain in the stomach. The woman will not be able to bear the sight or smell of food. Ice cold water will be vomited immediately and the retching may become violent enough to trigger labor. The vomiting will be accompanied by diarrhea.

IPECACUANHA Symptoms include excessive salivation as a signal that one is about to vomit. There is repeated and incapacitating vomiting throughout the pregnancy that reoccurs during the labor and may be accompanied by migraine. Vomit consisting of blood, bile, food, and mucous may trigger labor.

PHOSPHORUS Applicable symptoms include vomiting in labor if food is eaten and cravings for cold food and drinks but vomits them as soon as they are warmed in the stomach.

Chapter Seven

LATE LABOR, DELIVERY, AND POST-PARTUM

After Pains

ARNICA MONTANA Arnica will often prevent the worst of the pain from after pains if administered at the close of a labor in which the mother feels bruised or has strained a great deal during the pushing stage. There will often be heart palpitations.

CAULOPHYLLUM THALICTROIDES For the relief of spasmodic pains in the lower abdomen, even into the groin, back, and chest after a particularly long and exhausting labor.

CHAMOMILLA VULGARIS The after pains of Chamomilla are quite violent and distressing, making the woman irritable and touchy. Chamomila is one of the best remedies for after pains if the mental/emotional symptoms fit.

CIMICIFUGA RACEMOSA After pains with nausea, vomiting, and great tenderness if any pressure is applied to the abdomen are the keynotes of Cimicifuga.

COFFEA CRUDA Wtih Coffea the pain is out of proportion to the amount of contracting that is occurring in the uterus. The woman will be sleepy but unable to sleep.

FERRUM METALLICUM Ferrum is keynoted by violent, labor-like pains with discharge of both fluid and clotted blood.

KALI CARBONICUM Pains in the back shooting into gluteal muscles, thighs, and hips.

MAGNESIA PHOSPHORICA Magnesia is indicated by nerve pain of a cramping, spasmodic nature. Often used in conjunction with Calcarea phosphorica.

PULSATILLA NIGRICANS All symptoms, including labor pains, become worse toward evening with Pulsatilla. The woman desires warmth on her abdomen although other symptoms are generally worse for heat and warm stuffy rooms.

SABINA OFFICINALIS Sabina is keynoted by very severe cramping with pain from sacrum to pubis or moving into the thighs. The abdomen will be very sensitive. There is a discharge of blood and clots with each painful contraction.

SECALE CORNUTUM Secale is a remedy that is often useful for older women who have borne many children and whose tissues may be lax and out of tone.

SEPIA SUCCUS With Sepia there is a constant sensation of weight in anus with pains shooting upward from there into vagina. The painful spasms are also felt in the back.

Anesthesia, Reaction To

OPIUM The keynotes of Opium include heavy sleep, stupor, stertorous breathing, and sweaty skin. There may be delirium.

PHOSPHORUS Phosphorus symptoms include tightness in the chest, spacey, disconnected thoughts, fear, anxiety, and weakness—phosphorus is always a remedy with weakness in the picture.

Bleeding/Hemorrhage

More than a very little bleeding before the crowning of the baby's head is serious cause for concern. There are no good reasons for bleeding at this stage! A prompt and appropriate response is imperative.

ACONITUM NAPELLUS Symptoms of Aconitum include sudden active hemorrhage of bright red blood with faintness, panic, and shock. There will be sharp, shooting pains in the uterus.

ARNICA MONTANA Arnica is of benefit after any traumatic experience, mental or emotional shock, and bruised or traumatized tissues.

BELLADONNA Belladonna hemorrhage is gushing with bright red blood. The hemorrhage may be accompanied by violent bearing-down sensations and a rigid cervix.

CARBO VEGETABILIS The woman will be in a state of extreme collapse, almost lifeless. Her face will be blue and her body will be cold with cold sweat. The pulse may be almost imperceptible, and respiration very rapid. Her vitality will be low from extreme loss of blood and bodily fluids. ***This is a resuscitation remedy; medical intervention, if you are not already there, should be considered immediately.***

CINNAMONUM CEYLANICUM Hemorrhage after only a few pains—usually indicting placenta previa, a very dangerous situation. Immediate transport is necessary and Cinnamonum may be useful in slowing the hemorrhage. (Please see Placenta Previa)

CROCCUS SATIVUM With Croccus blood comes in large clots and may be indicative of a retained placenta. There will be ice-cold extremities. This is a life-threatening situation and must be dealt with by immediate extraction of the placenta by whatever means necessary.

CAULOPHYLLUM THALICTROIDES Caulophyllum symptoms include hemorrhage with uterine inertia, very weak, irregular, or no discernible contractions but with bearing-down pains, internal trembling, weakness, exhaustion, and general debility. Please understand, even memorize, the symptom picture of this polycrest remedy if you will have any responsibility for a pregnant or a laboring woman at any time.

HAMAMELIS VIRGINIANA Hemorrhage, dark in color, with bearing-down sensation in the lower back is the usual picture of Hamamelis. There will be exhaustion out of proportion to the amount of blood lost.

IPECACUANHA Ipecac is characterized by profuse gushes of bright red blood, which may indicate placenta previa—a dangerous situation for Mom and baby. There will be pain from the navel moving into the uterus with nausea Any hemorrhage seen will be bright red, foamy, gushing, profuse, and difficult to stop. This remedy will be used as an emergency remedy while medical assistance is sought.

PHOSPHORUS Insidious onset, gradually increasing to profuse, bright red blood is a keynote of Phosphorus, which is considered a remedy mostly for tall, slim women who are overly sensitive, excitable, and impressionable.

PULSATILLA NIGRICANS This remedy is for post-partum hemorrhage from retained placenta when other typical Pulsatilla symptoms, including the need for reassurance even after the crisis is over, are present.

SABINA OFFICINALIS Sabina is indicated when there is bright red blood containing dark clots—the uterus is attempting to fold down and blood is trying to coagulate.

SECALE CORNUTUM Secale hemorrhages are flows of dark, thin blood from a low-lying placenta. The uterus will feel relaxed and soft, even during contractions. Uterine inertia may have presented problems earlier in the pregnancy, during the labor, or at the time of delivery.

TRILLIUM PENDULUM Trillium is a remedy for women who habitually hemorrhage after delivery. There will be gushes of blood at the slightest motion.

BIOPLASMA Bioplasma is all twelve tissue salts together in the same bottle and is the very best first-aid remedy for bleeding of any kind that I know of.

Braxton Hicks (False Labor Pains)

CAULOPHYLLUM THALICTROIDES Caulophyllum is indicated for pains in all directions except effective downward pressure—a near perfect description of false labor. These types of contractions are usually related to a slight hormone irregularity.

CHAMOMILLA VULGARIS Abdominal pains with the passing of large quantities of pale urine.

KALI CARBONICUM Kali carb is indicated by pains in the back spreading down over the buttocks and thighs instead of moving around the abdomen.

SECALE CORNUTUM Secale is usually a remedy for older women who have borne several children. The uterus is weakened and pains often come with bloody discharge.

SEPIA SUCCUS Sepia labor-like pains come complete with bearing-down sensations and the feeling that everything is just going to fall out through the pelvic floor. The woman will be uneasy about the state of her own and the baby's health. She will annoyed or overwhelmed by family responsibilities.

VIBURNUM OPULUS Abdominal pain that shoots down the legs during any month of pregnancy and labor may be interrupted by ineffective contractions.

Catheterization—Negative Effects Of

CANTHARIS VESICATORIA Terrible burning pains from being catheterized accompanies by constant, but usually ineffective, desire to urinate.

CAUSTICUM Paralysis of bladder, loss of muscle tone, relaxation of muscles and tissues, trembling and sensitivity to both heat and cold following catheterization.

STAPHYSAGRIA The negative effects of catheterization include pain, squeezing, or stinging. There are feelings of humiliation or embarrassment from the procedure.

Cesarean Section (See Chapter on Cesarean Section)

Hematoma

ARNICA MONTANA Arnica acts on the blood and the veins—especially venous congestion or abnormal collecting of blood. Arnica is thought of mostly as an injury and trauma remedy and has a wide usefulness—and not just with blood related or bruising issues.

BELLIS PERENNIS Bellis acts very much like Arnica, but with a more pronounced effect after traumatic childbirth. Bellis acts on the muscular fibers of the blood vessels and speeds repair of these vessels after congestion due to trauma or blows. At the same time, Bellis is excellent for injuries to deeper tissues.

Overexertion

ARNICA MONTANA The woman usually feels sore and bruised and does not want to be touched. Shock may be imminent or has just been a problem. A keynote of Arnica is the woman claiming they are fine when they obviously are not, usually with some degree of confusion.

BELLIS PERENNIS Bellis acts on deeper tissues than Arnica and is specific to childbirth. Bellis may relieve bruised soreness after childbirth where the more commonly reached for Arnica has not been effective.

RHUS TOXICODENDRON Like Arnica and Bellis, Rhus is a remedy for the after-effects of over-doing it physically. A keynote here is that the aches and pains are actually improved by a little bit of gentle exercise—after the initial aggravation on beginning to move has passed. Restlessness is brought on by physical pain and there may be mild depression.

Paraplegia Following Childbirth

CAULOPHYLLUM THALICTROIDES Caulophyllum is one of the leading polycrest remedies for anything to do with childbearing. A unique keynote of this remedy is numbness or paralysis of the legs following a difficult childbirth. Other Caulophyllum keynotes should be present, as always with homeopathy, but I know of no other remedy with paralysis of the legs following childbirth in the symptom picture.

Perineal Trauma

ARNICA MONTANA Arnica is the leading first aid remedy for trauma and bruising to muscles and soft tissues. There will be a great sense of weariness with the woman insisting that she is really OK when she obviously is not.

CALENDULA OFFICINALIS Calendula is almost always added to a gel and used topically. It promotes healing of fissures and tears without scarring and stops bleeding and reduces pain.

Post-Partum Depression

CIMICIFUGA RACEMOSA This is an important remedy for extreme depression and exhaustion. A keynote is a feeling of a black cloud over everything with irrational fears and forebodings of death. The woman may talk incessantly, jumping from one subject to another or she may sit and mope with great sadness. She will burst into tears when questioned about what the problem may be.

IGNATIA AMARA Ignatia symptoms are usually the result of grief, emotional shock, or disappointment—perhaps even disappointment with the way the birth went. There will be sadness and sighing and an empty feeling in the pit of the stomach. The woman desires to be alone and is worse from consolation and sympathy. Ignatia should always be considered for a miscarriage or if the child did not survive birth.

NATRUM MURIATICUM The picture of this remedy will have been present in their life before this pregnancy and will include severe depression and feelings of isolation. She is typically offended easily, can hold grudges for years, is emotionally shut down and closed off and completely unable to cry in front of other people. Suicide is a possibility any time there is a Nat mur picture and should be watched for carefully.

PULSATILLA NIGRICANS Pulsatilla is keynoted by changeable moods, being emotional and tearful, and feeling ignored or forsaken. Pulsatilla personalities crave affection and sympathy. Their basic nature is submissiveness with silent grief and resentment.

SEPIA SUCCUS Sepia is the leading remedy for post-partum depression in women at any stage of life. They feel mentally and physically worn out and over-whelmed by responsibilities of family. She often feels unappreciated for her efforts. Her weeping becomes worse for sympathy or explaining how she feels.

PHOSPHORUS Phosphorus depression is driven by imaginary fears for their own health or over-identification with the suffering of others. There is extreme thirst for cold drinks. Emotional symptoms include fear of being alone and over-sensitivity to noise, odors, and light. She will have difficulty focusing or keeping her mind on any one thing. There will be aggravation of all symptoms in the evening just as the sun goes down.

Post-Hemorrhage Fainting & Weakness

(These two remedies help strengthen and build the blood)

CHINA OFFICINALIS Symptoms of China include debility, great weakness, and delirium from loss of blood or fluids. There will be ringing in the ears with the least noise or excitement being stressful, even intolerable. There may be continued off-and-on bleeding from retained membranes following a miscarriage.

FERRUM PHOSPHORICUM Ferrum increases hemoglobin and the blood's ability to carry oxygen and nutrients to cells. The phosphoricum is indicated by great prostration with physical and mental lassitude. Loss of blood will have made the face and lips abnormally pale with trembling and extreme weakness.

Resuscitation

ACONITUM NAPELLUS Symptoms of Aconitum includes fear of impending death and a pronounced fear of doctors. This remedy is for emergency situation contributed to or brought on by fright or alarming circumstances. The development of Aconite symptoms is sudden and alarming in intensity.

ANTIMONIUM TARTARICUM The woman becomes increasingly weak with a pale bluish face and cold sweat. She will be drowsy with lack of reaction and her chin and lower jaw will be quivering.

ARNICA MONTANA Arnica is the first remedy for physical, mental, and emotional shock. If it is administered in a timely manner, the situation may improve so dramatically that the deeper remedies may not be needed. Unlike some of the other remedies listed here, the situation need not be extremely serious for Arnica to be called for.

With Arnica, the woman will claim she is fine when, obviously, she is not and cannot even remember what has happened.

ARSENICUM ALBUM One of the distinctive keynotes of Arsenicum is sudden great weakness which seems to be out of proportion to the amount of trauma suffered. Arsenicum is restorative and stabilizing to all systems of the body (digestive, circulatory, lymphatic, glandular). Other indicative symptoms of Arsenicum include shortness of breath with extreme restlessness, or restlessness alternating with anxiety.

CARBO VEGETABILIS Carbo veg is a *VERY* strong acting resuscitation remedy. Symptoms will include lack of reaction following violent trauma or shock, icy coldness, laborious breathing, shortness of breath, paleness, and a blue tinge to the skin. Carbo veg is also useful in many septic conditions.

LAUROCERASUS OFFICINALIS Failure of an infant to breathe after birth is a horrible thing to see, especially if the responsibility for the child's welfare is your. This remedy is specific for situations like this, especially where there is no cord wrap or other explanation visible by the time the baby is fully born.

Laurocerasus is a well-known heart remedy so heart/chest issues in the infant should be checked carefully. The infant will most likely gasp for breath after being given the remedy. More than one dose will likely be needed and follow-up remedies utilized according to the symptoms that the child displays as it is recovering. This is an amazing remedy in these situations! Medical diagnostics may not be needed unless further signs of trouble develop. If the situation that created the trauma occurred during the birth process (a cord wrap, for example) and is now resolved with the baby doing well, the crisis has passed and all is well.

OPIUM Opium is characterized by stupor and obstructed, slow respiration. The face will be deeply flushed and mottled with red or purple coloring. The eyes will be heavy and half closed, constricted, staring, and unresponsive to light. The skin will be sweaty and the limbs will be twitching limb. Eventually, if the pattern is not broken, there will be loss of consciousness.

Each of these remedies has many uses outside of serious and life-threatening situations. If the symptoms listed above are seen however, quick action to save life will be needed. The remedies, while part of those life-saving measures because of their dramatic and amazing action, will be acting to buy you sufficient time to get medical assistance.

Retained Placenta

CANTHARIS VESICATORIA The picture of Cantharis always contains burning somewhere. A retained placenta situation is no exception. The painful burning sensation is what determines that this is the remedy, among the many choices available, that would be best. Historical information claims that this remedy aids in the expulsion of dead fetal tissue and membranes following a miscarriage.

CAULOPHYLLUM THALICTROIDES This is a much valued remedy for anything related to hormones and uterine inertia. The retained placenta that calls for Caulophyllum will have come about because of lack of uterine tone and uterine inertia. There will be unusual rigidity of the cervix with internal trembling and weakness.

CIMICIFUGA RACEMOSA Sometimes used alternately with Caulophyllum when there is uterine inertia. For this remedy to be indicated there will be great tenderness of the uterine region. The labor pains will have been displaced to the back, hips, and thighs and be causing a great deal of sciatic pain.

GOSSYPIUM HERBACEUM With the Gossypium picture, there are bearing-down pains as there should be but the placenta does not deliver.

PULSATILLA NIGRICANS The Pulsatilla pattern of weak labor pains with insufficient downward force is an indication that the uterus will not contract sufficiently to expel the placenta. This situation is not always easily identified because the woman will be tired and so sensitive to pain that the pains of labor and the contractions necessary to dislodge the placenta look more intense than they really are. Post-partum hemorrhage from a retained placenta is likely unless this remedy has been given earlier and the Pulsatilla mental/emotional symptoms have disappeared during the labor and delivery.

SABINA OFFICINALIS Bleeding from the retained placenta is bright red with dark clots and is worse for the slightest motion when Sabina is needed. The flow of blood occurs in paroxysms and is accompanied by contractions.

SEPIA SUCCUS The keynote of Sepia is that everything feels like it is "falling out the bottom" and, after birth, this may really become true sometimes. When the placenta is finally felt at the oz but does not finish coming through and will not pull away even with manual assistance, it is likely that the uterus has inverted and is following the placenta out. This is a serious situation and will require either medical assistance or intervention by a well-trained midwife.

Scar Tissue

GRAPHITES NATURALIS Graphities is known for aiding in the absorption of scar tissue and will help heal tears (small ones) that may otherwise lead to infection. There will be burning pain in the old scars that this remedy will be of assistance with.

SILICA TERRA Silica stimulates the system to reabsorb fibrotic conditions and scar tissue and promotes the expulsion of any foreign objects from the body. silica eliminates the need for injuries and scars to fester, creating the pus and pressure usually necessary to expel foreign objects.

THIOSINAMINUM Thiosinaminum is considered a solvent, both internally and externally, for scar tissue and keloids. It is also indicated for wounds that are slow to heal or are forming scar tissue or granulations and may improve inelasticity of the skin.

Shock

ACONITUM NAPELLUS Shock for which Aconitum is indicated is accompanied by, or brought on by, great fear. Aconite symptoms always come on suddenly and with intensity and usually include palpitations and rapid pulse. There is fear of the future and a pronounced fear of doctors with people needing Aconitum.

ARNICA MONTANA Arnica is the first remedy for physical and emotional shock. The woman will claim she is OK or tell you that she will be OK when she is obviously not doing well at all. There will be some degree of mental confusion and, usually, heart palpitations.

BELLIS PERENNIS Bellis is much like Arnica and is indicated when the shock results from injury to deeper internal tissues. Bellis may ay relieve any bruised soreness after childbirth better than Arnica.

CARBO VEGETABILIS Carbo veg is a strong acting resuscitation remedy. Symptoms will include lack of reaction following violent trauma or shock, icy coldness, laborious breathing, shortness of breath, paleness, a blue tinge to the skin and very low vitality. Carbo veg has often been useful when the person has fainted from weakness caused by loss of blood and body fluids. Carbo veg should be considered when bleeding from varicosities of the vulva are present. *Carbo Vegetabilis is a first-aid remedy of great effectiveness, especially in extreme situations.*

CHINA OFFICINALIS China is a remedy for shock brought on from excessive loss of blood or bodily fluids. This is a serious situation and there will be faintness with low or absent blood pressure which was preceded by a very rapid but thready pulse.

IPECACUANHA Ipecec is for arterial bleeding from partial premature separation of the placenta. The hemorrhage seen will be bright red, foamy, gushing, profuse, and difficult to stop. While these remedies are amazing, every other possible remedy, herbal and otherwise, should be employed immediately in an attempt to control the bleeding. Transport to a hospital will probably be necessary. There will be persistent nausea and vomiting.

RESCUE REMEDY and ER911 (RESCUE REMEDY with ARNICA added) Rescue Remedy is a Flower Essence Remedy (Bach) and is a polycrest for shock. The addition of Arnica dds to its effectiveness, especially if the labor has been long and the woman is feeling bruised and beaten up.

BIOPLASMA Bioplasma is all twelve tissue salts (cell salts) together in the same bottle. This is the very best first-aid remedy for bleeding of any kind that I have ever seen. It may be used with Rescue Remedy or ER911 whenever the shock is blood or body fluid related. I have seen both internal hemorrhages and localized bleeding stop suddenly when Bioplasma has been used. I administer the remedy orally and apply it topically when the bleeding is from an external injury.

Urine Retention

ACONITUM NAPELLUS With Aconitum the genital area is dry and tender. Urinating is painful and difficult and comes drop by drop. There will be burning at the neck of the bladder. Thye woman will be nervous and excitable with anxiety on attempting to pass urine. There is fear of death or that something is going to go terribly wrong.

APIS MELLIFICA Apis is characterized by the opposing symptoms of scanty or suppressed urine and urine output being much more profuse than the quantity of fluid consumed accounts for. The urine will have a deep color and there will be burning when urinating. The burning sensation will be worst as the last drops are passed.

Apis is a very useful remedy for urine retention in the newborn.

ARNICA MONTANA Arnica, in this situation as in all others it is indicated for, is a tissue trauma remedy. The retention of urine in the bladder will follow exertion and bruising during labor. There will be an aching, pressing feeling in the bladder and the bladder will feel full and sore. There is constant dribbling of urine after labor but when the woman attempts to pass urine into the toilet, the flow stops altogether. A very annoying pattern since the woman will probably be reluctant to just dribble into her padding instead of try to continually return to the bathroom.

CANTHARIS VESICATORIA Cantharis is indicated for severe cystitis with intense, burning pain in the neck of bladder. An excellent remedy for atony or paralysis of the bladder from long retention of urine during the labor. The bladder pains are worse from drinking even a small quantity of water.

CAUSTICUM Causticum is indicated for retention of urine after labor, surgical procedures, or just from failure to void urine for too long a time. The urine may dribble or pass very slowly.

GELSEMIUM SEMPERVIRENS The keynote of this remedy is the inability to pass urine while attendants are in the room (bashful bladder). The woman often retains urine after the delivery, is too weak to be left alone in the bathroom, but cannot pass urine when the midwives or nurses are present. Tricky!

LYCOPODIUM CLAVATUM With Lycopodium, the urge to urinate is strong, but the woman must wait a long time for any urine to pass. There is a bearing-down sensation over bladder area from retained urine.

OPIUM Opium is for use after a frightening delivery experience which has resulted in either retained urine or involuntary urination. There may be paralytic atony of bladder.

Uterine Inertia (See Chapter on Labor)

Uterine Infections (Sepsis)

ARSENICUM ALBUM Arsenicum is a remedy for more advanced cases where there is very great weakness and extreme chilliness. Other keynotes of Arsenicum are anxious restlessness, shortness of breath, burning pains that are—oddly— relieved by heat. The liver and spleen are usually enlarged. Emotional symptoms may include fear of death, which may be justified, as uterine infections are serious business!

BELLADONNA The sepsis for which Belladonna is indicated is often from retained placenta. While Belladonna hemorrhages involve bright red blood and profuse bleeding, the bleeding of a sepsis condition calling for Belladonna may manifest with the blood coagulating and being dark colored and very offensive smelling. There will be blood flow between after-pain contractions. Symptoms aggravated by light, motion, and noise will always be seen with Belladonna situations.

BAPTISIA TINCTORIA Sepsis, following childbirth or in the blood, with (usually) low-grade fever Extreme prostration. All secretions and fluids are offensive—breath, stool, urine, sweat. Foul odor of the body. Since all of these symptoms are pretty basic to Sepsis, the choice of the remedy will be guided by the emotional patterns.

BRYONIA ALBA Bryonia is indicated for all forms of peritoneal infection with severe pain that is aggravated by the least movement. There will be a bursting splitting headache that makes the woman irritable and bad tempered.

PYROGENIUM Pyrogen is particularly indicated for infectious conditions of any type in which the temperature rises rapidly, then oscillates up and down. The fever begins with pains in the limbs. There is great heat with profuse sweat, followed by chilliness with cold sweat over body. The sweating does not cause a fall in temperature as one would expect it to. The pulse is slow, even when the fever is very high. Urine will be as clear as water.

Chapter Eight

POST CESAREAN DELIVERY

Homeopathic remedies do not enter the bloodstream through the digestive system. Rather, they move through the body in a direct route from cell to cell, tissue to tissue. Homeopathics may work poorly in normal use if a drug is hiding a symptom from the vital force. However pain medications and drugs used during surgery usually do not create an anti-dote situation with the homeopathics recommended below. Homeopathic remedies return the body to as near a state of stasis as is possible in whatever circumstances the person may be in. The energy system of the body seems to automatically adjust the homeopathic remedy's action to whatever the drug is doing in the body. Use of these remedies following the trauma of a C-section usually proves very helpful.

Immediately Post-Op

ARNICA MONTANA As always, Arnica is a trauma remedy and indicated for tenderness, soreness, bruising, and trauma to any tissues.

BELLIS PERENNIS Bellis is much like Arnica, but acts on deeper tissues and on the fibrous tissues of veins and arteries. Bellis is considered to be an even better choice than the more popular and well-known Arnica for surgical situations as its specialty is trauma to deep tissues.

PHOSPHORUS Phosphorus helps the body to eliminate anesthesia residue more quickly and is especially useful for post-surgical vomiting.

HYPERICUM PERFORATUM Hypericum is a remedy for injuries to nerves and is very useful for pain relief after operations. A keynote indication will be shooting pains originating from the surgical site.

STAPHYSAGRIA Staphysagria's keynote symptom is lacerated tissues with pain at the incision site. Abdominal gas pains will be quite intense. There will be sadness and feelings of failure because a C-section was required.

A Few Days After Surgery

CALCAREA FLUORATA This remedy is for the prevention of scar tissue, granulations, or adhesions, especially following surgery.

CALENDULA OFFICINALIS The most common use for Calendula is topically for poor wound healing.

Chapter Nine

INFANT CARE

Asphxia (Difficulty breathing)

ACONITUM NAPELLUS Aconite is a very potent emergency resuscitation remedy for oxygen deprivation and impending shock. There will almost always be a rapid pulse and the tiny heart will be beating frantically. There may be what look like, and maybe even are, stroke-like symptoms.

The most important keynote of the Aconitum picture is the suddenness and the intensity with which the emergency, and the accompanying frightening symptoms, came on. The infant may be doing fine and then, very suddenly, serious signs of distress are seen. It is never wise to leave a newborn completely unattended, even with attendants close by, while caring for the mother during the first hour or more.

ANTIMONIUM TARTARICUM The Antimonium picture is as different from Aconite as it can be. The baby becomes increasingly weak with the face becoming pale and bluish. The infant will be drowsy with lack of reaction to attempts to stimulate or interact with him. The body will be covered with a cold sweat and the chin and lower jaw will quiver.

ARNICA MONTANA Arnica should be administered to the baby whenever the pushing stage of birth has been long and traumatic. If there is even a slight mal-presentation, the baby may be developing bruising and trauma from pushing against the bony structures of the mother's pelvis. In this case, giving Arnica to the mother during the labor will help the baby immensely. The mother will be benefited by a better emotional state and less trauma to her own sensitive tissues.

Arnica may be applied directly to a hematoma on the baby's head if one has developed. The baby may have a hot head with a colder than normal body if Arnica is indicated.

BELLADONNA Belladonna has a very distinctive, and frightening, picture. Birth trauma will have created cerebral congestion with violent pulsing of the carotid arteries. The child's eyes will be fixed and dilated. The child may be only semi-conscious or unconscious altogether.

LAUROCERASUS OFFICINALIS The symptoms displayed when Laurocerasus is indicated are frightening indeed. There will have been some degree of neonatal asphyxia (oxygen deprivation) during the birth process. The baby will be cold, blue and gasping for breath. Breathing may be especially difficult, ineffective and tiring due to stiffness or paralysis of lung tissue. Heart and chest issues may have developed or these issues may be congenital and have been the cause of the baby's distress. More often than not, this baby will spend some time in a neonatal care unit. Laurocerasus is true *resuscitation* remedy and has been responsible for saving life and creating a good quality of life in what was a very traumatized infant.

Birth Defects

Possible miasms and other inherited family traits used to be the first thing to look for when there are birth defects present at birth. In today's world, we must also factor in exposure to drugs and chemicals by the mother, not just during pregnancy but during the months before conception.

The belief of previous generations that the placenta protects the child from exposure to drugs taken by the mother is unrealistic in today's world of the ever increasing "sophistication" of man-made chemicals. Personally, I doubt very much that the placenta *ever* provided that kind of protection. It only takes a glimpse at statistics such as those for babies born to mothers who took Thalidomide to realize that a fetus can be harmed in irreversible ways by the drugs ingested by the mother.

CALCAREA CARBONICA This is the polycrest remedy for the Psora miasm, which is characterized by a range of birth defects, multiple allergies, extreme sensitivity to the environment, and assimilation problems.

LAUROCERASUS OFFICINALIS The most common things seen with Laurocerasus have to do with the muscles. Symptoms include spasms of the limbs with muscular weakness and epileptic-type convulsions. It should be remembered that the heart is also a muscle and may be struggling. If it is, there will be accompanying lung disorders.

CIMICIFUGA RACEMOSA The birth defects for which Cimicifuga is useful are wide and varied. They include epilepsy, heart disorders, spinal and muscular disorders and displacement issues with the hip, sacrum, and lumbar vertebrae.

LYCOPODIUM CLAVATUM Lycopodium defects involve the heart and the liver and are usually quite serious. Homeopathic treatment may help a great deal and will, at least, buy time to seek medical intervention. The heart may be enlarged at birth or enlarge as it struggles to get circulation going in the newborn. Water in the pericardium (fibrous sac in which the heart is contained), jaundice from a struggling liver and chronic hepatitis may become an issue as the child grows.

TUBERCULINUM BOVINUM The symptoms of Tuberculinum are those of the Tuberculosis miasm and, since they involve behavioral disorders such as ADHD and hyperactivity, they may not be noticed for awhile. Heart disorders and paralysis of muscles may be seen more quickly.

Breast Milk in Newborn

PULSATILLA NIGRICANS Found only one reference in homeopathic literature for this phenomenon. The suggested remedy was Pulsatilla nigricans. I experienced this situation with one of my own children—a boy. I took Pulsatilla myself (because I matched many of the symptoms of the Pulsatilla picture). I quit nursing the baby on the advice of a mid-wife, although I am not sure that doing so was completely necessary. The problem in the baby cleared up immediately and I felt much better, too.

Colic

CHAMOMILLA VULGARIS Chamomilla is a polycrest remedy for cross babies who suffer greatly from colic. The baby will be very sensitive to the mood of the mother, especially if she is nursing her infant.

Chamomilla is particularly indicated for Mom and baby if there is an intolerance for milk. This includes a baby who gets colic if the nursing mother ingests cheese or other milk products and for the bottle-fed baby who becomes intolerant of cow's milk. The infant is fussy and peevish and draws its legs up toward its chest in an attempt to relieve the pain. One cheek may be red and the other cheek pale.

COLOCYNTHIS Distinctive symptoms of Colocynthis include gastric distress that is better by pressure on tummy. The infant prefers to lie on its abdomen and screams from pain when moved. If the baby must be held or carried about, it likes to be facing away from the carrier person's body with their hand or arm placed firmly across the poor little tummy. The baby with a Colocynthis tummy aches also wiggles about in an attempt to find relief from the tummy pain.

MAGNESIA PHOSPHORICA The baby who will be benefitted by Mag phos experiences painful spasmodic cramping with a great deal of colic. The pain can sometimes be relieved by warmth and the baby hiccups and passes gas more than is normal as the body tries to deal with the flatulence.

NUX VOMICA Nux is for the fussy, colicky baby whose colic and constipation are the result of rich or stimulating foods eaten by the nursing mother. The remedy will bring the baby much relief but the only real "cure" is for Mom to simplify her diet.

STAPHYSAGRIA The baby will have a swollen abdomen with a great deal of flatulence. The distress seems to be tied to the emotions of the nursing mother more than with other remedy pictures—except for Chamomilla which has a similar connection between mother and baby.

Constipation

ALUMINUM OXYDATA Constipation can have many causes but the type that is helped by Aluminum oxydata is usually the result of an intolerance to formulas or processed baby foods.

BRYONIA ALBA Bryonia is indicated for constipation issues or nursing babies more often than for similar issues with bottle fed babies. There will be inflammation and dryness of mucous membranes elsewhere in the baby's body and the passing of very hard stool after much straining.

CALCAREA CARBONICA The baby for whom Calcarea carb is indicated will be constipated but there will be very little discomfort unless pressure is applied to the abdomen. The cause and the concern here is that there may be poor assimilation of nutrients.

NATRUM MURIATICUM The constipation of the Nat mur picture alternates with diarrhea. The abdomen is swollen with rumbling flatulence and the colic comes with nausea. It is likely that there was, or is, some sort of grief or loss issue going on with the mother. It may have been present during the pregnancy and still unresolved as she nurses her child.

NUX VOMICA Nux is indicated if the baby's problems are the result of rich or stimulating foods eaten by the nursing mother. There will be frequent, unproductive attempts to pass stool with the baby. While the remedy may be helpful to a large degree, the only real solution is for the mother to remove irritating to the baby foods from her diet.

OPIUM Opium is an infrequently used remedy for infants but is exactly what is needed if there is obstinate constipation with the stool passing as round, hard balls. The stool first protrudes and then recedes in a very annoying and painful manner.

Convulsion

CICUTA VIROSA Cicuta is specific for use when, during an illness, the baby seems to finally be doing better but then suddenly goes into spasmodic convulsions and becomes very rigid.

Cradle Cap

CALCAREA CARBONICA Indications other than the crustiness and itchiness of the scalp will include diarrhea from the poor assimilation of nutrients.

Cyanosis

LACHESIS MUTA The symptoms of Lachesis include breathing appearing to almost stop—and the baby's skin tones becoming a little bit bluish, when baby falls asleep. The infant breathes better in an upright position.

LAUROCERASUS OFFICINALIS Laurocerasus is a remedy for the after effects of oxygen deprivation during birth. The baby will be cold, blue tinged and gasping for breath. There may be heart and chest disorders and stiffness or paralysis of lung tissue that are the underlying cause of the cyanosis.

Delayed Development

CALCAREA CARBONICA and CALCAREA PHOSPHORICA These two remedies are useful for delayed development due to nutritional insufficiency or inability to absorb nutrients. The diet of the nursing mother should be carefully checked or a different formula used.

SILICA TERRA Silica is indicated for slow bone growth due to nutritional deficiency.

Diaper Rash

CALCAREA CARBONICA This remedy is an anti-psoric and very useful for a variety of skin problems in persons of any age.

Diarrhea

BRYONIA ALBA The diarrhea to which Bryonia applies is slimy green and occurs immediately after the baby nurses. It usually alternates with constipation and there is passage of smelly flatus.

CHAMOMILLA VULGARIS Chamomilla is a polycrest remedy for infants who are cross, peevish, whiney, and intolerant of mother's milk and formula alike. There will be frequent green, slimy, watery stools that smell like rotten eggs.

CALCAREA PHOSPHORICA Calcarea phos is indicated by a soft stool that passes with difficulty, most often in the morning or just after nursing.

COLOCYNTHIS Chronic watery diarrhea, yellowish in color, that passes while the baby is nursing or taking any kind of liquid typifies Colocynthis.

Emergencies

ACONITUM NAPELLUS As stated on a previous page in a discussion of this remedy, Aconite is a very potent emergency resuscitation remedy for oxygen deprivation and impending shock. The most important keynote of the Aconitum picture is the suddenness and the intensity with which the emergency, and the accompanying frightening symptoms, came on. There will almost always be a rapid pulse and the tiny heart will be beating frantically. There may be what look like, and may are, stroke-like symptoms.

Eye Infection (conjunctivitis)

ARGENTUM NITRICUM The need for this remedy is recognized by the great amount of swelling and the abundance of the discharge going on in the body. Argentum is also indicated for chronic inflammation, soreness, and swelling of the margins of the eyelids.

ARSENICUM ALBUM The picture of Arsenicum, as far as eyes are concerned, is hot burning eyes with excessive watering and tears. The tears will be acidic and make the cheeks and eyelids sore. The eyes will also be extremely sensitive to light.

CALCAREA CARBONICA This remedy is for eyes that water first thing in the morning—in babies or anyone else. The eyes also water in open air. The eyelids are most often swollen and itchy and there is sensitivity to light. When there is a cold, the inflammation of eyes is very pronounced.

CHAMOMILLA VULGARIS With Chamomilla the eyes will be full of a yellowish colored puss and there will be spasmodic closing of the eyelids. This remedy is mentioned for bloody water running from the eyes of newborn babies. This is a situation that I have never actually seen. The baby will show the typical Chamomilla disposition, including wanting to be held and comforted all of the time.

EUPHRASIA OFFICINALIS Euphrasia is a polycrest for anything to do with the eyes. Its symptoms picture includes inflammation with discharge of thick acrid matter, eyes that water all the time, and burning and swelling of the eyelids.

NITRICUM ACIDUM Fatigue is always part of the picture of acid remedies and this will be seen, to a lesser degree and more difficult to recognize, even with children. The infant's eyelids will be stiff—the upper lid appearing almost paralyzed—and there will be sharp, sticking pains that make the baby fuss and cry a lot.

PULSATILLA NIGRICANS A Pulsatilla eye infection is unique in that the inflammation, which is yellow, thick and copious, is very bland. With a Pulsatilla child, inflammation comes on with cold symptoms. The eyes will burn and itch and the infant will rub at them constantly.

SILICA TERRA Since Silica's function is to remove obstructions, it is indicated to remove the swelling and blockage of tear ducts that may accompany a head cold or eye infection.

Failure to Thrive

AETHUSA CYNAPIUM The baby will display projectile vomiting or diarrhea immediately after nursing, often due to pyloric stenosis. The baby becomes dehydrated and exhausted. She will sleep a few moments after nursing a little bit, wake hungry and nurse for another few moments. Then the cycle begins again, to continue until the infant becomes too weak and exhausted to nurse. This remedy, clear liquids and electrolytes—given intravenously if necessary—may be needed to turn things around. This is a serious and frightening situation.

CALCAREA CARBONICA Failure to thrive situations with children are always alarming and this one is no exception. There will be malnutrition from digestive difficulties with all that a shortage of nutrients creates in a growing body. The infant's abdomen will be large, hard, and sensitive to any pressure and the skin appears dry and wrinkled.

CALCAREA PHOSPHORICA Unless there are birth defects such as heart problems, nutritional issues due to digestive problems are at the core of failure to thrive situations. With Calcarea phos, the primary manifestation is an impact on the bones and teeth. The child's mental development may be slower than average with temper tantrums and extreme irritability being common.

CHAMOMILLA VULGARIS Chamomilla is not a remedy of serious failure to thrive issues but things are certainly not quite right, easy, or enjoyable for the baby or the baby's family. Chamomilla babies are fussy and colicky. They wants to be held and carried about all of the time, although they are not very happy with that situation either. They rarely nurse well, with many things in the mother's diet that seem to disagree with them. There is almost always diarrhea and, in the newborn, mild jaundice.

LYCOPODIUM CLAVATUM As always, there is poor absorption of nutrients with many food allergies creating all of the disasters of malnutrition. The Lycopodium baby is thin and withered looking, always cold and lacking in vital heat. The baby's tummy is bloated due to much gas.

NATRUM MURIATICUM A child needing Nat mur is sleepy more of the time than is normal, irritable when awake and cries from the slightest cause. The baby will be weak with skin that is dry and appears chapped all the time. The baby will be very thin, particularly through the buttocks and the limbs will be cold. The child is usually late in talking.

SARSAPARILLA OFFICINALIS The difficulties associated with Sarsaparilla may be connected to kidney issues, with the blood having imbalances of nutrients and containing impurities as a result of kidney insufficiency. Sarsaparilla is also specific for cleaning the blood of toxins that are the result of problems in the last few inches of the colon. Symptoms, besides not thriving well, include gas, colic with backache, and diarrhea.

SILICA TERRA The Silica picture, once again, is arrested development due to poor assimilation of nutrients. There is speculation (and science to back it up) that at least some of the cause is the ill effects of vaccinations. The abdomen becomes distended, hard, and hot and there is often an intolerance to milk, even the mother's milk. The child will have exceptionally thin legs, especially in comparison with the tummy, and spinal curvature is occasionally seen. The baby appears to feel hungry all the time and cries to nurse, but loses interest in the breast of the bottle very quickly.

Heart

DIGITALIS Digitalis is specific for non-closure of the foramen ovale at birth. This is one of the valves, or shunts, that is designed to close at birth as the baby's circulatory system moves from appropriate to in the womb to appropriate for the world in which he will be breathing air and on his own, separate from the mother. The only other solution for this problem is surgery, although Digitalis in homeopathic form will increase the oxygen carrying capacity of the blood until the surgery can take place. The results of homeopathics are often impressive and usually instantaneous. That will be the case here as the baby's color improves. This is remarkable but must not be mistaken for cure until medical diagnostic procedures have shown that the valve has closed properly.

Hernia

CALCAREA CARBONICA Calcarea carbonica is an anti-psoric remedy with many skin issues. The common occurrence of hernias in babies who fit this picture seems to be tied to the general patterns of poor digestion and poor nourishment as a result. The infant sleeps poorly and wakes easily. (Compare to Bell. Puls. and Rhus-t.)

LYCOPODIUM CLAVATUM Lycopodium is another anti-psoric remedy but operates at a deeper level—quite a bit deeper than is usual with an anti-psoric. There may be an enlarged heart, perhaps with water in pericardium (the sac around the heart), and liver issues manifesting with jaundice of varying degrees. The hernia with this pattern is more likely to be on the right side of the body than on the left side.

NUX VOMICA The hernia of Nux is usually on the left side of the baby's body while, with Lycopocium above, the hernia is usually on the right side. The baby seems chilly and likes to be warmly wrapped. The abdomen will be sensitive to touch with nausea, indigestion, and colic more pronounced in the morning, although it runs throughout the day to some degree. A distinctive symptom is that the baby's stools are small, hard balls that only pass with difficulty.

Jaundice

A little bit of jaundice is common to newborns as their tiny, immature livers begin to process impurities and break down the excess blood that was stored in the spleen to be available from there should the need arise due to hemorrhage (Isn't God good?). Jaundice may also occur if there was any bruising from a difficult birth because the little liver must process the damaged red blood cells and then either repair or replace them.

These common "physiological" jaundices are not considered dangerous but must be watched in case they represent a more serious Rh or ABO incompatibility. In Rh and ABO incompatibility (both serious conditions) the jaundice usually comes on quite rapidly (Aconitum napellus) and the baby may appear sickly and unable to nurse from birth. Blood tests can easily determine these incompatibilities.

If the placenta takes a little bit of time to deliver and the baby is not separated from the oxygen and nutrients being provided by it by the immediate cutting of the cord, babies are less likely to develop jaundice as the mother's liver is still helping to filter the blood and deal with excess red blood cells that are breaking down.

The remedies below are, for the most part, meant to support the tiny liver in common types of jaundice, not with Rh or ABO incompatibilities.

ACONITUM NAPELLUS The jaundice of Aconite, like all Aconite symptoms, comes on rapidly. I would consider Aconite for use with conventional methods of treatment for Rh and Abo incompatibilities.

ARNICA MONTANA If the birth was at all difficult with any possibility of bruising, Arnica should be employed to assist the tiny liver in the breaking down of the damaged red blood cells in the bruised tissues.

CHAMOMILLA VULGARIS Chamomilla, as mentioned before, is a polycrest remedy for babies. The baby will be fretful, wanting to be held and carried about. Chamomilla might be best used in conjunction with another jaundice remedy.

CHELIDONIUM MAJUS Chelidonium is an outstanding organ remedy with particular affinity for the liver and gallbladder, making it an important remedy to consider for jaundice. Lyc. is complementary.

LYCOPODIUM CLAVATUM The primary action of Lycopodium, like Chelidonium above, is on digestive organs, liver, and large intestine. Jaundice after first week of life, believed to be connected to a bilirubin-like pigment present in the milk of some nursing mothers, responds well to this remedy. This type of jaundice is considered harmless (annoying as people comment on the baby's jaundice and provide you with advice). This remedy has a reputation for speeding the clearing of the jaundice through its support of the baby's liver and digestive organs.

NATRUM SULPHURICUM Nat sulph is a remedy that is indicated for liver disorders and difficulties arising from trauma to the head. Certainly birth can produce trauma to the head. Liver damage may also occur when a careless birth attendant grips the newborn too tightly around the stomach as it emerges from its mother. Nat sulph balances the water in the blood and aids the cells in staying properly hydrated.

Nasal Congestion

CALCAREA CARBONICA When Calcarea carbonica is needed it will be for a child that catches cold easily and with every change in the weather. The baby seems hungrier than normal and is never really well as colic alternates with stuffiness. When the child is stuffy, there will be swelling of the nose and upper lip.

KALI BICHROMICUM Some keynotes of Kali bichromicum is profuse, watery discharges or, alternatively, thick, sticky, greenish-yellow, ropy, and acrid discharges that obstruct the nose. Post-nasal drip down the back of throat creates coughing out of thick mucus, sometimes triggering vomiting. Sometimes there will be pain at the root of the nose and dark red blood from the nose.

LYCOPODIUM CLAVATUM The child has difficulty breathing—breathes entirely through his mouth which makes nursing difficult. Catarrh with swelling of the nose. Some connection with kidney difficulties exists as the child cries just before urinating. If the mother attempts to clear the nose she will find lots of crusts and stiff elastic type plugs.

SAMBUCUS NIGRA The Sambucus picture is characterized by inflammation and ***dryness*** of mucous membranes of nose and sinus cavities.

Respiratory Ailments Pneumonia

ANTIMONIUM TARTARICUM Some of the specific symptoms of Antimonium include rattling of mucous in the chest with little expectoration and the infant lets go of the nipple and cries out as if out of breath. Immature lungs, with resultant labored heart action, should be looked for as a causative factors. The baby wants to be carried about in an upright position.

BRYONIA ALBA Respiratory keynotes of Bryoia include difficult, quick respiration, dry, hacking, painful cough with difficult, quick and shallow respiration and croup with fever also responds to this remedy.

IPECACUANHA Although predominantly thought of as a digestive aid, Ipecacuanha is useful for attacks of difficult shortness of breath—the baby literally gasps in an attempt to get enough air. There will be a loose, hoarse rattle in the chest but with no expectoration. The cough is so suffocative that the child becomes blue in the face and stiffens his whole little body. The cough may become so intense as to produce vomiting.

KALI CARBONICUM Kali carbonicum is another remedy where the child feels better when sitting up or leaning forward. If put to bed lying down, shortness of breath will wake the baby (and the parents) during the night. The child will have a tendency for colds to go in to the chest.

LYCOPODIUM CLAVATUM Lycopodium is a wonderful remedy for those times when something like pneumonia is neglected or, in spite of treatment, becomes protracted. There will be rattling breathing with shortness of breath. The breathing will be worse when the child is lying on its back. Expectoration is distinctive shades of greenish, yellow, or gray.

PHOSPHORUS All Phosphorus remedies include weakness and fatigue is their symptom pictures. The child will be displaying the typical symptoms of bronchitis, pneumonia of lower *left* lung that is worse from lying on left side. Suffocative breathing and cough, irritated and inflamed mucous membranes, and pale face with blue rings under eyes are some other symptoms to watch for.

SAMBUCUS NIGRA Child wakes suddenly, feeling as though he is suffocating, sits up, and then turns blue if he is not already that color. Paroxysms of suffocative coughs during the night with crying and shortness of breath. Nose so stuffed up that nursing is difficult. Whistling sound when breathing.

SULPHUR Sulphur symptoms include shortness of breath in the middle of the night that is better for sitting up, loose cough with much rattling of mucous and a lot of heat in the chest. There will be violent coughs which come in sets of two or three bouts at a time with the cough being worse when the child is laid on its back or on its side.

Teething

I have found that the Calcarea remedies, applied to the gums, bring a lot of relief to teething children. I usually use homeopathics in a liquid form but for applying topically to an infant's gums I like to remake the remedy using very soft granules that stay against the gums for a few minutes while dissolving.

ACONITUM NAPELLUS With Aconite the baby's gums are hard, hot, and inflamed. There will be slimy, greenish stools and diarrhea alternating with constipation.

BELLADONNA Belladonna is always keynoted by heat and redness. The poor child's gums will be hot and red with painful swelling. The pain is probably throbbing (like all Belladonna pains) and the child's face may be quite red.

CALCAREA CARBONICA The picture of Calcarea carb is difficult and, usually, delayed teething that comes *with fever*.

CALCAREA PHOSPHORICA With Calcarea carb teething is delayed and the teeth come through slowly. Sometimes there are mild convulsions (if such a word as mild can be used for convulsions in a child) *without fever* when the teeth are breaking through.

CHAMOMILLA VULGARIS Chamomilla is best used in conjunction with other remedies for teething and is only indicated if the child is peevish, cross, and wants to be carried about all day.

FERRUM PHOSPHORICUM There is much achiness and pain with the delayed teething of the Ferrum phos picture. The pain may be so great that the child become frantic and hysterical from it.

GELSEMIUM SEMPERVIRENS The Gelsemium child startles awake in the night with sudden fits of screaming. The gums are swollen and tender and the child becomes very upset when someone examines or even touches them.

IGNATIA AMARA Ignatia is not polycrest but it is useful if there are convulsion during the teething months.

KREOSOTUM The need for Kreosotum indicates that teething is a very painful process for this child. The gums will be puffy with a bluish color and it will feel like, to the parents, that the child is never going to sleep through the night ever again.

PHYTOLACCA DECANDRA The teething difficulties of Phytolacca are why there are so many teething rings for sale in the world—the baby's gums feel better for biting on something firm. Infants and children tend to clench the teeth tightly together.

SILICA TERRA Silica may help move teeth upward and through the gum if they do not seem to know how to complete the process on their own.

Thrush

There really is a wide range of symptoms with thrush; no one remedy will work for every child. What is going on and what it looks like inside the mouth are the guiding characteristics, of course.

BORAX VENETA The Borax thrush fills the mouth with *white fungus-like growth.* The child will experience intense pain while nursing and will cry and refuse to nurse.

KALI CHLORICUM The Kali chloricum thrush is conspicuously different from other thrushes because the entire mouth is r*ed with gray-based ulcers* everywhere. The tongue will be swollen and there will be profuse acidic saliva that causes the skin around the baby's mouth to chap and peel.

MERCURIALIS CORROSIVUS Lots of *albuminous mucous with ulcers* on the gums and tongue are characteristic of a thrush that will respond well to Mercurialis corrosivus. (This is a different remedy that Mercurius solublis/vivus.) There will be a very burning, scalding sensation in the mouth and the child will be very unhappy.

NATRUM MURIATICUM There will be *ulcers all over the mouth* and on the tongue burns painfully with food and nursing when Nat mur is called for.

Umbilicus

ABROTANUM ARTEMISIA This is a remedy for the oozing of blood and moisture from the umbilicus of a newborn long after it should have healed up. Abrotanum is also a "failure to thrive" remedy with emaciation of the lower limbs only.

CALCAREA PHOSPHORICA With Calcarea phos the slow healing umbilicus is matched by fontanelles that are also slow to close.

SILICA TERRA Silica is used when there is inflammation and infection that needs to be pushed out. There will be only a little bit of pus formation, making the situation look less urgent than it probably is.

Urine retention (in infant)

APIS MELLIFICA Apis is distinguished by the dark color of the urine when some does pass. As an insect remedy, the need for Apis will always be when there is burning upon urination making the baby cry out.

ARNICA MONTANA Urine is retained due to trauma and bruising at birth. Arnica has probably already been given—if the midwives are paying attention—and this entire situation is already on the way out. If not, the infant will be screaming from pain in the bladder. The mother will often be experiencing urine retention problems of her own at the same time. Both mother and baby should be given a dose or two of Arnica.

OPIUM There will be spasms in the neck of the bladder (You probably won't know that unless your are a foot zonist or reflexologist). A clue will be that the urine starts with a very slow, small stream.

Chapter Ten

BREAST FEEDING

There is a wonderfully amazing herbal pack recipe to be used as a poultice on the breast for mastitis infections to be found in Butterfly Miracles with Herbal Remedies. Most breast infections are fairly minor and go away without much concern but when they become nasty they are truly nasty indeed. Ignore one and you could be in for a serious illness. I have known women to lose part of a breast to stop a mastitis infection and my own worst memories of my childbearing years center around the suffering I experienced with mastitis infections.

General Problems/Pain/Infection/Cracked Nipples

As always in homeopathy, the entire person should be factored in, both in treatment and in choosing the remedy. The keynotes of the remedy should match the woman's symptoms, with an especially heavy emphasis on the emotional aspects.

ARSENICUM ALBUM This type of mastitis infection manifests with burning pains in the breast. The emotional picture of Arsenicum includes extreme nervousness, restlessness, anxiety, and fear. Nursing requires a certain degree of calm and the ability to sit patiently while the baby nurses. Calmness and patience are hard attributes to attain for people in a pronounced Arsenicum pattern.

A keynote of Arsenicum is that symptoms, both physically and emotionally are worse between 11 pm and 2 am, making middle of the night feedings a particular trial for some women. Arsenicum may help with the discouragement and despair at the lack of sleep that nursing a baby engenders.

BELLADONNA As with all things Belladonna, there will be redness, heat, and throbbing pain. Red streaks will radiate outward from the nipple and the glands will be swollen and hot. Belladonna is primarily a right-sided remedy and this will be reflected in the breast that develops the most severe symptoms. One of the Calcarea remedies of often required after Belladonna has cleared away the heat and swelling.

BORAX VENETA Usually, in the days before the infection really gets rolling, the woman's milk, if pumped for later use, curdles very rapidly. An odd symptom of an infection that will respond to Borax is pain in *opposite* breast when nursing.

After the baby has nursed, there will be stitching pain in the empty breasts that is better for applied pressure or compression. The milk is thick, tastes bad, and creates sores in baby's mouth that make nursing difficult. A new plan for feeding the baby should probably be sought until the infection has cleared.

BRYONIA ALBA Bryonia symptoms are often brought on by fear or a fright of some kind. The breast will be hot, painful, swollen, and *stony hard*. The infection will likely be accompanied by a splitting headache and the woman will be irritable and hard to please and will probably desire to be left alone. Bryonia is a chilly remedy but during an infections there may be dry, burning heat that makes all symptoms worse.

CALCAREA CARBONICA The basic symptoms will be hot, swollen breast with stitching pain when nursing. The pain will be accentuated by the milk being too abundant. As with most mastitis infections, the milk will be disagreeable to the baby. The nipples will be cracked, ulcerated, and very tender. An odd keynote is that, although there is a lack of milk supply, the breasts will be distended and painful.

The emotional symptoms of Calcarea carbonica are the typical picture of an exhausted new mother who worries constantly about all of her duties and responsibilities. The worry and apprehension become worse towards evening.

CALCAREA PHOSPHORICA As with all remedies that contain Phosphorus, there will be weakness. This weakness usually occurs after prolonged months of nursing while keeping up other responsibilities. The nipples will be aching and sore, and feel overly large. The milk seems disagreeable to the baby—the infant either nurses frequently and then vomits or refuses to nurse at all even though there is no obvious infection. Perhaps the time for weaning has arrived.

CASTOR EQUI One unique aspect of this remedy is that the nipples are cracked and ulcerated and are so tender the woman cannot even bear the touch of clothing. The breasts will swell and itch violently. ***This remedy is an almost classic symptom picture for this condition and has a reputation for being effective even in advanced cases where other remedies and treatments have failed.***

CHAMOMILLA VULGARIS The breasts are sore and the nipples are inflamed and very tender. Although the condition is not serious enough to be termed mastitis and is mainly inflammation instead of infection, there is the unique symptom of cramping whenever the baby nurses, much like the first days after the baby was born.

The mother will display at least some of the emotional characteristics of the Chamomilla picture. These symptoms include being discontented and dissatisfied, being overly sensitive to pain and to noise around them, and being irritable and quarrelsome.

DULCAMARA When Dulcamara is indicated the sore breasts will be very engorged and extra sensitive to cold. Throughout her nursing time, she will have found her milk supply suppressed somewhat if she gets chilled or catches a cold or some such thing. The mother is likely to quit nursing early because of pain in the breasts but, unfortunately, the nipples will tend to be sore long after weaning. Dulcamara is especially useful when there is thrush on the breasts of the nursing woman.

LAC CANINUM This remedy is for painful breast infections that are worse from the least movement. There is constant pain in the breasts and the nipples, and the breast feels as if it is full of hard lumps. This picture includes the decline of loss of adequate milk supply for no obvious reason. There may be headaches that alternate sides of the head. The headaches may affect the vision to the extent that they can properly be called migraines.

A keynote of this remedy is a craving for milk and milk products which greatly irritates the digestion.

LAC VACCINUM DEFLORATUM A strong keynote for this remedy is that there was a decrease in the size of breasts during pregnancy with scanty flow of milk after the baby is born. This remedy can do much to restore the milk supply and flow as needed. This is not a common remedy when an infection occurs as it more a remedy for keeping up the milk supply.

Emotional symptoms include listlessness and being quite disinclined toward any mental or physical exertion. The woman may also become averse to company, not wanting to see or talk to anyone

LYCOPODIUM CLAVATUM Lycopodium is not a mastitis remedy; it is more for bleeding nipples that are raw and sore. There is a discharge of blood and water from the nipples that this remedy is likely to help clear up. The child vomits blood after sucking from the bleeding nipples so it is important to act quickly with the remedy if the mother wishes to continue nursing the baby.

An odd keynote of this remedy is milk in the breast without being pregnant. Confusion, indecision, and loss of confidence are keynotes of the emotional pattern of Lycopodium.

NUX VOMICA Nipples are painful only during suckling with little or no soreness in between. The nipples may have a distinctive white spot in the center. There is a *painless* gathering of milk in the breasts between nursing or when time is lengthened out between nursings. Other Nux symptoms, especially those having to do with being irritable and impatient, are usually present. The woman with these physical symptoms will almost always have been, and still is, a dynamic and driven person who is ambitious and competitive in nature.

PHOSPHORICUM ACIDUM Phosphoricum acidum is keynoted by sharp pressure in the *left* breast. Phosphorus and acid in homeopathic remedies always indicate frail health and physical weakness. The milk will be scanty and the woman's overall health impacted negatively from nursing. The infant vomits the milk constantly and there is never enough to nurse the baby again after it has vomited.

PHOSPHORUS Phosphorus is indicated if there is irregular bleeding from the uterus when nursing, even long after the baby is born. Great debility and fatigue are always part of the Phosphorus pattern. In this case, there will be a sudden increases in the milk supply that will be followed by extreme fatigue.

The emotional pattern of this remedy is being over-sensitive to external impressions, noises, odors, lights, and the opinions of others.

PHYTOLACCA DECANDRA ***Phytolacca is far and away the leading polycrest for mastitis with Belladonna and Bryonia accounting for a good percentage of the rest of the cases.*** The breasts that will respond to Phytolacca will be lumpy and hard and tender only in spots. An interesting and unusual keynote with Phytolacca is the pains frequently change location or wander to other areas of the chest or even to more distant parts of the body, indicating that the infection may be in the blood rather than limited only to the breast tissue.

None of the mental and emotional symptoms are very pronounced but they are many and varied. The woman my be irritable and nervous or she may become gloomy and indifferent to life.

PULSATILLA NIGRICANS The Pulsatilla woman often weeps for no reason when the child is at the breast (and often when it is not!). After weaning, the breasts swell, feel stretched, intensely sore, and milk continues to be secreted off and on, from time to time. Sometimes there was a little dripping of milk during the pregnancy, even with the first pregnancy.

SEPIA SUCCUS With Sepia, the nipples are often bleeding and sore, with the strange symptom of the soreness being preceded by itching. *The nipples crack across the top side.* There will be the keynote symptoms of the woman feeling overwhelmed by the responsibilities of family.

SILICA TERRA The pains of Silica are sharp and are often felt in the uterus and in the back at the same time that they are felt in the breasts. There will be great itching and the breasts will be swollen and hard The milk supply is often suppressed and the woman constantly wonders if she is getting a mastitis infection. *The nipples crack around the base.*

The emotional symptoms of Silica include anxiousness and loss of self-confidence with an anticipation of failure when something must be undertaken.

Milk Supply Insufficient

Many of the remedies for increasing milk supply are discussed previously in the breast feeding section. Two more are mentioned below.

IGNATIA AMARA Ignatia is indicated by diminished milk supply with sharp pains in nipples *only* when breathing in deeply. Ignatia situations are often associated with grief and the depletions of the milk supply will have occurred following some sort of grief or disappointment.

SECALE CORNUTUM With Secale there is suppression of milk with stinging in the breasts and the breasts do not fill with milk properly.

Drying Up Milk Supply (involution)

Belladonna, Lac Canninum, and Urica Urens These are 3 remedies that are indicated for arresting the flow of milk when weaning. The choice should be made based on the emotional patterns of the remedies and the emotional symptoms that the woman is displaying at the time.

Chapter Eleven

BASIC DOSAGE GUIDELINES

Homeopathic remedies are meant to act as a healing catalyst in the body. The purpose of taking the remedy is to stimulate the body's own mechanisms to re-establish a state of balance and health. Unlike antibiotics, homeopathic remedies are **not** taken until the bottle is empty.

A Very Important and Very Basic Rule

A homeopathic remedy is a catalyst. It stimulates the body to begin healing itself. ***Once you see a marked improvement from the remedy, give it less often—or not any more at all.*** A muscle test is the best indication of frequency and when to stop. If you don't muscle test follow the traditional rules. How often and when to take a remedy is a judgment call, at best, so follow the norms outlined in homeopathic philosophy and pay attention to your common sense and intuition.

Do not take, or allow others to take, a remedy until the bottle is empty. This is a serious mistake. If you feel better for a time but now the same symptoms are back, perhaps worse than ever, you have probably taken the remedy for too long and for too often.

- Always stop on improvement.
- Start again if the same symptoms return and then repeat dosages as needed.
- If you have given several doses and have had no response, stop and reassess. It is very likely that you have chosen the wrong remedy entirely. In reality, this rarely happens.
- Change the remedy if the symptom picture changes. If the same symptoms return, repeat the remedy you have given or move to a higher potency for a dose or two.
- An improvement in mood and feelings of well-being is often the first and most accurate indication that you have the right remedy and it is working.

I like to think of a homeopathic remedy as a pebble which, when thrown into a pond, simply goes plop. It is the ripples created within the body that are the healing responses. The closer the symptoms match the remedy picture, the closer you have come to hitting the center of the pond with your rock and the more beautiful—and beneficial—will be the results.

Potency

The remedies in the first section of this book are low potency remedies. Recommendations for how and how often to take these remedies are found in the Introduction, Some Homeopathic Philosophizing.

Low potencies (30C, possibly 200C, Tissue Salts, and Flower Essences) are advised for use in most instances for pregnant women and infants, , unless you are quite experienced with homeopathic remedies. A 200C is usually strong enough for even emergency situations. Tissue salt remedies, Flower Essences, and low potency combination remedies are usually given 3 or 4 times a day for up to 4 weeks, depending on the severity of the symptoms and the progress of the healing. Remedies in 30C and 200C potency are given as needed or as recommended by a homeopathic physician or as recommended in accepted and common literature. This will rarely be more than once a day and, with a 200C will probably not be every day.

For further information, please see Basic Dosage Guidelines, in Butterfly Miracles with Homeopathic Remedies by LaRee Westover

Index of Remedies

Absinthium artemisia 59, 90
Acetaldehyde 52
Aconitum napellus 10, 23, 56, 107, 132, 137, 138, 141, 147, 150, 153, 154, 155, 159, 162, 164, 166
Aethusa cynapium 107, 163
Allium cepa 7, 23
Aloe socotrina 73, 103
Aluminum oxydata 73, 86, 103, 161
Aluminum phosphorica 16
Aluminum silicata 48
Anacardium orientale 36, 108, 128, 131
Antimonium crudum 51, 103
Antimonium tartaricum 108, 142, 145, 153, 159, 165
Apis mellifica 7, 20, 51, 53, 67, 71, 74, 108, 130, 134, 143, 155, 167
Arnica montana 38, 39, 57, 85, 87, 108, 109, 110, 128, 137, 138, 139, 142, 145, 147, 149, 150, 151, 153, 154, 155, 157, 159, 164, 167
Arsenicum album 8, 23, 26, 34, 35, 42, 45, 51, 58, 62, 66, 67, 69, 70, 73, 74, 75, 76, 78, 80, 109, 116, 128, 129, 130, 131, 137, 141, 144, 145, 147, 153, 156, 162, 169
Asparagus officinalis 63
Aspartyl-phenylalanine 12, 30, 31
Aurum metallicum 66, 79, 81, 109
Avena sativa 49
Baryta carbonica 33, 66, 73, 77
Belladonna 20, 46, 52, 58, 68, 69, 80, 83, 96, 109, 121, 128, 132, 138, 142, 143, 145, 150, 156, 159, 166, 169, 171
Bellis perennis 110, 127, 151, 154, 157
Berberis vulgaris 26, 32, 37, 70, 71, 72
Borax veneta 110, 166, 169
Bryonia alba 45, 52, 57, 70, 73, 84, 85, 110, 132, 156, 161, 162, 165, 169
Cactus grandiflorus 66, 81
Cadmium bromatum 27
Cadmium metallicum 7
Cadmium oxidatum 3
Caffeine 18, 53, 95, 128, 129, 130
Calcarea carbonica 6, 21, 35, 67, 69, 75, 77, 79, 80, 99, 110, 128, 129, 130, 133, 134, 135, 160, 161, 162, 163, 164, 165, 166, 169
Calcarea fluorata 13, 15, 100, 111, 133, 157
Calcarea iodata 46
Calcarea muriatica 22
Calcarea phosphorica 15, 94, 96, 111, 127, 131, 149, 161, 162, 163, 166, 167, 170
Calcarea sulphurica 15
Candida albicans nosode 14, 16, 17, 45
Cantharis vesicatoria 33, 43, 71, 72, 111, 134, 138, 151, 153, 155
Capsicum annuum 17
Carbo vegetabilis 73, 74, 84, 103, 111, 128, 131, 132, 134, 135, 144, 145, 150, 153, 154
Carduus benedictus 40
Carduus marianus 9, 69, 70, 76
Cassia acutifolia 90
Castor equi 111, 170
Causticum 53, 86, 89, 99, 112, 134, 142, 145, 147, 151, 155
Ceanothus americanus 76
Cell Salts/Tissue Salts (see Biochemic in General Index)
Cetraria islandica 55
Chamomilla vulgaris 31, 48, 71, 86, 87, 95, 96, 112, 128, 130, 141, 142, 145, 146, 149, 151, 160, 162, 163, 164, 166, 170
Chelidonium majus 29, 32, 35, 49, 91, 103, 112, 128, 164
China officinalis (See Cinchona) 46, 70, 76, 80, 97, 112, 137, 147, 152, 155
Chionanthus virginica 16
Cimicifuga racemosa 13, 28, 32, 38, 85, 113, 131, 133, 137, 139, 141, 143, 144, 145, 147, 149, 151, 154, 160
Cinchona (See China officinalis) 70, 76, 80, 97, 137
Citrus limonum 99
Cocculus indicus 113, 130, 132
Coffea cruda 58, 96, 113, 130, 133, 142, 149
Colchicum autumnale 113, 132, 134
Colocynthis 38, 69, 113, 160, 162
Conium maculatum 33, 46, 68, 114, 138
Crataegus oxyacantha 17, 49
Crocus sativus 5, 114, 128
Crotalus horridus 62
Croton tiglium 88

Index of Remedies

Cuprum metallicum 31, 48, 86, 87, 102
Cuprum sulphuricum 86, 87
Cypripedium pubescens 63
Damiana aphrodisiaca 52
Digitalis purpurea 75, 81, 145, 163
Di-methyl formamide 32
Echinacea augustfolia/purpurea 20, 23, 42, 46, 51, 56
Elaps corallinus 44
Ephedra vulgaris 16, 43, 95
Epigea repens 54
Equisetum hyemale 9, 24, 40, 50, 71, 94
Erigeron canadensis 114
Eryngium aquaticum 26, 55
Eupatorium perfoliatum 45
Euphorbia ipecacuanhae 14
Euphorbia pilulifera 6
Euphorbium officinarum 7, 53, 63, 102
Euphrasia officinalis 8, 9, 14, 23, 41, 47, 64, 91, 95, 162
Fagopyrum esculentum 99
Ferrum metallicum 15, 68, 89, 102, 149
Ferrum muriaticum 44
Ferrum phosphoricum 15, 20, 31, 40, 41, 42, 43, 53, 58, 91, 100, 114, 127, 152, 166
Filix mas 25, 33, 34, 46, 55, 59, 90, 92
Ficus religiosa 64
FLOWER ESSENCES
- **Agrimony** 4, 101
- **California Poppy** 4
- **Cherry Plum** 31, 44, 92, 97
- **Chicory** 24
- **Clematis** 92
- **Crab Apple** 101
- **Eucalyptus Globulus** 101
- **Gentian** 5, 9
- **Impatiens** 92
- **Larch** 10
- **Larkspur** 10
- **Mimulus** 101
- **Morning Glory** 4, 64, 100
- **Mountain Iris** 4
- **Pine** 93
- **Red Chestnut** 14, 44, 97
- **Red Poppy** 4
- **Rock Rose** 92, 101
- **Self-heal** 4
- **Star of Bethlehem** 92
- **Vervain** 14
- **Walnut** 4
- **White Oleander** 101
- **Willow** 97

Foeniculum sativum 61, 90
Fucus vesiculosus 40, 100
Fumaria officinalis 94
Galega officinalis 88
Gambogia morella 103
Gaultheria procumbens 90
Gelsemium sempervirens 7, 28, 32, 42, 45, 57, 83, 84, 86, 114, 141, 143, 144, 145, 147, 155, 166
Ginkgo biloba 95
Ginseng 43, 52
Glonoinum 79, 83, 115
Glycyrrhiza glabra 26
Gossypium herbaceum 115, 138, 146, 154
Graphites naturalis 103, 115, 123, 124, 133, 154
Grindelia robusta 6, 7
Guaco mikania 5, 6, 14
Guarana 62
Gunpowder 6
Gymnocladus canadensis 50
Hamamelis virginiana 115, 132, 135, 150
Helianthus annuus 87
Hepar sulphuris calcareum 21, 47, 65, 95, 115, 135
Histaminum muriaticum 8, 94
Homeria collina 40, 54
Hydrangea arborescens 100
Hydrastis canadensis 36, 95, 115, 135
Hydrazine 32
Hydrophyllum virginicum 6
Hyoscyamus niger 87, 116
Hypericum perforatum 10, 13, 21, 57, 116, 143, 157

Index of Remedies

Ignatia amara 6, 21, 75, 116, 130, 131, 132, 137, 141, 143, 144, 152, 166, 171

Iodum purum 5, 77, 93

Ipecacuanha 14, 16, 35, 36, 116, 130, 137, 147, 150, 155, 165

Ipomoea purpurea 64, 100

Iridium metallicum 32

Iris versicolor 9, 24, 26, 52, 55, 84, 91

Juglans nigra 59, 90

Juniperis communis 28

Kali bichromicum 72, 74, 76, 95, 134, 135, 165

Kali carbonicum 71, 80, 116, 127, 130, 134, 138, 141, 148, 151, 165

Kali cyanatum 61

Kali hypophosphoricum 5

Kali iodatum 43, 77

Kali muriaticum 3, 15, 47, 54, 132

Kali nitricum 36

Kali phosphoricum 15, 22, 27, 40, 49, 53, 58, 96, 117, 144

Kali silicicum 34, 64

Kali sulphuricum 14, 15, 27, 44, 98, 101

Kali telluricum 86

Kalmia latifolia 36, 89

Kola Nut 50, 87, 96

Kousso 91

Kreosotum 117, 135, 166

Lac caninum 117, 170

Lac vaccinum defloratum 117, 128, 129, 132, 170

Lachesis muta 68, 77, 135, 161

Lactuca virosa 117

Lappa arctium 27, 39, 90

Laurocerasus officinalis 118, 153, 159, 160, 161

Ledum palustre 38, 44

Leptandra virginica 59

Lilium tigrinum 118

Ligusticum porteri 54, 93

Lobelia inflata 49, 50, 60, 61, 79, 88, 118, 143, 146

Lobelia purpurascens 60

Lomatium dissectum 54

Lonicera xylosteum 43

Lupulus humulus 96

Lycopodium clavatum 5, 13, 26, 63, 67, 69, 71, 75, 76, 80, 104, 110, 118, 129, 132, 134, 143, 155, 160, 163, 164, 165, 170

Magnesia muriatica 118

Magnesia phosphorica 15, 85, 119, 127, 131, 144, 149, 160

Magnesia sulphurica 24

Mahonia aquifolium 55, 56

Malathion 94

Malva neglecta 28

Mancinella venenata 16, 41, 54, 63

Medicago sativa 42

Medorrhinum 82, 119, 129, 134, 135

Mentha piperita 44, 61, 95

Mercurius solublis/vivus 21, 33, 47, 67, 68, 81, 89, 81, 95, 129, 167

Millefolium achillea 52, 56, 107, 119

Morbillinum 87

MSG 27, 30, 31

Myrrh 26, 31, 48, 55

Myrtus communis 43, 93

Naja tripudians 79, 81, 99

Narcotinum 98

Nasturtium aquaticum 39, 94

Natrum arsenicum 15

Natrum lacticum 29

Natrum muriaticum 8, 15, 16, 24, 26, 41, 53, 72, 82, 91, 96, 100, 119, 127, 128, 129, 131, 134, 139, 152, 161, 163, 167

Natrum nitricum 31, 96

Natrum phosphoricum 15, 119, 129, 131

Natrum salicylicum 92

Natrum silicicum 64

Natrum sulphuricum 15, 16, 27, 28, 34, 35, 46, 64, 67, 69, 84, 86, 87, 91,94, 99, 120, 131, 132, 135, 165

Nepeta cataria 61

Niccolum carbonicum 48

Nitricum acidum 120, 133, 162

Nux vomica 26, 28, 32, 35, 52, 70, 71, 80, 83, 86, 120, 127, 128, 129, 130, 132, 134, 141, 143, 144, 146, 160, 161, 164, 170

Oleander 83

Opium 35, 98, 120, 149, 153, 155, 161, 167

Index of Remedies

Paris quadrifolia 61
Penicillinum 29, 34, 55, 63
Penthorum sedoides 59, 63
Phosphoricum acidum 42, 51, 78, 84, 171
Phosphorus 5, 8, 13, 40, 71, 72, 74, 75, 76, 79, 80, 82, 96, 97, 100, 117, 120, 127, 129, 130, 134, 144, 147, 149, 150, 152, 157, 165, 170, 171
Phytolacca americana 56
Phytolacca decandra 26, 47, 121166, 171
Pinus sylvestris 3, 7
Piscidia erythrina 88
Platinum metallicum 60, 121, 146
Plumbago littoralis 62
Plumbum metallicum 48, 74, 77, 121
Podophyllum peltatum 35
Polygonum sagittatum 63
Populus candicans 98
Prozac 88
Pseudo-narcissus 9
Psorinum 7, 13, 40, 60, 82
Pulmonaria officinalis 93
Pulsatilla nigricans 36, 47, 53, 58, 68, 76, 82, 95, 121, 131, 132, 133, 134, 135, 137, 138, 139, 141, 144, 146, 147, 149, 150, 152, 154, 160, 162, 171
Pulsatilla nuttaliana 14, 82
Pyrogenium 14, 74, 80, 122, 156
Quassia amara 59
Radium bromatum 63, 64
Radon 28
Ranunculus bulbosus 40, 41, 49, 77
Ranunculus sceleratus 8, 9, 16, 23, 54, 87, 88, 93
Reserpinum 22, 41, 42, 94
Rheum palmatum 28, 39
Rhus aromatica 40
Rhus toxicodendron 57, 72, 73, 85, 88, 122, 130, 131, 133, 134, 137, 151
Ricinus communis 122
Rumex acetosa 39
Ruta graveolens 85, 122, 131, 133, 137, 138
Sabina officinalis 122, 137, 138, 149, 150, 154
Sacharinum 12
Sambucus nigra 44, 123, 165
Sanguinaria canadensis 35, 57, 84
Sanicula aqua 123, 135
Sarcoma nosode 102
Scutellaria laterifolia 4, 41, 87
Secale cornutum 10, 123, 138, 143, 146, 147, 149, 150, 151, 171
Sepia succus 6, 13, 21, 68, 70, 72, 78, 110, 123, 127, 128, 129, 132, 133, 135, 137, 138, 139, 147, 149, 151, 152, 154, 171
Silica terra 3, 7, 15, 51, 86, 102, 104, 123, 133, 154, 162, 163, 166, 167, 171
Solidago virgaurea 47
Spongia tosta 21, 78
Staphysagria 124, 141, 146, 151, 157, 160
Stillingia sylvatica 26
Strontium nitricum 31, 100
Sulphur 38, 45, 74, 75, 80, 83, 110, 124, 129, 130, 134, 166
Sulphur iodatum 47
Sulphuricum acidum 9
Syphilinum 82
Syzygium aromaticum 60, 91
Tabacum nicotiana 8
Tanacetum vulgare 90
Taraxacum officinale 21, 27, 55
Tartaricum acidum 27
Teplitz aqua 93
Terebinthiniae oleum 32, 34, 64, 73, 95
Thallium sulphuricum 32
Thiosinaminum 33, 36, 64, 93, 94, 115, 123, 124, 133, 154
Thuja occidentalis 16, 23, 24, 28, 29, 30, 31, 41, 48, 51, 64, 68, 73, 83, 88, 91, 99, 124, 129
Thymus serpyllum 26
Thyroidinum 26, 78
Tissue salts (See Biochemic in General Index. Tissue Salts are also made as individual homeopathic remedies. Bioplasma on page 15 provides a list of all tissue salts.) 173
Trichloroethylene 32
Trifolium pratense 26, 27, 39, 56
Trigonella foenum graecum 43
Trillium pendulum 124, 150

Index of Remedies

Tuberculinum bovinum 10, 13, 82, 125, 160
Ulmus fulva 39
Uranium nitricum 100
Urtica urens 6, 41, 63, 125
Ustilago maydis 125
Uva ursi 13
Valeriana officinalis 49, 58, 85
Valium 34
Venus mercenaria 87
Veratrum album 7, 36, 125, 128
Veratrum viride 125, 143
Verbascum thapsus 61
Vespa crabro 50, 51, 60, 93
Viburnum opulus 48, 54, 125, 151
Viburnum prunifolium 126, 138, 146
Vinca minor 60, 88, 98
Viola odorata 14, 24, 78,91
Wyethia helenoides 8, 41, 43
Zincum bromatum 59
Zincum metallicum 86
Zincum muriaticum 22
Zincum phosphoricum 9, 15, 43, 98
Zingiber officinale 23
Zizia aurea 13

General Index

Abscess 3, 9, 51, 55, 99, 104, 123

Abuse 4, 38, 108, 124, 141

Acne 3, 47

ADHD 37, 82, 160

Adhesions 33, 94, 111, 124, 157

Adrenal cortex 6, 18, 21

Allergies 3, 5, 7, 8, 9, 11, 17, 22, 24, 29, 41, 47, 51, 60, 62, 67, 69, 71, 75, 76, 77, 80, 82, 95, 102, 104, 118, 125, 143, 160, 163

Amenorrhea 47

Anorexia 45, 101

Amennorrhea 47

Amniotic fluid 119, 127, 131

Anal fissures 120

Anus 34, 60, 90, 91, 128, 129, 135, 147, 149

Anaphylactic shock 6, 8, 29, 34

Anemia 5, 17, 20, 31, 38, 40, 41, 42, 47, 58, 78, 88, 97, 98, 100, 102, 127

Anesthesia 5, 116, 120, 149, 157

Aneurysm 66, 69, 71, 81

Anger 3, 5, 9, 10, 38, 67, 68, 69, 70, 74, 81, 88, 93, 97, 101, 11, 114, 124, 126, 141, 150

Anxiety 3, 5, 8, 10, 12, 17, 18, 20, 22, 23, 34, 38, 40, 42, 44, 45, 53, 57, 58, 59, 63, 64, 67, 69, 70, 72, 73, 75, 76, 78, 82, 83, 85, 88, 94, 96, 97, 98, 101, 102, 113, 114, 118, 119, 127, 130, 131, 133, 137, 141, 149, 153, 155, 169

Asthma 6, 7, 8, 9, 12, 17, 24, 26, 66, 74, 78, 83, 91, 94

Baby 811, 96, 107, 108, 109, 110, 111, 113, 114, 115, 116, 117, 119, 121, 122, 123, 124, 126, 128, 131, 133, 138, 142, 144, 145, 146, 147, 150, 151, 153, 159, 160, 161, 162, 163, 164, 165, 166, 167, 169, 170, 171

Back 13, 17, 21, 24, 28, 51, 57, 58, 59, 60, 64, 70, 72, 73, 74, 78, 85, 86, 87, 88, 89, 100, 101, 102, 103

Backache 13, 15, 16, 17, 51, 53, 63, 85, 88, 94, 98,

Bearing-down 109, 110, 123, 125, 127, 128, 133, 135, 137, 138, 146, 150, 151, 154, 155

Bed-wetting 14, 24, 53, 71, 72, 77, 91, 100

Bee stings 6, 51, 60, 74

Behavioral disorders 160

Belching 35, 45, 63, 75, 76, 79, 91, 114, 129

Bell's palsy 112

Bile 35, 55, 62, 64, 75, 91, 116, 147

Biochemic cell salts 15

Bioplasma 15, 150, 155

Birth defects 125, 159, 160, 163

Bladder 6, 11, 12, 13, 14, 15, 21, 24, 26, 27, 28, 33, 48, 53, 55, 62, 63, 64, 65, 68, 71, 72, 73, 78, 94, 100, 11, 112, 114, 118, 123, 134, 142, 145, 151, 155, 167

Bleeding 15, 24, 40, 58, 63, 64, 73, 84, 93, 95, 109, 119, 121, 122, 124, 125, 126, 137, 150, 152, 155, 156

Bleeding, during menses 24, 125

Bleeding, during pregnancy 102, 103, 108, 109, 113, 138, 142, 146, 150, 154

Bleeding, nipples 170, 171

Bleeding, postpartum 93, 102, 171

Bleeding gums 88, 119, 127

Blood clotting 98

Blood pressure 8, 17, 27, 49, 50, 66, 79, 81, 83, 88, 93, 100, 108, 112, 127, 137, 155

Blood sugar 6, 12, 17, 41, 43, 55, 56, 63, 96

Bone 13, 33, 34, 38, 45, 77, 88, 89, 94, 100, 116, 161

Brain 11, 16, 20, 22, 25, 27, 35, 40, 42, 43, 46, 48, 49, 50, 57, 54, 68, 84, 85, 86, 87, 95, 97, 98, 143

Braxton Hicks 127, 146, 151

Breast feeding 117, 169, 171

Breast milk (see also Nursing)

- **Breast milk, excessive** 121
- **Breast milk, drying up production** 171
- **Breast milk, insufficient** 171
- **Breast milk, let down response** 109
- **Breast milk, in newborn** 160

Breathing difficulties (see respiratory distress)

Bronchitis 7, 46, 56, 57, 78,108, 165

Bruises 56, 85, 110

Bulimia 5, 88, 101

Calcium 40, 50, 111, 124, 127, 129, 144

Cancer 11, 12, 17, 22, 26, 28, 36, 37, 39, 46, 56, 62, 102, 117

Candida albicans 15, 17

Catarrh 7, 15, 47, 91, 93, 95, 100, 165

Cell salts/Tissue salts (see Biochemic)

Cervix 51, 103, 108, 111, 113, 114, 118, 123, 125, 141, 142, 143, 145, 146, 147, 150, 153

Cesarean 151, 157

Chemical poisoning 5, 17, 30, 32,

General Index

Mercury poisoning 27
Ch'i (see energy)
Chicken Pox 95
Childbirth 13, 42, 47, 91, 105, 107, 110, 112, 116, 119, 122, 127, 138, 144, 145, 151, 152, 154, 156
Chills 3, 26, 45, 56, 60, 61, 79
Chronic Fatigue Syndrome (CFS) 17, 18, 19, 20, 21, 22
Circulation 5, 17, 27, 38, 42, 50, 54, 65, 68, 78, 79, 81, 87, 99, 100, 107, 111, 113, 115, 132, 144, 160
Colds 7, 17, 23, 24, 44, 45, 56, 82, 165
Colic 5, 20, 24, 27, 31, 36, 44, 46, 54, 59, 60, 61, 63, 70, 73, 76, 79, 80, 90, 91, 102, 110, 112, 113, 118, 121, 124, 125, 160, 161, 163, 164
Colon 3, 18, 22, 36, 60, 61, 93, 101, 103, 163
Compassion 10, 69, 70, 81, 97
Confidence 3, 4, 10, 19, 33, 66, 68, 71, 72, 76, 81, 83, 101, 102, 108, 109, 118, 123, 143, 170, 171
Congestive Heart Failure 17
Contentment 75
Contractions 7, 86, 93, 109, 111, 112, 113, 114, 116, 118, 119, 125, 127, 137, 139, 142, 143, 144, 145, 146, 147, 150, 151, 154, 156
Convulsions 11, 12, 28, 31, 32, 33, 39, 48, 59, 61, 82, 83, 85, 88, 89, 96, 102, 109, 115, 116, 143, 160, 161, 166
Coryza 7, 8, 9, 23, 95
Cough 7, 11, 12, 16, 23, 24, 25, 26, 27, 41, 44, 45, 46, 48, 52, 53, 56, 57, 58, 73, 74, 78, 82, 84, 93, 94, 97, 99
Courage 4, 43, 92, 101
Cramping 34, 35, 36, 44, 46, 58, 62, 69, 75, 80, 85, 91, 102, 160, 170, 125, 126, 138, 143, 144, 146, 149
Cravings 4, 5, 18, 35, 70, 75, 79, 80, 110, 119, 130, 133, 147
Cystitis 40, 54, 63, 64, 65, 71, 72, 73, 108, 111, 119, 123, 155
Cheek 60, 112
Chicken pox 95
Cure 1, 5, 23, 45, 89, 160, 163
Dehydration 35, 62, 70, 76, 80, 88, 107, 144
Depression 4, 5, 10, 12, 15, 18, 21, 22, 24, 28, 29, 32, 34, 38, 40, 43, 53, 58, 66, 67, 68, 74, 77, 79, 80, 81, 82, 83, 84, 88, 91, 94, 96, 98, 113, 116, 119, 120, 121, 124, 151, 152
Despondency 5, 43, 77, 93, 97, 118
Detoxifying 8, 9, 12, 20, 26, 27, 37
Diabetes 17, 25, 27, 37, 40, 51, 64, 67, 69, 71, 75, 80, 88, 91, 94, 104
Diaper rash 110, 119, 161
Diarrhea 4, 5, 12, 14, 15, 16, 22, 23, 26, 28, 29, 33, 34, 35, 36, 39, 40, 42, 44, 46, 52, 54, 55, 57, 59, 60, 61, 62, 66, 70, 72, 74, 75, 76, 80, 90, 91, 97, 100, 101, 103
Digestive system 13, 26, 36, 42, 69, 71, 75, 76, 117, 157
Dioxins 37
Dust 7
Dyslexia 5, 69, 75, 7
Dystocia 107, 116
Edema 7, 8, 39, 66, 71, 74, 79, 91, 94, 108, 111, 113, 124, 134
Emergency 38, 92, 107, 132, 147, 150, 153, 159, 162, 173
Esophagus 27, 36, 39, 44, 61, 76
Endocrine 50, 134
Endometriosis 122, 124
Energy 65
Epilepsy 12, 89, 160
Epithelioma 64
Epstein-Barr 17, 18, 22
ER911 38, 155
Exercise 3, 13, 15, 24, 29, 122, 123, 134, 135, 151
Exhaustion 19, 20, 21, 24, 32, 39, 40, 41, 42, 43, 44, 48, 49, 51, 57, 58, 62, 74, 77, 78, 80, 87, 91, 96, 97, 99, 100, 102, 107, 109, 110, 111, 113, 114, 117, 124, 125, 130, 135, 136, 137, 144, 145, 147, 150, 152
Eyes 6, 7, 8, 39, 41, 43
- **Allergy** 6, 7, 8, 9, 23, 41, 59, 95
- **Blindness** 41
- **Dark circles** 21, 33, 34, 40, 51, 55, 59
- **Itching** 6, 7, 8
- **Sensitive** 7, 8, 16, 24, 84
- **Strain** 41, 84, 85
- **Watering** 9, 64, 95

Failure to thrive 111, 123, 163, 167
Fainting 5, 8, 40, 79, 97, 109, 113, 152
Faith 4, 5, 19, 66, 71, 76
False labor 113, 125, 139, 143, 146, 151

General Index

Fatigue 3, 5, 10, 11, 14, 15, 16, 17, 18, 19, 20, 21, 22, 27, 28, 29, 32, 34, 38, 40, 41, 42, 43, 44, 45, 47, 49, 50, 52, 53, 57, 58, 62, 78, 83, 84, 87, 88, 89, 90, 91, 95, 96, 98, 100, 101, 102, 112, 114, 117, 118, 119, 120, 128, 129, 137, 145, 147, 162, 165, 171

Fear 4, 5, 10, 14, 20, 21, 23, 39, 42, 44, 45, 53, 56, 57, 58, 59, 63, 65, 66, 67, 68, 71, 72, 76, 79, 80, 81, 87, 92, 97, 98, 101, 102, 103, 104, 107, 109, 110, 113, 118, 119, 120, 130, 131, 137, 139, 141, 145, 149, 152, 153, 154, 155, 156, 169

Fetal distress 108, 145

Fever 3, 7, 14, 18, 23, 25, 28, 29, 34, 44, 45, 46, 55, 56, 57, 58, 62, 70, 74, 76, 80, 82, 96, 110, 114, 122, 125, 156, 165

Fever, pregnancy 145

Fever, newborn 107, 112, 166

Fibroid 27, 56, 111, 115, 119, 125, 135

Flatulence 21, 27, 31, 34, 36, 46, 51, 53, 59, 60, 61, 63, 75, 90, 94, 100, 103, 118, 160, 161

Flu 25, 35, 44, 45, 56, 62, 70, 75, 80, 100

Food allergies 5, 51, 60, 67, 69, 71, 75, 76, 80, 104, 118, 125, 163

Food poisoning 8, 23, 42, 45, 62, 70, 128

Gallbladder 27, 35, 46, 49, 59, 62, 69, 70, 71, 72, 75, 76, 91, 128, 164

Gastroenteritis 35, 36, 73

Glands 6, 8, 13, 17, 21, 25, 27, 33, 34, 41, 45, 46, 47, 48, 49, 50, 55, 56, 57, 59, 65, 69, 77, 82, 90, 92, 93, 94, 99, 103, 122, 125, 129, 142, 169

Gout 6, 29, 63, 64, 88, 89, 91, 93, 125

Gonorrhea 82, 119

Greed 75

Grief 6, 21, 26, 38, 39, 42, 44, 49, 51, 53, 75, 76, 78, 82, 84, 92, 94, 109, 116, 119, 127, 129, 130, 132, 137, 141, 143, 144, 147, 152, 161, 171

Guilt 67, 73, 75, 88, 93

Gums 3, 25, 74, 85, 88, 96, 120, 127, 166, 167

Hay fever 7, 8, 23, 24, 39, 41, 74, 82, 95

Headache 2, 4, 7, 9, 11, 12, 13, 14, 16, 21, 23, 24, 25, 28, 31, 32, 35, 36, 40, 41, 43, 44, 46, 50, 51, 52, 54, 57, 59, 61, 62, 64, 70, 76, 79, 83, 84, 86, 87, 89, 91, 94, 95, 96, 99, 100, 101, 103, 108, 112, 114, 115, 116, 117, 118, 120, 122, 128, 129, 134, 137, 143, 145, 156, 169

Heart 6, 7, 8, 11, 16, 17, 26, 33, 36, 37, 39, 42, 43, 49, 50, 59, 60, 61, 62, 63, 66, 67, 69, 72, 74, 75, 78, 79, 81, 82, 83, 85, 87, 88, 89, 90, 93, 97, 100, 101, 110, 115, 118, 125, 132, 145, 153

Heart palpitations 5, 10, 12, 13, 14, 36, 78, 98, 109, 128, 129, 130, 146, 149, 154

Heart, newborn 11, 145, 147

Heartburn 5, 35, 46, 53, 54, 58, 59, 75, 79, 100, 109, 114, 118, 119, 129

Heat exhaustion 100

Hemorrhage 15, 40, 42, 62, 74, 99, 102, 107, 108, 111, 113, 114, 115, 116, 119, 120, 123, 124, 125, 142, 146, 150, 152, 154, 155, 164

Hepatic (see liver)

Hepatitis 17, 69, 70, 71, 76, 160

Hernia 110, 164

Herpes 39, 45, 63, 99, 119, 129, 135

Hiccups 44, 53, 61, 75, 76, 160, 118, 132

Hives 6, 8, 50, 130

Hormones 3, 6, 37, 50, 52, 68, 70, 72, 78, 128, 131, 139, 153

Humility 74

Hunger 5, 29, 35, 36, 59, 70, 76

Hypertension 12, 97, 124, 134

Hypoglycemia 5, 12, 17, 36, 42, 67, 69, 71, 72, 75, 80, 89, 103, 120

Immune system 1, 4, 6, 17, 18, 20, 21, 22, 23, 25, 26, 37, 38, 42, 45, 46, 54, 56, 62, 77, 78, 94, 101

Auto-immune 12, 77

Impatience 21, 27, 49, 82, 101

Impetigo 99

Indigestion 5, ,36, 46, 53, 54, 60, 61, 67, 80, 91, 97, 100, 111, 119, 129, 132, 164

Industrial solvents 32

Infant 11, 12, 22, 44, 65, 77, 82, 89, 90, 99, 107, 108, 110, 112, 115, 118, 119, 120, 127, 142, 153, 159, 160, 161, 162, 163, 164, 165, 166, 167, 170, 173

Infection 3, 6, 12, 14, 17, 18, 20, 23, 24, 25, 26, 28, 41, 45, 46, 53, 54, 55, 56, 57, 62, 70, 71, 83, 93, 95, 103, 104, 110, 115, 122, 134, 138, 154, 156, 162, 167, 169, 170, 171

Influenza 8, 23, 26, 39, 42, 50, 56, 57, 62, 75, 80, 101

Insomnia 10, 20, 21, 43, 49, 58, 59, 85, 97, 120, 122, 141

Iron deficiency 31, 58, 102, 103
Iron absorption 42, 58, 102, 114
Irritability 3, 4, 11, 12, 14, 18, 21, 27, 36, 38, 40, 41, 48, 59, 65, 67, 82, 84, 86, 87, 93, 96, 97, 103, 108, 110, 112, 113, 116, 120, 128, 137, 141, 147, 163
Itch 6, 7, 8, 9, 10, 23, 24, 31, 34, 41, 46, 47, 49, 50, 51, 54, 58, 61, 63, 64, 65, 73, 74, 82, 90, 91, 95, 98, 99, 103, 108, 109, 111, 115, 117, 124, 125, 128, 129, 130, 135, 161, 162, 170, 171
Jaundice 39, 49, 71, 80, 99, 112, 118, 120, 160, 163, 164
Joint pain 6, 113, 130
Keloids 33, 36, 93, 94, 102, 124, 154
Kidneys 3, 9, 12, 14, 26, 28, 31, 32, 34, 39, 40, 42, 48, 53, 55, 59, 63, 64, 65, 66, 67, 69, 70, 72, 73, 82, 94, 100, 101, 113, 133, 134, 135
Kidney stones 14, 32, 52, 63, 64, 89, 125
Labor (see also Contraction) 108, 125, 138, 141, 149, 159
Labor, anxiety/fear of 107, 109, 111, 124, 139, 141
Labor, arterial pulse hard 125
Labor, back pain 13, 116, 118, 126, 142, 146
Labor, exhaustion 112, 113, 117, 144, 149
Labor, false 113, 125, 146, 151
Labor, flow of blood 108, 112, 125, 146, 150
Labor, failure to dialate 108, 111, 114, 118, 125
Labor, fever 145
Labor, headache 115
Labor, lack of progress 108, 109, 111, 112, 113, 115, 121, 122, 124, 131, 143, 145, 146, 147, 154
Labor, pains 85, 108, 109, 113, 138, 146, 149
Labor, premature 109, 147
Larynx 7, 48, 74
Law of similars 1, 12, 18, 25, 88
Learning disabilities 10, 66, 75, 76
Leg cramps 88, 111, 119, 131
Limbs 5, 12, 14, 16, 23, 24, 28, 29, 32, 38, 40, 43, 44, 46, 54, 58, 59, 64, 67, 72, 83, 84, 86, 89, 99
Liver 3, 8, 16, 18, 20, 21, 23, 25, 26, 27, 28, 29, 31, 32, 34, 39, 43, 48, 50, 54, 55, 56, 59, 62, 66, 69, 70, 71, 72, 75, 76, 78, 80, 84, 89, 90, 98, 103, 109, 112, 113, 114, 115, 116, 118, 120, 122, 124, 125, 126, 133, 139, 142, 145, 146, 149, 150, 154, 155, 157, 160, 164, 165
Low potency 1, 2, 3, 135, 137, 139, 173
Lungs 3, 23, 25, 27, 42, 45, 46, 50, 54, 56, 57, 74, 92, 93, 94
Lupus 12, 32, 94
Lyme disease 44
Lymph 3, 20, 21, 23, 25, 26, 33, 34, 46, 47, 48, 50, 54, 55, 56, 59, 62, 66, 69, 75, 77, 78, 80, 90, 92, 93, 94, 99, 129, 153
Malaria 45
Malnutrition 5, 13, 35, 39, 74, 75, 80, 163, 110
Mastitis 47, 109, 110, 115, 117, 121, 169, 170, 171
Materia Medica 107
Measles 87
Meningitis 25, 83
Menstrual problems 6, 16, 37, 38, 48, 88, 98, 99, 103, 117, 125
Meridians 65, 66, 67, 68, 69, 70, 71, 72, 73, 74, 75, 76, 77, 78, 79, 80, 81
Methanol 11, 30
Miasms 7, 10, 24, 32, 69, 71, 77, 82, 99, 102, 110, 119, 125, 159, 160
Migraine 16, 27, 41, 52, 67, 72, 82, 83, 84, 88, 95, 170, 116, 117, 129, 147
Milk (see nursing, breast milk) 46, 88, 91, 107, 109, 111, 113, 116, 117, 121, 122, 124, 125, 160, 162, 163, 164, 169, 170, 171
Miscarriage 37, 107, 109, 111, 114, 116, 119, 121, 122, 123, 124, 125, 126, 127, 137, 138, 144, 146, 152, 153
Mold 7, 8, 45, 54,
Mood 4, 5, 6, 11, 17, 18, 21, 22, 38, 43, 47, 49, 64, 68, 76, 87, 88, 108, 115, 141, 152, 160, 173
Morning sickness 91, 108, 109, 115, 116, 118, 120, 131, 132,
Mucous 135, 147, 165, 166, 167
Mucous membranes 129, 161, 165
Mumps 56
Muscle 3, 7, 27, 40, 42, 45, 47, 48, 64, 72, 73, 77, 83, 85, 89, 94, 95, 99, 100, 102, 103
Muscle, facial 58, 71, 83
Muscle pain (ache, stiff, spasm, weak) 7, 10, 11, 14, 15, 17, 18, 21, 25, 26, 27, 32, 33, 34, 39, 49, 57, 59, 64, 77, 85, 86, 87, 88, 89, 97
Muscle test 65, 91
Muscle tone 11, 12, 13
Nasal congestion 45
Nephritis 63, 65

Nerves 4, 13, 15, 20, 22, 26, 27, 29, 30, 31, 42, 43, 48, 49, 57, 58, 59, 65, 67, 70, 71, 77, 84, 85, 86, 87, 88, 97, 98, 100, 102

Nervous system 5, 6, 12, 31, 41, 46, 49, 54, 66, 67, 68, 78, 85, 86, 87, 88, 94, 96, 101

Neuralgia 10, 43, 45, 57, 61, 62, 63, 67, 69, 77, 83, 88

Newborn 25, 107, 108, 109, 112, 118, 120, 121, 123, 155, 159, 160, 162, 163, 164, 167

Nipples 46, 108, 110, 111, 115, 121, 123, 165, 169, 170, 171

Nose 7, 8, 9, 23, 26, 41, 46, 54, 56, 57, 63, 74, 77, 83, 84, 95, 99, 103, 125, 143, 165

Nosebleed 100, 114, 123

Nosode 7, 10, 12, 13, 16, 25, 32, 35, 40, 57, 60, 62, 82, 87, 89, 90, 102, 119, 125, 129

Never the Same Since 39, 47, 48, 70, 73, 76, 79, 81, 83, 84

Nursing 88, 94, 39, 44, 107, 108, 110, 111, 117, 1118, 119, 121, 123, 125, 147, 160, 161, 162, 163, 164, 165, 166, 167, 169, 170, 171

Nutrients, lack of absorption 35, 36, 39, 48, 51, 61, 67, 69, 75, 80, 102, 107, 110, 111, 114, 118, 129, 163

Osteoporosis 25

Overexertion 102

Ovarian 46, 103

Pancreas 11, 21, 24, 70, 76, 89, 92

Paralysis 6, 32, 33, 42, 53, 64, 68, 82, 85, 86, 89, 98, 103, 112, 122, 134, 142, 145, 151, 152, 155, 159, 160, 161

Parasites 3, 14, 17, 33, 34, 44, 46, 55, 59, 62, 66, 70, 75, 80, 89, 90, 91

Panic attacks 5, 10, 34, 51, 67, 69, 82, 119, 141

PCP 37

Perineal 152

Pica 35

Polycrest 5, 6, 10, 13, 16, 20, 26, 28, 30, 32, 34, 38, 42, 45, 46, 49, 50, 51, 56, 57, 58, 62, 66, 68, 69, 70, 73, 74, 75, 76, 77, 78, 79, 80, 83, 85, 86, 87, 96, 97, 99, 102, 108, 109, 110, 111, 113, 115, 116, 118, 120, 121, 122, 123, 127, 128, 129, 130, 131, 133, 134, 138, 139, 143, 144, 150, 152, 155, 162, 164, 166, 171, 181

Post-partum 91, 93, 96, 109, 110, 111, 116, 117, 120, 121, 124, 142, 149, 150, 152, 154

Potency 1, 2, 107, 173

Prevention of miscarriage 111, 137, 139

Prevention of scar tissue 157

Process of cure 5

Prostate 3, 46, 65, 73, 100

Psora 7, 61, 69, 71, 77, 82, 99, 110, 160

Realms 139

Rectum 33, 91, 103, 110, 114, 115, 118, 125, 128, 135

Repertory (See Materia Medica)

Respiratory 6, 7, 8, 18, 26, 29, 32, 33, 44, 52, 54, 55, 90, 92, 93, 94, 108, 109, 165

Samuel Hahnemann 1, 28, 70, 78, 99, 119

Sarcodes 78

Scar tissue 33, 36, 56, 58, 64, 93, 94, 115, 123, 124, 133, 154, 157,

Schuessler cell salt (See Biochemic Cell Salts) 15

Sensitivities 13, 18

Skin (itchy) 3, 7, 8, 9, 11, 12, 24, 27, 30, 34, 36, 39, 40, 41, 45, 46, 47, 48, 51, 58, 60, 61, 63, 64, 71, 72, 73, 77, 82, 83, 88, 90, 94, 95, 97, 99, 103, 104, 108, 120, 124, 125, 128, 130, 133, 144, 147, 149, 153, 154, 161, 163, 164, 167

Sodium 30

Spiritual 4, 72, 92, 93, 188

Stomach 10, 14, 15, 21, 22, 26, 27, 28, 34, 35, 36, 39, 40, 42, 44, 45, 46, 51, 53, 54, 55, 60, 61, 62, 66, 70, 71, 75, 76, 80, 82, 84, 88, 90, 93, 97, 120, 128, 130, 131, 132, 147, 152, 165

Stretch marks 111, 133

Succussion 1

Suicide 61, 66, 79, 81, 84, 152

Suppression 171

Sycotic (Sycosis) 24

Syphilis 82

Tailbone 13, 57, 143

Tissue cell salt (See Biochemic Cell Salts)

Tongue 7, 8, 9, 14, 16, 23, 25, 54, 55, 59, 63, 70, 76, 88, 97, 167, 119

Trauma 38, 39, 57, 66, 81, 85, 92, 97, 101, 108, 116, 120, 124, 137, 139, 144, 145, 147, 150, 151, 152, 153, 154, 155, 159, 165, 167

Trust 71, 92

Tuberculosis 10, 46, 82, 94, 160, 125

Typhoid Fever 62

Vaccines 29, 51, 62, 82, 83

Vaccinosis 82

Vital force 157

Whooping Cough 26, 27, 56, 57, 74

Meet the Author

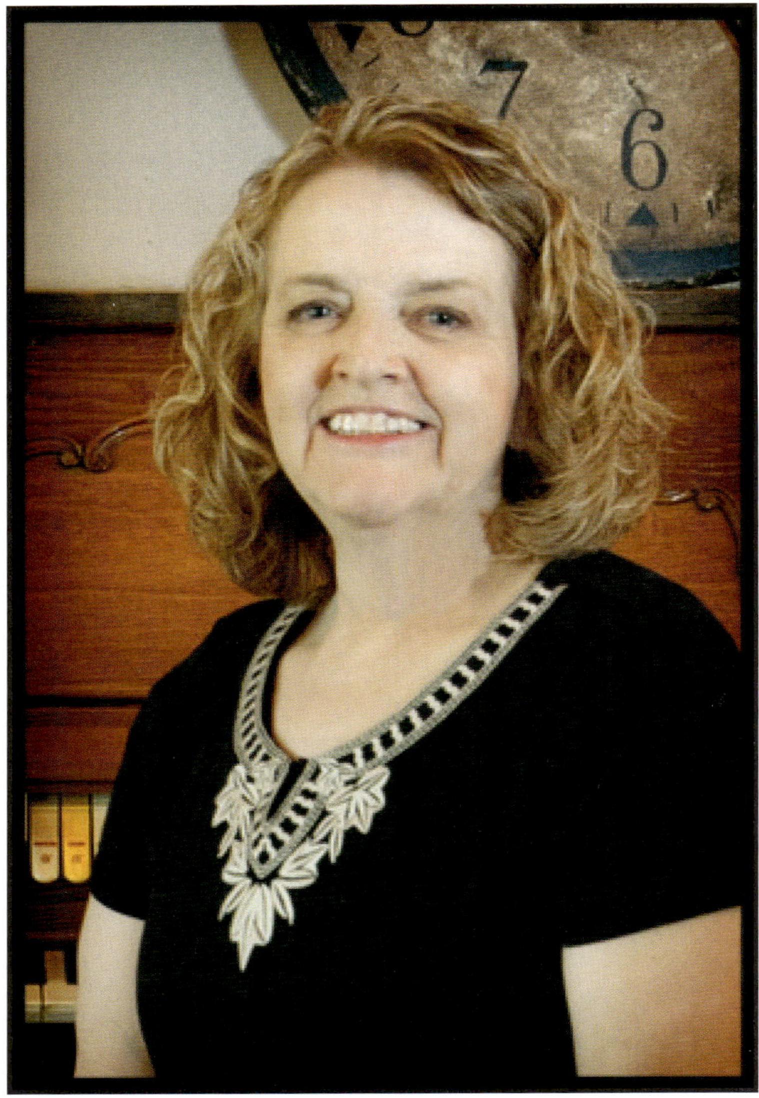

LaRee Westover has been studying and living various natural medicine modalities for over thirty years. Her experience includes the use of essential oils, herbals, and homeopathy, as well as energy work. She has an extensive knowledge of plants, their family groups, and their individual medicinal qualities.

Using this knowledge as a springboard, LaRee has been able to relate the specific energies of each plant and how each is utilized within its specific modality as she has compiled the information for each of her four books. Her practical, no nonsense, hands-on approach has inspired countless people to make the leap to natural healing.

LaRee teaches, "To feel the living spirit and intelligence of each plant is the true foundation of alternative medicine. Just as each plant can exemplify the attributes of our loving Father, so can the plants personify some lessons about the operation of the body and the soul. The possibilities for learning are endless. To think 'alternatively' is to think differently; we must think as nature does—holistically. Nature emphasizes the whole, rather than the precise piece, and nature has an inherent logic and wisdom. .

Whether it is through essential oils, herbs , homeopathics, or energy, LaRee's insight into the natural world is precise and helpful to the novice as well as the more advanced practitioner.